Liver Surgery: From Basics to Robotics

Guest Editor

DAVID A. GELLER, MD

SURGICAL CLINICS
OF NORTH AMERICA

www.surgical.theclinics.com

Consulting Editor
RONALD F. MARTIN, MD

August 2010 • Volume 90 • Number 4

SAUNDERS an imprint of ELSEVIER, Inc.

W.B. SAUNDERS COMPANY

A Division of Elsevier Inc.

1600 John F. Kennedy Blvd., Suite 1800, Philadelphia, PA 19103-2899

http://www.theclinics.com

SURGICAL CLINICS OF NORTH AMERICA Volume 90, Number 4

August 2010 ISSN 0039–6109, ISBN-13: 978-1-4377-2614-5

Editor: Catherine Bewick

Surgical Clinics of North America (ISSN 0039–6109) is published bimonthly by Elsevier Inc., 360 Park Avenue South, New York, NY 10010-1710. Months of publication are February, April, June, August, October, and December. Business and Editorial Offices: 1600 John F. Kennedy Blvd., Suite 1800, Philadelphia, PA 19103-2899. Periodicals postage paid at New York, NY and additional mailing offices. Subscription prices are $291.00 per year for US individuals, $475.00 per year for US institutions, $145.00 per year for US students and residents, $356.00 per year for Canadian individuals, $590.00 per year for Canadian institutions, $401.00 for international individuals, $590.00 per year for international institutions and $200.00 per year for Canadian and foreign students/residents. To receive student/resident rate, orders must be accompanied by name of affiliated institution, date of term, and the *signature* of program/residency coordinator on institution letterhead. Orders will be billed at individual rate until proof of status is received. Foreign air speed delivery is included in all *Clinics* subscription prices. All prices are subject to change without notice. POSTMASTER: Send address changes to *Surgical Clinics*, Elsevier Health Sciences Division, Subscription Customer Service, 3251 Riverport Lane, Maryland Heights, MO 63043. **Customer Service (orders, claims, online, change of address): Telephone: 1-800-654-2452 (U.S. and Canada); 314-447-8871 (outside U.S. and Canada). Fax: 314-447-8029. E-mail: journalscustomerservice-usa@elsevier.com (for print support); journalsonlinesupport-usa@elsevier.com (for online support).**

Reprints. For copies of 100 or more, of articles in this publication, please contact the Commercial Reprints Department, Elsevier Inc., 360 Park Avenue South, New York, New York 10010-1710. Tel. (212) 633-3812, Fax: (212) 462-1935, e-mail: reprints@elsevier.com.

The *Surgical Clinics of North America* is also published in Spanish by McGraw-Hill Interamericana Editores S.A., P.O. Box 5-237 06500 Mexico D.F. Mexico; and in Portuguese by Interlivros Edicoes Ltda., Rua Comandante Coelho 1085, CEP 21250, Rio de Janeiro, Brazil; and in Greek by Paschalidis Medical Publications, Athens Greece.

The *Surgical Clinics of North America* is covered in *MEDLINE/PubMed (Index Medicus)*, *EMBASE/Excerpta Medica*, *Current Contents/Clinical Medicine*, *Current Contents/Life Sciences*, *Science Citation Index*, and *ISI/BIOMED*.

Printed and bound by CPI Group (UK) Ltd, Croydon, CR0 4YY

Transferred to Digital Print 2011

Contributors

CONSULTING EDITOR

RONALD F. MARTIN, MD
Staff Surgeon, Department of Surgery, Marshfield Clinic, Marshfield, Wisconsin; Clinical Associate Professor, University of Wisconsin School of Medicine and Public Health, Madison, Wisconsin; Colonel, Medical Corps, United States Army Reserve

GUEST EDITOR

DAVID A. GELLER, MD, FACS
Richard L. Simmons Professor of Surgery; Department of Surgery, Starzl Transplant Institute; Co-Director, UPMC Liver Cancer Center, University of Pittsburgh, Pittsburgh, Pennsylvania

AUTHORS

SHERIF R.Z. ABDEL-MISIH, MD
Surgical Oncology Fellow, Division of Surgical Oncology, The Ohio State University Medical Center, Arthur G. James Cancer Hospital, Richard J. Solove Research Institute, Columbus, Ohio

PETER ABRAMS, MD
Fellow in Abdominal Transplantation, Department of Surgery, Thomas E. Starzl Transplantation Institute, Montefiore Hospital, University of Pittsburgh School of Medicine, Pittsburgh, Pennsylvania

KAREEM M. ABU-ELMAGD, MD, PhD, FACS
Professor of Surgery, Intestinal Rehabilitation and Transplantation Center, Thomas E. Starzl Transplantation Institute, Department of Surgery, University of Pittsburgh Medical Center, UPMC Montefiore, Pittsburgh, Pennsylvania

DAVID L. BARTLETT, MD
Bernard Fisher Professor of Surgery and Chief, Division of Surgical Oncology, Department of Surgery, University of Pittsburgh Medical Center Cancer Pavilion, Pittsburgh, Pennsylvania

MARK BLOOMSTON, MD
Assistant Professor of Surgery, Division of Surgical Oncology, The Ohio State University Medical Center, Arthur G. James Cancer Hospital, Richard J. Solove Research Institute, Columbus, Ohio

CHERIF BOUTROS, MD, MSc
Department of Hepatobiliary and Surgical Oncology, Roger Williams Medical Center, Providence, Rhode Island

MATTHEW R. BOWER, MD
Division of Surgical Oncology, Department of Surgery, James Graham Brown Cancer Center, University of Louisville School of Medicine, Louisville, Kentucky

RUSSELL E. BROWN, MD
Division of Surgical Oncology, Department of Surgery, James Graham Brown Cancer Center, University of Louisville School of Medicine, Louisville, Kentucky

JOSEPH F. BUELL, MD, FACS
Professor of Surgery and Pediatrics, Director, Tulane Abdominal Transplant Institute; Section of Transplantation, Department of Surgery, Tulane University, New Orleans, Louisiana

ROBERT CANNON, MD
Tulane Abdominal Transplant Institute; Section of Transplantation, Department of Surgery, Tulane University, New Orleans, Louisiana

SCOTT A. CELINSKI, MD
Assistant Professor of Surgery, Division of Surgical Oncology, Baylor University Hospital, Dallas, Texas

MICHAEL A. CHOTI, MD, MBA, FACS
Jacob C. Handelsman Professor of Surgery, Division of Surgical Oncology, Johns Hopkins Medical Institutions, Baltimore, Maryland

BRYAN M. CLARY, MD
Department of Surgery, Duke University Medical Center, Durham, North Carolina

PIERRE-ALAIN CLAVIEN, MD, PhD
Swiss Hepato-Pancreatico-Biliary and Transplantation Center, Department of Surgery, University Hospital of Zürich, Zürich, Switzerland

GUILHERME COSTA, MD, FACS
Assistant Professor of Surgery, Intestinal Rehabilitation and Transplantation Center, Thomas E. Starzl Transplantation Institute, Department of Surgery, University of Pittsburgh Medical Center, UPMC Montefiore, Pittsburgh, Pennsylvania

RUY J. CRUZ JR, MD, PhD
Assistant Professor of Surgery, Intestinal Rehabilitation and Transplantation Center, Thomas E. Starzl Transplantation Institute, Department of Surgery, University of Pittsburgh Medical Center, UPMC Montefiore, Pittsburgh, Pennsylvania

IBRAHIM DAGHER, MD
Department of General Surgery, Paris-Sud School of Medicine, Antoine Beclere Hospital, Clamart, France

N. JOSEPH ESPAT, MD, MS
Professor and Chief, Surgical Oncology; Vice-Chair, Surgery, Department of Hepatobiliary and Surgical Oncology, Roger Williams Medical Center, Providence, Rhode Island

T. CLARK GAMBLIN, MD, MS
Associate Professor of Surgery, Chief, Divisions of Surgical Oncology, Medical College of Wisconsin, Milwaukee, Wisconsin

DAVID A. GELLER, MD
Richard L. Simmons Professor of Surgery; Department of Surgery, Starzl Transplant Institute; Co-Director, UPMC Liver Cancer Center, University of Pittsburgh, Pittsburgh, Pennsylvania

ALAN W. HEMMING, MD
Professor of Surgery, Chief of Transplantation and Hepatobiliary Surgery, Abdominal Transplant and Hepatobiliary Surgery, Department of Surgery, University of California San Diego School of Medicine, San Diego, California

DAVID A. IANNITTI, MD
Section of Hepato-Pancreatico-Biliary Surgery, Division of Gastrointestinal and Minimally Invasive Surgery, Department of Surgery, Carolinas Medical Center, Charlotte, North Carolina

KAMRAN IDREES, MD
Surgical Oncology Fellow, Division of Surgical Oncology, Department of Surgery, University of Pittsburgh Medical Center Cancer Pavilion, Pittsburgh, Pennsylvania

STEVEN C. KATZ, MD
Department of Hepatobiliary and Surgical Oncology, Roger Williams Medical Center, Providence, Rhode Island

SABOOR KHAN, MBBS, PhD, FRCS
Gastrointestinal and Hepatobiliary and Pancreas Fellow, Division of Gastroenterologic and General Surgery, Mayo Clinic, Rochester, Minnesota

AJAI KHANNA, MD, PhD
Professor of Surgery, Section of Transplantation and Hepatobiliary Surgery, Department of Surgery, University of California San Diego School of Medicine, San Diego, California

JOHN R. KLUNE, MD
Resident in General Surgery, Department of Surgery, UPMC Presbyterian Hospital, University of Pittsburgh Medical Center, Pittsburgh, Pennsylvania

KWAN N. LAU, MD
Section of Hepato-Pancreatico-Biliary Surgery, Division of Gastrointestinal and Minimally Invasive Surgery, Department of Surgery, Carolinas Medical Center, Charlotte, North Carolina

KUNO LEHMANN, MD
Swiss Hepato-Pancreatico-Biliary and Transplantation Center, Department of Surgery, University Hospital of Zürich, Zürich, Switzerland

DAVID C. LINEHAN, MD
Professor of Surgery and Chief, Section of Hepatobiliary Pancreatic and Gastrointestinal Surgery, Department of Surgery, Washington University School of Medicine, St Louis, Missouri

J. WALLIS MARSH, MD, MBA
Professor of Surgery, Department of Surgery, Thomas E. Starzl Transplantation Institute, Montefiore Hospital, University of Pittsburgh School of Medicine, Pittsburgh, Pennsylvania

JOHN B. MARTINIE, MD
Section of Hepato-Pancreatico-Biliary Surgery, Division of Gastrointestinal and Minimally Invasive Surgery, Department of Surgery, Carolinas Medical Center, Charlotte, North Carolina

ROBERT C.G. MARTIN, MD, PhD, FACS
Director, Division of Surgical Oncology, Department of Surgery, James Graham Brown Cancer Center, University of Louisville School of Medicine, Louisville, Kentucky

KEVIN TRI NGUYEN, MD, PhD
Department of Surgery, Starzl Transplant Institute, UPMC Liver Cancer Center, University of Pittsburgh, Pittsburgh, Pennsylvania

TIMOTHY M. PAWLIK, MD, MPH, FACS
Associate Professor of Surgery, Hepatobiliary Surgery Program Director, Johns Hopkins Medical Institutions, Baltimore, Maryland

ANDREW B. PEITZMAN, MD
Mark M. Ravitch Professor of Surgery, Executive Vice Chairman, Department of Surgery, University of Pittsburgh, Pittsburgh, Pennsylvania

GRETA L. PIPER, MD
Instructor, Department of Surgery, University of Pittsburgh, Pittsburgh, Pennsylvania

GEORGE A. POULTSIDES, MD
Assistant Professor of Surgery, Division of Surgical Oncology, Stanford University School of Medicine, Stanford, California

SRINEVAS K. REDDY, MD
Department of Surgery, Duke University Medical Center, Durham, North Carolina

KAYE M. REID-LOMBARDO, MD, FACS
Assistant Professor of Surgery, Division of Gastroenterologic and General Surgery, Mayo Clinic, Rochester, Minnesota

GUIDO SCLABAS, MD, MS
Gastrointestinal and Hepatobiliary and Pancreas Fellow, Division of Gastroenterologic and General Surgery, Mayo Clinic, Rochester, Minnesota

DAVID SINDRAM, MD, PhD
Section of Hepato-Pancreatico-Biliary Surgery, Division of Gastrointestinal and Minimally Invasive Surgery, Department of Surgery, Carolinas Medical Center, Charlotte, North Carolina

HADRIEN TRANCHART, MD
Department of General Surgery, Paris-Sud School of Medicine, Antoine Beclere Hospital, Clamart, France

ALLAN TSUNG, MD
Assistant Professor of Surgery, Divisions of Surgical Oncology and Transplantation, Department of Surgery, University of Pittsburgh Medical Center, Pittsburgh, Pennsylvania

YUHSIN V. WU, MD
Resident, Division of General Surgery, Department of Surgery, Washington University School of Medicine, St Louis, Missouri

ANDREW X. ZHU, MD
Associate Professor, Department of Medicine, Division of Medical Oncology, Massachusetts General Hospital Cancer Center; Director, Liver Cancer Research Program, Massachusetts General Hospital, Boston, Massachusetts

Contents

Understanding the complexities of the liver has been a long-standing challenge to physicians and anatomists. Significant strides in the understanding of hepatic anatomy have facilitated major progress in liver-directed therapies—surgical interventions, such as transplantation, hepatic resection, hepatic artery infusion pumps, and hepatic ablation, and interventional radiologic procedures, such as transarterial chemoembolization, selective internal radiation therapy, and portal vein embolization. Without understanding hepatic anatomy, such progressive interventions would not be feasible. This article reviews the history, general anatomy, and the classification schemes of liver anatomy and their relevance to liver-directed therapies.

This article describes the development of hepatic surgery from old anecdotes to spectacular progress achieved during the last 25 years. The door to this evolution was opened by anatomists who paved the way for a few courageous hepatic surgeons, who performed pioneering work between 1960 to 1980. Then, hepatic surgery and transplantation became widely accepted for the treatment of many diseases. Surgery on the liver has become safer with low postoperative mortality as a result of the creation of centers of excellence offering multidisciplinary expertise and technical innovation.

Hepatic ischemia/reperfusion (I/R) injury occurs in a variety of clinical contexts, including transplantation, liver resection surgery, trauma, and hypovolemic shock. The mechanism of organ damage after I/R has been studied extensively and consists of complex interactions of multiple inflammatory pathways. The major contributors to I/R injury include production of reactive oxygen species, release of proinflammatory cytokines and chemokines, and activation of immune cells to promote inflammation and tissue damage. Recent research has focused on the mechanisms by which these immune responses are initially activated through signaling molecules and their cellular receptors. Thorough understanding of the pathophysiology of liver I/R may yield novel therapeutic strategies to reduce I/R injury and lead to improved clinical outcomes.

emphasis on a recent consensus conference on laparoscopic liver resection in 2008, the learning curve for laparoscopic liver surgery, laparoscopic major hepatectomies, oncologic outcomes of laparoscopic liver resection for hepatocellular carcinoma and colorectal cancer liver metastases, and the comparative benefits of laparoscopic versus open liver resection. Current evidence suggests that minimally invasive hepatic resection is safe and feasible with short-term benefits, no economic disadvantage, and no compromise to oncologic principles.

> Hepatocellular carcinoma (HCC) accounts for 80% of all primary liver can-
> cers and ranks globally as the fourth leading cause of cancer-related
> death. Partial hepatectomy remains the best treatment option for select
> patients with HCC without cirrhosis. Liver transplantation is well estab-
> lished as the gold standard for patients with HCC and cirrhosis in the ab-
> sence of extrahepatic spread and macrovascular invasion. Local regional
> therapy is indicated in select patients who are not surgical candidates, and
> its role as adjuvant therapy remains to be clarified by prospective studies.

> Intrahepatic cholangiocarcinoma (ICC) is a primary cancer of the bile ducts,
> arising from malignant transformation of the epithelial cells that line the
> biliary apparatus. ICC is relatively uncommon, but its incidence is on the
> increase. ICC is frequently discovered as an incidental, indeterminate liver
> mass. Surgical resection of ICC represents the only potentially curative
> therapeutic option. The role of routine hilar lymphadenectomy is controver-
> sial, but should be considered to optimize staging. Although adjuvant che-
> motherapy and radiotherapy is probably not supported by current data,
> each should strongly be considered in patients with lymph node metastasis
> or an R1 resection. For those patients with inoperable disease, locoregional
> therapy with transarterial chemoembolization can be considered.

> Colorectal adenocarcinoma remains the third most common cause of can-
> cer death in the United States, with an estimated 146,000 new cases and
> 50,000 deaths annually. Survival is stage dependent, and the presence of
> liver metastases is a primary determinant in patient survival. Approximately
> 25% of new cases will present with synchronous colorectal liver metasta-
> ses (CLM), and up to one-half will develop CLM during the course of their
> disease. The importance of safe and effective therapies for CLM cannot be
> overstated. Safe and appropriately aggressive multimodality therapy for
> CLM can provide most patients with liver-dominant colorectal metastases
> with extended survival and an improved quality of life.

> This review summarizes regional strategies for management of neuroen-
> docrine liver metastases (NLM), including hepatic resection, ablation, liver
> transplantation, and hepatic arterial embolization/chemoembolization. De-
> spite early disease recurrence and/or progression, resection of NLM with
> or without combined ablation provides long-term survival and symptom
> improvement. When complete resection of gross liver disease is not feasi-
> ble, resection as a tumor debulking strategy should be considered in

patients with extreme hormonal symptoms refractory to other treatments or with tumors in locations that would affect short-term quality of life. Hepatic arterial embolization with or without local instillation of chemotherapy may induce disease response, symptomatic improvement, and prolonged survival in patients with unresectable NLM. Early disease recurrence, high postoperative mortality, the absence of extensive experience, and lack of universal indications for organ allocation preclude orthotopic liver transplantation as an option for most patients with unresectable NLM.

THE CLINICS ARE NOW AVAILABLE ONLINE!

Access your subscription at:
www.theclinics.com

Foreword

Liver Surgery: From Basics to Robotics

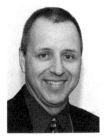

Ronald F. Martin, MD
Consulting Editor

In the late 1970s the British Broadcasting Corporation produced a documentary television series, entitled "Connections", hosted by science historian James Burke that endeavored to show how seemingly unrelated scientific discoveries were in fact related. The show was reprised in the mid-1990s with two more series. The pattern of Burke's entertaining delivery during each episode would come full circle in his discourse to the topic with which he began the show. Each show portrayed the continuity of science and showed how discovery comes full circle.

The discipline of surgery has its circles as well. This foreword is being written as we complete another academic year. Seasoned chief residents will leave for their futures and wary new first-year residents will arrive prepared to suffer catecholamine excess each time their pager goes off. Another cycle. This year, however, has a bit of a different feel though. The medical educational community, at least in the United States, is awaiting the opinion of the Accreditation Council for Graduate Medical Education (ACGME) on the new work-hours guidelines for residents learning in ACGME-accredited institutions. Many educators are worried about how the "work" will get done; some are concerned about the effect on work ethic and the length of training, and those are legitimate concerns. In my opinion, there is only one real concern: what represents the greater risk to surgical education (and eventually patient safety)—possible resident fatigue or loss of educational continuity?

Experts function by using pattern recognition. Pattern recognition is learned through long periods of sustained deliberate study and practice of patterns. The learning theorists tell us that one can show a series of chess games in midstage to chess experts and by judging how individual chess players respond to these midgame situations we can develop the same results that would occur if the chess players all played out a full scale chess tournament lasting many, many hours. This finding at least suggests that one really needs to focus primarily on the critical stages of the pattern

Surg Clin N Am 90 (2010) xv–xvi
doi:10.1016/j.suc.2010.06.002
0039-6109/10/$ – see front matter © 2010 Elsevier Inc. All rights reserved.
surgical.theclinics.com

and not necessarily the entire pattern start to finish each time—at least for experts. Resident learners, however, are generally not yet expert. Perhaps they need exposure to even the "given" parts of the game.

Another factor affecting our continuity is the way in which data arrive to all of us. About one generation ago there were three major television networks in the United States and a handful of prominent newspapers. This created a degree of synchronicity of thought and collective interest on many topics. Today almost all information is "random access information." Even materials delivered by large organizations are taken asynchronously with the use of digital recording devices, on-demand Internet access, and even podcasts. One can even order the Clinical Congress of the American College of Surgeons on DVD. There is really no absolute need for us to get any information synchronously. Perhaps the circle is broken, perhaps not; but, as stated previously, the new academic year is upon us and with that a regeneration of our hopes for the future. And what better topic for the hope of regeneration than hepatic surgery?

This is the first issue of the *Surgical Clinics of North America* since I accepted the role as Consulting Editor that revisits a recent topic. We had always intended for the cycle to repeat itself somewhat over a 5- to 6-year period—approximately the length of a surgical residency program. In 2004, Drs Khatri and Schneider wrote an excellent issue on liver surgery. Dr Geller has been kind enough to oversee the revision of this topic. At his request Professor Clavien has contributed an excellent article on the history of hepatic surgery that reminds us that knowledge of the liver's regenerative powers was known to the ancient Greeks and also reminds us that the first liver resection performed in the United States is credited to Dr William W Keen (1891). Dr William Williams Keen, the same, wrote the introduction to the inaugural issue of the *Surgical Clinics of North America* in February of 1921—62 years after beginning his career in surgery! It was Dr Keen's introduction that I quoted in my first foreword as the first Consulting Editor of this series, which brings us back to Dr Geller kindly agreeing to accept my request on behalf of our publishers to revisit this topic. The links between persons that I have described may not be as elegant as those Mr Burke would have described in his television show but they remind us all that we surgeons are not as far apart from one another as we sometimes may think.

The *Surgical Clinics of North America*, unlike many excellent journals, is not designed as a way to look at something necessarily new but, hopefully, as a platform to give us new ways to look at subjects both old and new. We aspire to provide perspective in the setting of content. That kind of perspective only comes from experts. Dr Geller and his associates have created an excellent review of liver surgery form its historical origins to the use of robotic devices. We are indebted to them and all their predecessors for their efforts.

Ronald F. Martin, MD
Department of Surgery
Marshfield Clinic
1000 North Oak Avenue
Marshfield, WI 54449, USA

E-mail address:
martin.ronald@marshfieldclinic.org

Preface

Liver Surgery: From Basics to Robotics

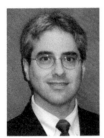

David A. Geller, MD
Guest Editor

It has been 122 years since the first elective hepatic resection was performed by Carl Langenbuch in 1888, yet the odyssey of liver surgery continues with a passion and thirst for further refinement. "Bloodless" liver surgery is now the norm, due in part to a better understanding of liver physiology, anesthesia techniques, and innovations in biomedical devices that facilitate liver parenchymal transection.

In this issue of *Surgical Clinics of North America*, a spectrum of liver surgery topics is summarized bringing the reader up to date with the era of modern hepatic resection surgery. The basics of liver anatomy and history are reviewed, along with the current molecular mechanisms of liver ischemia/reperfusion injury relevant to liver transplantation, hepatic trauma, and elective hepatic resections. Hepatic imaging techniques of ultrasound, CT, and MRI have improved and greatly facilitate our diagnostic capabilities for benign lesions and malignancies; however, the conundrum of the subcentimeter indeterminate liver lesion remains. The often confusing nomenclature of hepatic resection surgery was standardized at the 2000 Brisbane, Australia, International Heptao-Pancreato-Biliary Association meeting and is now known as the Brisbane 2000 terminology.

Advances in the past decade include the development of laparoscopic liver resection techniques, which have been reported in more than 3000 cases worldwide. Further, robotic liver resection surgery has been described but remains in its infancy. Repair of laparoscopic cholecystectomy injury remains an uncommon but important task for the hepatobiliary surgeon, as is the potentially life-saving emergency hepatic resection for traumatic liver injury.

Resection of hepatic colorectal cancer metastases has seen a paradigm shift from a prior emphasis on number of lesions to the present-day focus on sufficient liver remnant and invokes strategies of portal vein embolization and two-stage hepatectomies to increase resectability rates. Current approaches to management of

Surg Clin N Am 90 (2010) xvii–xviii
doi:10.1016/j.suc.2010.06.001
0039-6109/10/$ – see front matter © 2010 Elsevier Inc. All rights reserved.

surgical.theclinics.com

hepatocellular carcinoma continue to evolve, including live donor liver transplantation, selective hepatic resection, ablative techniques, regional liver therapies, and newer systemic chemotherapy. Intrahepatic cholangiocarcinoma is on the rise, and major hepatic resections have been advocated for metastatic neuroendocrine cancers.

Successful liver surgery requires a fundamental understanding of liver anatomy, disease pathophysiology, and modern hepatic resection techniques. Two questions always need to be addressed when contemplating hepatic resection surgery that requires both technical expertise and judgment: (1) Can the lesion technically be resected and (2) Should the lesion be resected?

I would like to thank all authors for their generous contribution and expertise in preparing their respective articles. They represent 10 of the leading institutions providing advanced hepatic surgery and contribute a broad knowledge base and diverse experience to the text. It is hoped that this edition will serve as a reference for hepatic surgery in 2010 and beyond and will inspire the next generation of hepatic surgeons to continue the quest for advances in liver surgery.

David A. Geller, MD
Department of Surgery
Starzl Transplant Institute
UPMC Liver Cancer Center
University of Pittsburgh
3459 Fifth Avenue
UPMC Montefiore, 7 South
Pittsburgh, PA 15213-2582, USA

E-mail address:
gellerda@upmc.edu

Liver Anatomy

Sherif R. Z. Abdel-Misih, MD, Mark Bloomston, MD*

KEYWORDS

• Liver • Anatomy • Surgery • Hepatic vasculature • Biliary tree

At present, liver resections are based upon the precise knowledge of the natural lines of division of the liver which define the anatomical surgery of the liver.
Henri Bismuth[1]

Although many of the advances in hepatic surgery have been linked to improvements in technology, there is no denying the impact of thorough knowledge of the internal anatomy of the liver on improved outcomes. This is largely due to the work of the French surgeon and anatomist, Claude Couinaud (1922–2008), who detailed his early work in *Le Foie: Études anatomiques et chirurgicales* (*The Liver: Anatomic and Surgical Studies*), in 1957, regarding segmental anatomy of the liver. Couinaud was able to closely examine the intrahepatic anatomy and demonstrated that hepatic functional anatomy is based on vascular and biliary relationships rather than external surface anatomy, improving the safety and feasibility of hepatic surgery today.[2]

GENERAL ANATOMY

The liver is the largest organ, accounting for approximately 2% to 3% of average body weight. The liver has 2 lobes typically described in two ways, by morphologic anatomy and by functional anatomy (as illustrated in **Fig. 1**).[1] Located in the right upper quadrant of the abdominal cavity beneath the right hemidiaphragm, it is protected by the rib cage and maintains its position through peritoneal reflections, referred to as ligamentous attachments (**Fig. 2**). Although not true ligaments, these attachments are avascular and are in continuity with the Glisson capsule or the equivalent of the visceral peritoneum of the liver.

Ligamentous Attachments

The falciform ligament is an attachment arising at or near the umbilicus and continues onto the anterior aspect of the liver in continuity with the umbilical fissure. The falciform ligament courses cranially along the anterior surface of the liver, blending into the hepatic peritoneal covering coursing posterosuperiorly to become the anterior portion of the left and right coronary ligaments. Of surgical importance, at the base

Division of Surgical Oncology, The Ohio State University Medical Center, Arthur G. James Cancer Hospital, Richard J. Solove Research Institute, 410 West, 10th Avenue, N-924 Doan Hall, Columbus, OH 43210, USA
* Corresponding author.
E-mail address: mark.bloomston@osumc.edu

Surg Clin N Am 90 (2010) 643–653
doi:10.1016/j.suc.2010.04.017   surgical.theclinics.com

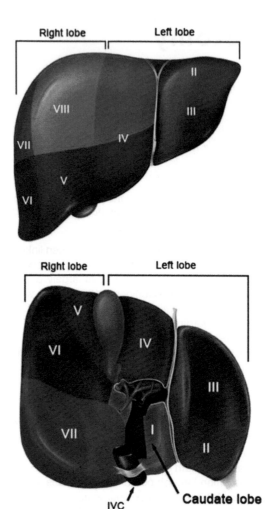

Fig. 1. Anterior and posterior surfaces of liver illustrating functional division of the liver into left and right hepatic lobes with Couinaud's segmental classification based on functional anatomy. *From* Brunicardi FC, Andersen DK, Billiar TR, et al. Schwartz's principles of surgery. 9th edition. New York: McGraw-Hill Publishing; 2010. p. 31–3; with permission.

of the falciform ligament along the liver, the hepatic veins drain into the inferior vena cava (IVC).[3] A common misconception associated with the falciform ligament is that it divides the liver into left and right lobes. Based on morphologic anatomy, this may be true; however, this does not hold true from a functional standpoint (discussed later).

Within the lower edge of the falciform ligament is the ligamentum teres (round ligament), a remnant of the obliterated umbilical vein (ductus venosus) that travels from the umbilicus into the umbilical fissure where it is in continuity with the ligamentum venosum as it joins the left branch of the portal vein. The ligamentum venosum lies within a fissure on the inferior surface of the liver between the caudate lobe posteriorly and the left lobe anteriorly, where it is also invested by the peritoneal folds of the lesser omentum (gastrohepatic ligament). During fetal life, the ductus venosus is responsible for shunting a majority of blood flow of the umbilical vein directly into the IVC,

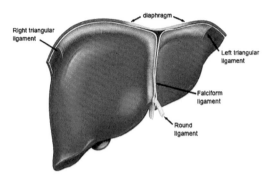

Fig. 2. Ligamentous attachments of the liver. *From* Brunicardi FC, Andersen DK, Billiar TR, et al. Schwartz's principles of surgery. 9th edition. New York: McGraw-Hill Publishing; 2010. p. 31–2; with permission.

transporting oxygenated blood from the placenta to the fetus. After birth, the umbilical vein closes as the physiologic neonatal circulation begins. In the presence of portal hypertension, the umbilical vein may recanalize to allow portasystemic collateralization through the abdominal wall, known as caput medusae.

At the cranial aspect of the liver is a convex area along the diaphragmatic surface that is devoid of any ligamentous attachments or peritoneum. This bare area of the liver is attached to the diaphragm by flimsy fibroareolar tissue. The coronary ligament lies anterior and posterior to the bare area of the liver comprised of peritoneal reflections of the diaphragm. These areas converge to the left and right of the liver to form the left and right triangular ligaments, respectively. The right coronary and right triangular ligaments course posterior and caudally toward the right kidney, attaching the liver to the retroperitoneum. All attachments help fixate the liver within the right upper quadrant of the abdomen. During hepatic surgery, mobilization of the liver requires division of these avascular attachments. In upper abdominal surgery, the liver has close associations with many structures and organs.

The IVC maintains an intimate relationship to the caudate lobe and right hepatic lobe by IVC ligaments.[4] These caval ligaments are bridges of broad membranous tissue that are extensions of the Glisson capsule from the caudate and right hepatic lobe. Of surgical importance, these ligaments are not simple connective tissue but rather contain components of hepatic parenchyma, including the portal triads and hepatocytes. Hence, during liver mobilization, these ligaments must be controlled in a surgical manner to avoid unnecessary bleeding or bile leakage during hepatic surgery.

Perihepatic Organs/Anatomy

The gastrointestinal tract has several associations with the liver (illustrated in **Fig. 3**). The stomach is related to the left hepatic lobe by way of the gastrohepatic ligament or superior aspect of the lesser omentum, which is an attachment of connective tissue between the lesser curvature of the stomach and the left hepatic lobe at the ligamentum venosum. Important neural and vascular structures may run within the gastrohepatic ligament, including the hepatic division of the vagus nerve and, when present, an aberrant left hepatic artery as it courses from its left gastric artery origin. The hepatic flexure of the colon where the ascending colon transitions to the transverse colon is in close proximity or sometimes in direct contact with the right hepatic lobe. Additionally, the duodenum and portal structures are in direct association with the liver through the hepatoduodenal ligament (inferior aspect of the lesser omentum) and porta hepatis.

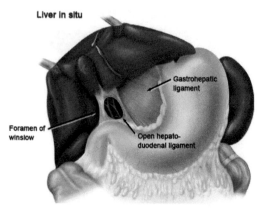

Fig. 3. Association of stomach, porta hepatis, and hepatic flexure to the Liver. *From* Bruni-cardi FC, Andersen DK, Billiar TR, et al. Schwartz's principles of surgery. 9th edition. New York: McGraw-Hill Publishing; 2010. p. 31–3; with permission.

Anatomic understanding of the portal anatomy is essential to hepatic resection and associated vascular and biliary reconstructions. Within the porta hepatis is the common bile duct, hepatic artery, and portal vein that course in a lateral, medial, and posterior configuration, respectively. The foramen of Winslow (epiploic foramen) has important relevance to the porta hepatis and hepato-pancreatico-biliary surgery. The foramen of Winslow, originally described by the Danish anatomist Jacob Winslow in 1732, is a communication or connection between the abdominal cavity and the lesser sac. During hepatic resection, need for complete control of the hepatic vascular inflow may be accomplished by a Pringle maneuver.[5,6] This maneuver, developed by an Australian surgeon, James Hogarth Pringle, while in Glasgow, Scotland, during the management of hepatic trauma, involves occlusion of the hepatic artery and portal vein inflow through control of the porta hepatis. This may be done by placement of a large clamp on the porta hepatis or more atraumatically with the use of a tourniquet passed through the foramen of Winslow and pars flaccida (transparent portion of lesser omentum overlying caudate lobe) encircling the porta hepatis.

The gallbladder resides in the gallbladder fossa at the posterior interface of segments IV and V. It establishes continuity with the common bile duct via the cystic duct. Additionally, the cystic artery most commonly arises as a branch off the right hepatic artery. Understanding of portal vasculature and biliary anatomy is crucial given its wide anatomic variability to avoid inadvertent injury during any hepatic, pancreatic, biliary, or foregut surgery.

Additionally, the right adrenal gland lies within the retroperitoneum under the right hepatic lobe. The right adrenal vein drains directly into the IVC; hence, care should be taken during hepatic mobilization so as to avoid avulsion of the vein or inadvertent dissection into the adrenal gland as this can result in significant hemorrhage.

LYMPHATIC AND NEURAL NETWORK

The liver possesses a superficial and deep lymphatic network through which lymph produced in the liver drains.[7] The deep network is responsible for greater lymphatic drainage toward lateral phrenic nodes via the hepatic veins and toward the hilum through portal vein branches. The superficial network is located within the Glisson capsule with an anterior and posterior surface. The anterior surface primarily drains to phrenic lymph nodes via the bare area of the liver to join the mediastinal and internal mammary lymphatic networks. The posterior surface network drains to hilar lymph nodes, including the cystic duct, common bile duct, hepatic artery, and peripancreatic as well as pericardial and celiac lymph nodes. The lymphatic drainage patterns have surgical implications with regard to lymphadenectomy undertaken for cancer of the gallbladder, liver, and pancreas.

The neural innervation and controls of liver function are complex and not well understood. However, like the remainder of the body, the liver does have parasympathetic and sympathetic neural innervation. Nerve fibers are derived from the celiac plexus, lower thoracic ganglia, right phrenic nerve, and the vagi. The vagus nerves divide into an anterior (left) and posterior (right) branch as they course from the thorax into the abdomen. The anterior vagus divides into a cephalic and a hepatic division of which the latter courses through the lesser omentum (gastrohepatic ligament) to innervate the liver and is responsible for the parasympathetic innervation. Sympathetic innervation arises predominantly from the celiac plexus as well as the thoracic splanchnic nerves.

HEPATIC VASCULATURE

The liver is a very vascular organ and at rest receives up to 25% of total cardiac output, more than any other organ. Its dual blood supply is uniquely divided between the hepatic artery, which contributes 25% to 30% of the blood supply, and the portal vein, which is responsible for the remaining 70% to 75%. The arterial and portal blood ultimately mixes within the hepatic sinusoids before draining into the systemic circulation via the hepatic venous system.[8]

Arterial Vasculature

Although the arterial vasculature of the liver is variable, the most common configurations are discussed in this article. As illustrated in **Fig. 4**, in the most common arterial configuration, the common hepatic artery originates from the celiac axis along with the left gastric and splenic arteries. The common hepatic artery proceeds laterally and branches into the proper hepatic artery and the gastroduodenal artery. The gastroduodenal artery proceeds caudally to supply the pylorus and proximal duodenum and has several indirect branches to the pancreas. The proper hepatic artery courses within the medial aspect of the hepatoduodenal ligament and porta hepatis toward

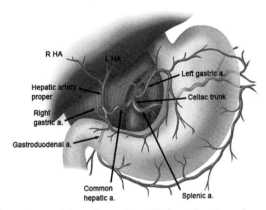

Fig. 4. Common hepatic arterial configuration. HA, hepatic artery. *From* Brunicardi FC, Andersen DK, Billiar TR, et al. Schwartz's principles of surgery. 9th edition. New York: McGraw-Hill Publishing; 2010. p. 31–4; with permission.

the liver to divide into left and right hepatic arteries to feed the respective hepatic lobes. Additionally, the right gastric artery has a variable origin arising from the hepatic artery as it courses laterally. The cystic artery to the gallbladder commonly arises from the right hepatic artery. In **Fig. 5**, common arterial variants are illustrated. The most common variants include aberrant (replaced) hepatic arteries in which the dominant hepatic arteries do not arise from the proper hepatic artery but rather from an alternate origin. An aberrant left hepatic artery typically arises from the left gastric artery and courses through the lesser omentum to supply the left liver and is seen in approximately 15% of patients. In spite of its alternate origin, the aberrant left hepatic artery still enters the liver through the base of the umbilical fissure in a medial orientation, similar to that of a native left hepatic artery. An aberrant right hepatic artery, seen in approximately 20% of patients, most commonly arises from the superior mesenteric artery. Unlike its left hepatic artery counterpart, the aberrant right hepatic artery often courses posterolateral in the hepatoduodenal ligament to enter the right liver.

Venous Vasculature

The portal vein provides the bulk of the nutritive blood supply to the liver. As illustrated in **Fig. 6**, the portal vein forms from the confluence of the superior mesenteric vein and splenic vein behind the neck of the pancreas. Additional venous branches that drain into the portal vein include the coronary (left gastric) vein, cystic vein, and tributaries of the right gastric and pancreaticoduodenal veins. The portal vein is valveless and is a low-pressure system with pressures typically 3 to 5 mm Hg. The coronary (left gastric) vein is of particular importance clinically as it becomes a major portasystemic shunt in the face of portal hypertension and feeds the gastroesophageal variceal complex. The main portal vein courses cranially toward the liver as the most posterior structure within the hepatoduodenal

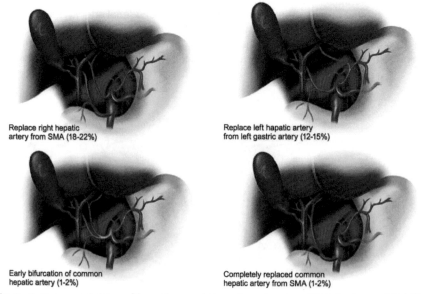

Replace right hepatic
artery from SMA (18-22%)

Replace left hapatic artery
from left gastric artery (12-15%)

Early bifurcation of common
hepatic artery (1-2%)

Completely replaced common
hepatic artery from SMA (1-2%)

Fig. 5. Common variations of hepatic vasculature. *From* Brunicardi FC, Andersen DK, Billiar TR, et al. Schwartz's principles of surgery. 9th edition. New York: McGraw-Hill Publishing. p. 31–4; 2010.

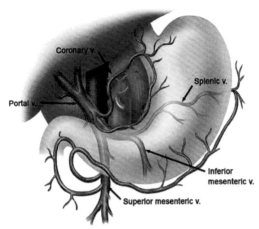

Fig. 6. Portal vein and the hepatic venous vasculature inflow. *From* Brunicardi FC, Andersen DK, Billiar TR, et al. Schwartz's principles of surgery. 9th edition; McGraw-Hill Publishing. p. 31–5; 2010.

ligament to divide into the left and right portal veins near the liver hilum. A small branch to the right side of the caudate is commonly encountered just before or after the main portal vein branching.

The left portal vein has two portions, an initial transverse portion and then an umbilical portion as it approaches the umbilical fissure. The left portal vein tends to have a longer extrahepatic course and commonly gives off a branch to the caudate lobe, but the caudate portal vein inflow is variable and may arise from the main or right portal vein also. The transverse portion of the left portal vein approaches the umbilical fissure and takes an abrupt turn toward it to form the umbilical portion as it enters the liver.

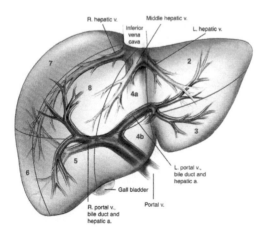

Fig. 7. Intrahepatic vascular and biliary anatomy, anterior view. *Adapted from* Cameron JL, Sandone C. Atlas of gastrointestinal surgery, vol. 1. 2nd edition. Hamilton (ON): BC Decker; 2007. p. 121 [**Fig. 1**]; the People's Medical Publishing House—USA, Shelton, CT; with permission.

Within the liver, the umbilical portion of the left portal vein commonly first gives off a branch to segment II before then dividing into branches to segment III and to segment IVa/IVb. The right portal vein often emerges closer to or within the hepatic parenchyma of the right liver itself. It quickly divides into anterior and posterior branches to segments V and VIII and segments VI and VII, respectively (see **Fig. 1**; **Figs. 7** and **8**).

The venous drainage of the liver is through the intrahepatic veins that ultimately coalesce into three hepatic veins that drain into the IVC superiorly. The left and middle hepatic veins may drain directly into the IVC but more commonly form a short common trunk before draining into the IVC. The right hepatic vein is typically larger, with a short extrahepatic course and drains directly into the IVC. Additional drainage occurs directly into the IVC via short retrohepatic veins and, on occasion, an inferior right accessory hepatic vein. The hepatic veins within the parenchyma are unique in that, unlike the portal venous system, they lack the fibrous, protective, encasing the Glisson capsule.[9] Ultrasonography facilitates intraoperative mapping of the internal anatomy of the liver. As seen in **Fig. 9**, by ultrasound, the portal venous anatomy can readily be identified by the echogenic, hyperechoic Glisson capsule surrounding the portal veins, whereas the hepatic veins lack this.

The IVC maintains an important and intimate association with the liver as it courses in a cranial-caudal direction to the right of the aorta. As the IVC travels cranially, it courses posterior to the duodenum, pancreas, porta hepatis, caudate lobe, and posterior surface of the liver as it approaches the bare area where it receives the hepatic venous outflow from the hepatic veins. Multiple small retrohepatic veins enter the IVC along its course, mostly from the right hepatic lobe. Hence, in mobilizing the

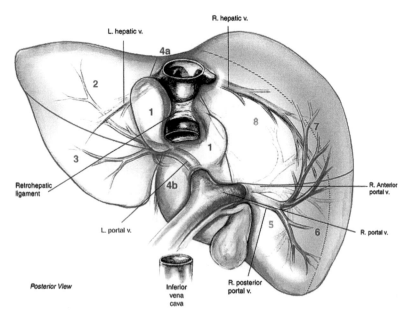

Fig. 8. Intrahepatic vascular and biliary anatomy. posterior view. *Adapted from* Cameron JL, Sandone C. Atlas of gastrointestinal surgery, vol. 1. 2nd edition. Hamilton (ON): BC Decker; 2007. p. 124 **[Fig. 2]**; the People's Medical Publishing House—USA, Shelton, CT; with permission.

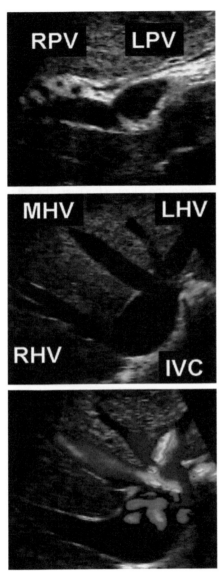

Fig. 9. Ultrasound appearance of hepatic venous vasculature. The top panel demonstrates the left and right portal vein branches (LPV, left portal vein; RPV, right portal vein) with the hyperechoic fibrous sheath of the Glisson capsule. The middle panel demonstrates the confluence of the right, middle, and left hepatic veins (LHV, left hepatic vein; RHV, right hepatic vein; MHV; middle hepatic vein) (note accessory left hepatic vein) with the IVC. The lower panel demonstrates vascular flow within the hepatic vein confluence and IVC. *From* Brunicardi FC, Andersen DK, Billiar TR, et al. Schwartz's principles of surgery. 9th edition. New York: McGraw-Hill Publishing; 2010. p. 14. Chapter 31; with permission.

liver or during major hepatic resections, it is imperative to maintain awareness of the IVC and its vascular tributaries at all times.

BILIARY TREE

The intrahepatic biliary tree is comprised of multiple ducts that are responsible for the formation and transport of bile from the liver to the duodenum and typically follows the portal venous system. The right hepatic duct forms from an anterior sectoral duct from segments V and VIII and a posterior sectoral duct from segments VI and VII. The anterior sectoral duct courses in an anterior, vertical manner whereas the posterior duct proceeds in a lateral, horizontal manner. The right duct typically has a short extrahepatic course with some branching variability. Surgeons should be mindful of this variable anatomy when operating at the hilum of the liver. The left hepatic duct drains the left liver and has a less variable course as it parallels the left portal vein with a longer extrahepatic course. The left and right hepatic ducts join near the hilar plate to form the common hepatic duct. As the common hepatic duct courses caudally, it is joined by the cystic duct to form the common bile duct. The common bile duct proceeds within the lateral aspect of the hepatoduodenal ligament toward the head of the pancreas to drain into the duodenum through the ampulla of Vater.

Biliary drainage of the caudate lobe is variable with drainage seen through left and right hepatic ducts in approximately 70% to 80% of cases.[8] In 15%, caudate drainage is seen through the left hepatic duct alone and the remaining 5% to 10% of cases drains through the right hepatic duct system alone. Hence, as discussed previously, surgical intervention involving the caudate lobe requires attention to biliary anatomy as well as vascular anatomy.

SUMMARY

Understanding of hepatic anatomy has evolved greatly over the past 50 years. Greater knowledge of vascular anatomy along with advancement of technologies for intraoperative mapping and parenchymal transection have made liver surgery safer and more efficacious. Recognition of the presence of a dual blood supply and dependence of hepatic tumors on arterial bloody supply have made feasible various interventional techniques allowing directed chemotherapy and radioactive particles via the hepatic artery with simultaneous embolization to minimize tumoral blood supply as treatment options for various tumor types. The complexities and nuances of liver anatomy require continual respect and lifelong learning by liver surgeons.

REFERENCES

1. Bismuth H. Surgical anatomy and anatomical surgery of the liver. World J Surg 1982;6(1):3–9.
2. Sutherland F, Harris J. Claude Couinaud: a passion for the liver. Arch Surg 2002; 137(11):1305–10.
3. Jamieson GG. The anatomy of general surgical operations. 2nd edition. Edinburgh (NY): Churchill Livingstone/Elsevier; 2006. p. 8–23.
4. Kogure K, Ishizaki M, Nemoto M, et al. Close relation between the inferior vena cava ligament and the caudate lobe in the human liver. J Hepatobiliary Pancreat Surg 2007;14(3):297–301.
5. Pringle JH. V. Notes on the arrest of hepatic hemorrhage due to trauma. Ann Surg 1908;48(4):541–9.

6. van Gulik TM, de Graaf W, Dinant S, et al. Vascular occlusion techniques during liver resection. Dig Surg 2007;24(4):274–81.
7. Skandalakis JE, Skandalakis LJ, Skandalakis PN, et al. Hepatic surgical anatomy. Surg Clin North Am 2004;84(2):413–35.
8. Blumgart LH, Belghiti J. Surgery of the liver, biliary tract, and pancreas. 3rd edition. Philadelphia: Saunders Elsevier; 2007. p. 3–30.
9. Ger R. Surgical anatomy of the liver. Surg Clin North Am 1989;69(2):179–92.

History of Hepatic Surgery

Kuno Lehmann, MD, Pierre-Alain Clavien, MD, PhD*

KEYWORDS

• Liver • Transplantation • Hepatic surgery • Resection

THE LIVER IS A FRAGILE BLEEDING MYSTERY

Many years lie between the first historical reports on hepatic anatomy and today's hepatic surgery. One of the first tales is the legend of Prometheus, written by Hesoid (750–700 BC), recounting ancient times. Prometheus stole fire from Zeus, the godfather of ancient Greece, and gave it to mankind. For this infringement, Zeus chained him to a rock and sent an eagle to devour his liver. The liver regenerated and gained its normal size overnight. Each morning the hungry eagle returned, and Prometheus was captured in eternal pain. Today, the amazing regenerative capacity of the liver is no longer an inspiration for mystical tales but is the basis for modern hepatobiliary surgery.[1]

An Alexandrian physician Herophilus (330–280 BC) was one of the first anatomists to describe the liver, although his written work is not available. The Greek physician Galen (AD 130–200) cited his work and accurately described the lobar anatomy and vasculature, interpreting the liver as the source of blood. However, in the following centuries of the Middle Ages, knowledge on hepatic anatomy moved forward very little.

More than 350 years ago, anatomists started exploring hepatic anatomy with clever ideas. In 1654, Glisson[2] from Cambridge, England, cooked the organ in hot water, removed the hepatic parenchyma, and explored the hepatic blood flow with colored milk. He discussed the intrahepatic anatomy and topography of the vasculature (**Fig. 1**). The growing knowledge of hepatic anatomy was one of the substantial preconditions for the development of hepatic surgery. However, this precondition was still far from realization, and the liver remained a fragile bleeding mystery.

ANATOMIC INSIGHTS PROVIDED THE FUNDAMENTAL BASIS FOR HEPATIC SURGERY

In the nineteenth century, two fundamental concepts enabling major surgery were introduced: anesthesia and asepsis. In 1842, Crawford W. Long used ether as

Swiss Hepato-Pancreatico-Biliary & Transplantation Center, Department of Surgery, University Hospital of Zürich, Rämistrasse 100, Zürich 8091, Switzerland
* Corresponding author.
E-mail address: clavien@access.uzh.ch

Surg Clin N Am 90 (2010) 655–664
doi:10.1016/j.suc.2010.04.018
0039-6109/10/$ – see front matter

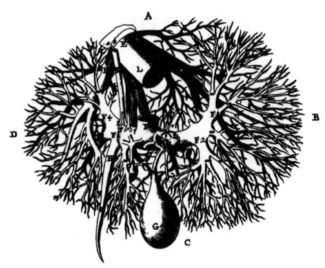

Fig. 1. Intrahepatic vasculature. (*From* Glisson F. Anatomia hepatis. London: Dugard; 1654.)

a surgical anesthetic for the first time in the United States. In 1867, Joseph Lister from Glasgow, Ireland, introduced antiseptic techniques against bacterial infections after Louis Pasteur from Paris, France, had discovered the dangers of bacteria.

Before this period, only anecdotal records of hepatic surgery existed. Usually, the surgeons described the removal of protruding hepatic tissue after trauma. Among these surgeons were Ambroise Paré from Paris, France, J.C. Massie from the United States, and Victor von Bruns from Germany. However, hepatic trauma at that time was generally managed without operation. It took many years before any courageous surgeon was successful in the first attempt of a planned hepatic resection.

Carl Langenbuch from Berlin, Germany (**Fig. 2**), performed the first cholecystectomy. He reported the first elective and successful hepatic resection in 1888.[3] In 1891, William W. Keen from Philadelphia performed the first resection in the United States. He used the "finger fracture" technique to divide the hepatic parenchyma. Intraoperative bleeding control remained the most striking challenge then. In 1896, Michel Kousnetzoff and Jules Pensky[4] suggested the use of a continuous mattress suture above the resection line for controlling bleeding. In 1908, Pringle[5] from Scotland, described a method of temporary compression of the portal ligament in a small series of patients. However, the major discoveries were still ahead.

It was again the fine work of anatomists that provided the key insights to overcome major bleeding. About 120 years ago, in 1888, Hugo Rex from Germany,[6] and in 1897, James Cantlie from Liverpool, England,[7] challenged the accepted anatomic division of the liver by the falciform ligament. Using corrosion studies, they separated the liver by the branches of the portal vein. Furthermore, they defined an avascular plane through the gallbladder bed toward the vena cava and through the right axis of the caudate lobe along the middle hepatic vein. Today, this plane is known as the Rex-Cantlie line. At the beginning of the twentieth century, Walter Wendell from Magdeburg, Germany,[8] and Hansvon Haberer from Graz, Austria,[9] were the first surgeons to perform resections along this anatomic plane.

Hepatic anatomy was further refined by the description of the intrahepatic biliary duct system and the vascular tree by Carl-Herman Hjortsjo[10] from Lund, Sweden, and John Healey and colleagues[11] from Houston, Texas. In 1954, Claude Couinaud[12]

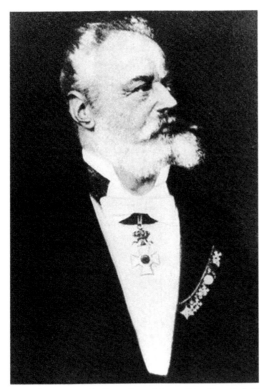

Fig. 2. Carl Langenbuch (1846–1881). (*Reprinted from* The Royal College of Surgeons of England; with permission.)

from Paris, France, published his seminal work on the segmental architecture of the liver (**Fig. 3**).[13] Based on the branches of the portal vein, he separated the liver into 8 well-described segments. The systematic descriptions of Carl-Herman Hjortsjo, John Healey, and Claude Couinaud had a major effect on surgical technique and related mortality.

In 1950, Ichio Honjo ki[14] from Kyoto, Japan, reported the first anatomic resection. The first resections in Europe and the United States were reported by Jean-Louis and Lortat-Jacob[15] from Paris, France in 1952, followed by Julian. K. Quattlebaum,[16] from Georgia in 1953. In the following years, many surgeons reported their experience, including Alexander Brunschwig[17] and George T. Pack and colleagues[18] in New York and later, William P. Longmire and Samuel A. Marable[19] in Los Angeles, California.

Over the years, serious concern was growing over hepatic nomenclature. Throughout the world, liver surgeons used different, sometimes confusing, terms.[20] Only a few years ago, in 2000, a group of international liver surgeons proposed a standardized nomenclature. This terminology was introduced at the biannual meeting of the International Hepato-Pancreato-Biliary Association in Brisbane, Australia. Subsequently, the terminology was called the Brisbane nomenclature.[21]

LIVER TRANSPLANTATION: A HARD SUCCESS

The transplantation era was an important period and driving force for the development of hepatobiliary surgery. In 1955, Cristopher S. Welch[22] from Albany, New York,

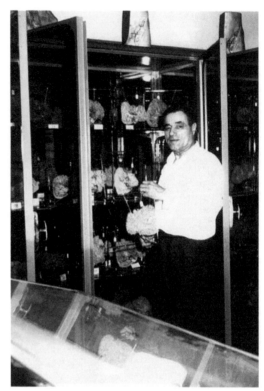

Fig. 3. Claude Couinaud working with his collection of liver casts at the School of Medicine in Paris, France, in 1988. (*From* Sutherland F, Harris J. Claude Couinaud: a passion for the liver. Arch Surg 2002;137(11):1305–10. Copyright (2002) American Medical Association. All rights reserved; with permission.)

published the first report of heterotopic liver transplantation in a dog. J. A. Cannon, Thomas E. Starzl, and Francis D. Moore and colleagues[23] continued with orthotopic liver transplantations (OLTs) in dogs and established the basis for transplantation in humans. In 1963, Starzl and colleagues[24] (**Fig. 4**) made the first attempt to transplant a human liver in Denver, Colorado. However, the young patient died during the operation due to uncontrollable bleeding. Another attempt by Moore[25] in Boston, Massachusetts, also did not succeed. It was again Starzl and colleagues[26] who reported the first series of successful OLT in 1968. Shortly after, Sir Roy Calne and colleagues[27] performed the first OLT in Europe in Cambridge, England. At that time, most patients did not survive OLT longer than a few weeks or months, although many patients initially tolerated the surgery well.

The solution to this problem was the discovery of cyclosporine A (CyA) by Hartmann F. Stähelin and Jean-Francois Borel from Basel, Switzerland, in 1972. Seven years later, Calne and colleagues[28] reported the first use of CyA in patients undergoing OLT. The result was a dramatic improvement in long-term survival. Before the introduction of CyA, the 5-year survival rate after OLT was less than 20%. But the survival rate improved to 60% or more with the introduction of CyA.[29] In the late 1980s, Tom E. Starzl introduced FK-506 (tacrolimus) as a new and promising immunosuppressant at the University of Pittsburgh. In the following years, immunosuppression was refined,

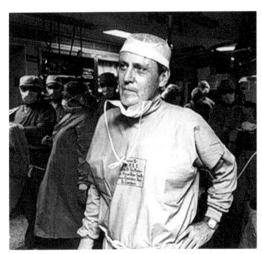

Fig. 4. Tom E. Starzl performed the first successful OLT in 1968. (*Reprinted from* the PittChronicle, University of Pittsburgh, October 15, 2007; with permission.)

and the introduction of effective drugs such as polyclonal antilymphocyte antibodies, anti-CD3 antibodies in the 1980s, mycophenolate mofetil in the early 1990s, and rapamycin in the late 1990s offered further alternatives in the management of patients after OLT.

Surgeons already recognized the critical role of adequate preservation in the early stage of solid-organ transplantation. Cold preservation technique was described in 1912 by the French surgeon Alexis Carrel, who preserved and transplanted vessels, skin, and connective tissues in dogs.[30] Together, Carrel and Charles A. Lindberg,[31] the famous aviator and engineer, constructed a perfusion pump and successfully preserved thyroid glands. The relevance of cooling the donor organ was recovered years later during animal experiments by Moore and colleagues.[23] For many years, storage in cold Collins solution was the standard for organ procurement.[32] A landmark advance was the development of the University of Wisconsin (UW) solution by Folkert O. Belzer and James H. Southard[33] in 1988. The UW solution represents an important gain of knowledge in the pathophysiology of ischemia and reperfusion injury. The UW solution contains colloids to prevent cell swelling, oxygen scavengers like allopurinol and glutathione for cell protection, and adenosine to facilitate adenosine triphosphate production.[34]

Nearly 30 years ago, in 1983, the National Institutes of Health Consensus Conference accepted liver transplantation as a therapy for patients with end-stage liver disease. Consequently, the number of patients on waiting lists increased massively in the following years, resulting in a dramatic shortage of available donor organs for transplantation. The mortality of patients waiting for an organ stimulated the development of new concepts.

This shortage was more accentuated in pediatric patients. Because children require size-matched organs, there was a high death rate in the pediatric waiting list for cadaveric organs. This high death rate stimulated the development of technical innovations based on the segmental anatomy of the liver. In 1984, Henri Bismuth,[35] from Paris, France, performed the first OLT using only the left hemiliver. In 1988, Rudolf Pichlmayr and colleagues,[36] from Hannover, Germany applied the concept of partial liver graft transplantation. They reported the use of a split graft, in which the right hemiliver was transplanted to an adult and the left to a child. Christoph E. Broelsch and colleagues[37] published the first patient series on split liver transplantation in Chicago, Illinois. Living donor liver transplantation was first reported in Brazil, in 1989, by Silvano Raia and colleagues.[38] A year later, Russel W. Strong and colleagues,[39] from Brisbane, Australia, published the next case of a mother donating the left hemiliver to her son. In 1994, Yoshio Yamaoka and colleagues,[40] from Kyoto, Japan, used the right hemiliver for transplantation and enabled living donor liver transplantation in adults. The report on first series of patients was published by Broelsch and colleagues[41] in Chicago, Illinois and later by Chung-Mau Lo and colleagues[42] in Hong Kong.

A potential approach to solve the shortage of donor organs was shown with a favorable outcome by the use of steatotic donor organs.[43] Donor risk scores and appropriate matching to selected recipients may further improve the outcome of these organs.[44] Today, liver transplantation is a great success and has become a standard procedure with excellent outcomes.[45]

HEPATIC SURGERY BECOMES SAFE AND EFFECTIVE

In the sixties, perioperative mortality rates up to 50% were common after right hemihepatectomy. Parallel to the progress in liver transplantation, hepatic surgery, mostly for oncologic diseases, became more sophisticated. In 1983, William P. Longmire and colleagues[46] from Los Angeles, California, published the results of 138 patients after major resections with a 30-day mortality of 10%. A few years later, in the 1990s, Jacques Belghiti and colleagues[47] from Paris, France, in a large series of 747 patients, reported a mortality of 1% in patients with normal liver parenchyma. Leslie H. Blumgart[48] from New York and Sheung Tat Fan and colleagues[49] from Hong Kong published similar results. However, the presence of cirrhosis,[50] portal hypertension,[51] and liver steatosis[52] were identified as important risk factors for perioperative morbidity and mortality. Because of the complexity of the diseases, and the perioperative care, these patients required specialized teams. An important step for the improved outcomes was the promotion of specialized, interdisciplinary centers.[53] A higher caseload in such hepato-pancreatico-biliary (HPB) centers translates into more experience, which is an important factor for favorable outcomes.[54,55]

Many technical tools further refined hepatic surgery. Masatoshi Makuuchi and colleagues[56] from Tokyo, Japan, introduced the concept of routine intraoperative ultrasonography for liver surgery. These investigators were also among the first to use portal vein embolization to increase the future liver remnant before major resection.[57] However, the concept of selective portal occlusion and subsequent contralateral hypertrophy was known since 1920.[58] Radiofrequency was introduced as a treatment for unresectable tumors.[59–61] For further details and an in-depth coverage of hepatic surgery in the twentieth century, the authors recommend the comprehensive overviews by Joseph G. Fortner and Lesilie H. Blumgart[62] and James H. Foster.[63]

The complex treatment strategies for metastatic liver disease are illustrative examples for the progress and success of HPB surgery.[1] In 1940, Richard B. Cattell,[64] in Boston, Massachusetts, performed the first resection of a metastatic tumor. However, still in the early eighties, resection of colorectal liver metastases remained controversial because of the high operative mortality.[65] Today, resection for liver metastasis provides favorable outcomes compared with the natural history.[66] In a series of 1001 consecutive patients, the 5-year survival rate was 37%.[67] Multistage procedures are currently recognized as effective strategies for patients with otherwise unresectable tumors.[1]

SUMMARY

Surgical experience and outcomes after major surgery have improved as a result of progress in many fields. Consequently, hepatic surgery has enjoyed a dramatic development during the last 3 decades. Today, liver surgery has lost the threat of the early years. In experienced hands, hepatic surgery has become reliable and effective and has consequently saved the life of many patients.

REFERENCES

1. Clavien PA, Petrowsky H, DeOliveira ML, et al. Strategies for safer liver surgery and partial liver transplantation. N Engl J Med 2007;356(15):1545–59.
2. Glisson F. Anatomia hepatis. London: Dugard; 1654.
3. Langenbuch C. Ein fall von resection eines linksseitigen schnurlappens der leber. Heilung Klin Wochenschr 1888;25:37 [in German].
4. Kousnetzoff M, Pensky J. Sur la resection partielle du foie. Rev Chir 1896;16: 501–21 [in French].
5. Pringle JH. V. Notes on the arrest of hepatic hemorrhage due to trauma. Ann Surg 1908;48(4):541–9.
6. Rex H. Beiträge zur morphologie der säugerleber. Morphol Jahrb 1888;14:517 [in German].
7. Cantile J. On a new arrangement of the right and left lobes of the liver. J Anat Physiol 1897;32:4–9.
8. Wendell W. Beiträge zur chirurgie der leber. Arch Klin Chir 1911;95:887 [in German].
9. von Haberer H. Zur frage der nicht parasitären leberzysten. Wien Klin Wochenschr 1909;22:1788 [in German].
10. Hjortsjo CH. The topography of the intrahepatic duct systems. Acta Anat (Basel) 1951;11(4):599–615.
11. Healey JE Jr, Schroy PC, Sorensen RJ. The intrahepatic distribution of the hepatic artery in man. J Int Coll Surg 1953;20(2):133–48.
12. Couinaud C. Lobes des ségments hépatiques: notes sur architecture anatomique et chirurgicale du foie. Presse Med 1954;62(33):709–12 [in French].
13. Sutherland F, Harris J. Claude Couinaud: a passion for the liver. Arch Surg 2002; 137(11):1305–10.
14. Honjo I, Araki C. [Total resection of the right lobe of the liver: report of a successful case]. Shujutsu 1950;4:345–9 [in Japanese].
15. Lortat-Jacob J, Robert H. Hepatectomie droite reglée. Presse Med 1952;60:549 [in French].
16. Quattlebaum JK. Massive resection of the liver. Ann Surg 1953;137(6):787–96.
17. Brunschwig A. The surgical treatment of primary and secondary hepatic malignant tumors. Am Surg 1954;20(10):1077–85.
18. Pack GT, Miller TR, Brasfield RD. Total right hepatic lobectomy for cancer of the gallbladder; report of three cases. Ann Surg 1955;142(1):6–16.
19. Longmire WP Jr, Marable SA. Clinical experiences with major hepatic resections. Ann Surg 1961;154:460–74.
20. Strasberg SM. Terminology of liver anatomy and liver resections: coming to grips with hepatic babel. J Am Coll Surg 1997;184(4):413–34.
21. Belghiti J, Clavien P, Gadzijev E, et al. The Brisbane 2000 terminology of liver anatomy and resections. HPB Surg 2000;2:333–9.
22. Welch C. A note on transplantation of the whole liver in dogs. Transplant Bull 1955;2:54.

23. Moore FD, Wheele HB, Demissianos HV, et al. Experimental whole-organ transplantation of the liver and of the spleen. Ann Surg 1960;152:374–87.

24. Starzl TE, Marchioro TL, Vonkaulla KN, et al. Homotransplantation of the liver in humans. Surg Gynecol Obstet 1963;117:659–76.

25. Moore FD. A miracle and a privilege: recounting a half-century of surgical advance. Washington, DC: Joseph Henry Press; 1995.

26. Starzl TE, Groth CG, Brettschneider L, et al. Orthotopic homotransplantation of the human liver. Ann Surg 1968;168(3):392–415.

27. Calne RY, Williams R, Dawson JL, et al. Liver transplantation in man. II. A report of two orthotopic liver transplants in adult recipients. Br Med J 1968;4(5630):541–6.

28. Calne RY, Rolles K, White DJ, et al. Cyclosporin A initially as the only immunosuppressant in 34 recipients of cadaveric organs: 32 kidneys, 2 pancreases, and 2 livers. Lancet 1979;2(8151):1033–6.

29. Iwatsuki S, Starzl TE, Todo S, et al. Experience in 1,000 liver transplants under cyclosporine-steroid therapy: a survival report. Transplant Proc 1988;20(1 Suppl 1):498–504.

30. Dutkowski P, de Rougemont O, Clavien PA. Alexis Carrel: genius, innovator and ideologist. Am J Transplant 2008;8(10):1998–2003.

31. Carrel A, Lindbergh CA. The culture of whole organs. Science 1935;81(2112):621–3.

32. Benichou J, Halgrimson CG, Weil R 3rd, et al. Canine and human liver preservation for 6 to 18 hr by cold infusion. Transplantation 1977;24(6):407–11.

33. Kalayoglu M, Sollinger HW, Stratta RJ, et al. Extended preservation of the liver for clinical transplantation. Lancet 1988;1(8586):617–9.

34. Southard JH, van Gulik TM, Ametani MS, et al. Important components of the UW solution. Transplantation 1990;49(2):251–7.

35. Bismuth H, Houssin D. Reduced-sized orthotopic liver graft in hepatic transplantation in children. Surgery 1984;95(3):367–70.

36. Pichlmayr R, Ringe B, Gubernatis G, et al. [Transplantation of a donor liver to 2 recipients (splitting transplantation)–a new method in the further development of segmental liver transplantation]. Langenbecks Arch Chir 1988;373(2):127–30 [in German].

37. Broelsch CE, Emond JC, Whitington PF, et al. Application of reduced-size liver transplants as split grafts, auxiliary orthotopic grafts, and living related segmental transplants. Ann Surg 1990;212(3):368–75 [discussion: 375–7].

38. Raia S, Nery JR, Mies S. Liver transplantation from live donors. Lancet 1989; 2(8661):497.

39. Strong RW, Lynch SV, Ong TH, et al. Successful liver transplantation from a living donor to her son. N Engl J Med 1990;322(21):1505–7.

40. Yamaoka Y, Washida M, Honda K, et al. Liver transplantation using a right lobe graft from a living related donor. Transplantation 1994;57(7):1127–30.

41. Broelsch CE, Whitington PF, Emond JC, et al. Liver transplantation in children from living related donors. Surgical techniques and results. Ann Surg 1991; 214(4):428–37 [discussion: 437–9].

42. Lo CM, Fan ST, Liu CL, et al. Adult-to-adult living donor liver transplantation using extended right lobe grafts. Ann Surg 1997;226(3):261–9 [discussion: 269–70].

43. McCormack L, Petrowsky H, Jochum W, et al. Use of severely steatotic grafts in liver transplantation: a matched case-control study. Ann Surg 2007;246(6):940–6 [discussion: 946–8].

44. Cameron AM, Ghobrial RM, Yersiz H, et al. Optimal utilization of donor grafts with extended criteria: a single-center experience in over 1000 liver transplants. Ann Surg 2006;243(6):748–53 [discussion: 753–5].

45. Busuttil RW, Farmer DG, Yersiz H, et al. Analysis of long-term outcomes of 3200 liver transplantations over two decades: a single-center experience. Ann Surg 2005;241(6):905–16 [discussion: 916–8].
46. Thompson HH, Tompkins RK, Longmire WP Jr. Major hepatic resection. A 25-year experience. Ann Surg 1983;197(4):375–88.
47. Belghiti J, Hiramatsu K, Benoist S, et al. Seven hundred forty-seven hepatectomies in the 1990s: an update to evaluate the actual risk of liver resection. J Am Coll Surg 2000;191(1):38–46.
48. Jarnagin WR, Gonen M, Fong Y, et al. Improvement in perioperative outcome after hepatic resection: analysis of 1,803 consecutive cases over the past decade. Ann Surg 2002;236(4):397–406 [discussion: 397].
49. Poon RT, Fan ST, Lo CM, et al. Improving perioperative outcome expands the role of hepatectomy in management of benign and malignant hepatobiliary diseases: analysis of 1222 consecutive patients from a prospective database. Ann Surg 2004;240(4):698–708 [discussion: 710].
50. Nagasue N, Yukaya H, Ogawa Y, et al. Human liver regeneration after major hepatic resection. A study of normal liver and livers with chronic hepatitis and cirrhosis. Ann Surg 1987;206(1):30–9.
51. Bruix J, Castells A, Bosch J, et al. Surgical resection of hepatocellular carcinoma in cirrhotic patients: prognostic value of preoperative portal pressure. Gastroenterology 1996;111(4):1018–22.
52. McCormack L, Petrowsky H, Jochum W, et al. Hepatic steatosis is a risk factor for postoperative complications after major hepatectomy: a matched case-control study. Ann Surg 2007;245(6):923–30.
53. Clavien PA, Mullhaupt B, Pestalozzi BC. Do we need a center approach to treat patients with liver diseases? J Hepatol 2006;44(4):639–42.
54. Dimick JB, Wainess RM, Cowan JA, et al. National trends in the use and outcomes of hepatic resection. J Am Coll Surg 2004;199(1):31–8.
55. Glasgow RE, Showstack JA, Katz PP, et al. The relationship between hospital volume and outcomes of hepatic resection for hepatocellular carcinoma. Arch Surg 1999;134(1):30–5.
56. Makuuchi M, Hasegawa H, Yamazaki S. Intraoperative ultrasonic examination for hepatectomy. Ultrasound Med Biol 1983;(Suppl 2):493–7.
57. Makuuchi M, Thai BL, Takayasu K, et al. Preoperative portal embolization to increase safety of major hepatectomy for hilar bile duct carcinoma: a preliminary report. Surgery 1990;107(5):521–7.
58. Rous P, Larimore L. Relation of the portal blood to liver maintenance. J Exp Med 1920;31:609–70.
59. Curley SA, Izzo F, Delrio P, et al. Radiofrequency ablation of unresectable primary and metastatic hepatic malignancies: results in 123 patients. Ann Surg 1999;230(1):1–8.
60. Elias D, Debaere T, Muttillo I, et al. Intraoperative use of radiofrequency treatment allows an increase in the rate of curative liver resection. J Surg Oncol 1998;67(3):190–1.
61. Siperstein AE, Rogers SJ, Hansen PD, et al. Laparoscopic thermal ablation of hepatic neuroendocrine tumor metastases. Surgery 1997;122(6):1147–54 [discussion: 54–5].
62. Fortner JG, Blumgart LH. A historic perspective of liver surgery for tumors at the end of the millennium. J Am Coll Surg 2001;193(2):210–22.
63. Foster JH. History of liver surgery. Arch Surg 1991;126(3):381–7.
64. Cattell R. Successful removal of a liver metastasis from carcinoma of the rectum. Lahey Clin Bull 1940;2:7–11.

65. Foster JH. Survival after liver resection for secondary tumors. Am J Surg 1978; 135(3):389–94.
66. Wagner JS, Adson MA, Van Heerden JA, et al. The natural history of hepatic metastases from colorectal cancer. A comparison with resective treatment. Ann Surg 1984;199(5):502–8.
67. Fong Y, Fortner J, Sun RL, et al. Clinical score for predicting recurrence after hepatic resection for metastatic colorectal cancer: analysis of 1001 consecutive cases. Ann Surg 1999;230(3):309–18 [discussion: 318–21].

Molecular Biology of Liver Ischemia/ Reperfusion Injury: Established Mechanisms and Recent Advancements

John R. Klune, MD[a], Allan Tsung, MD[b,c],*

KEYWORDS

- Liver • Hepatic • Ischemia/reperfusion
- Reactive oxygen species • HMGB1 • TLR4

Ischemia/reperfusion (I/R) injury is a phenomenon whereby damage to a hypoxic organ is accentuated following the return of oxygen delivery. Liver I/R injury can be categorized into warm and cold ischemia. Warm ischemia occurs in settings of transplantation, trauma, shock, and elective liver surgery in which hepatic blood supply is temporarily interrupted. Cold storage ischemia occurs during organ preservation before transplantation. The pathophysiology of liver I/R injury includes direct cellular damage as the result of the ischemic insult as well as delayed dysfunction and further damage resulting from activation of the immune system. The distal interacting elements in the cascade of inflammatory responses resulting in organ damage following hepatic I/R injury have been studied extensively. Activation of Kupffer cells with production of reactive oxygen species (ROS), up-regulation of the inducible nitric oxide synthase (iNOS) in hepatocytes, and up-regulation of proinflammatory

No financial support was required for this work.
[a] Department of Surgery, F675 UPMC Presbyterian Hospital, University of Pittsburgh Medical Center, 200 Lothrop Street, Pittsburgh, PA 15213, USA
[b] Division of Surgical Oncology, Department of Surgery, F1200 Presbyterian Hospital, University of Pittsburgh Medical Center, 200 Lothrop Street, Pittsburgh, PA 15213, USA
[c] Division of Transplantation, Department of Surgery, F1200 Presbyterian Hospital, University of Pittsburgh Medical Center, 200 Lothrop Street, Pittsburgh, PA 15213, USA
* Corresponding author. UPMC Liver Cancer Center, MUH 7 South, 3459 Fifth Avenue, Pittsburgh, PA 15213.
E-mail address: tsunga@upmc.edu

cytokines, chemokines, and adhesion molecules resulting in neutrophil-mediated injury are contributing events to the inflammation-associated damage.[1–5] These events, among others, are reviewed in depth in this article. Although there is much overlap in the mechanisms contributing to warm and cold I/R injury, the pathways are not interchangeable and clear differences do exist. More recent advancements and current research in ischemia reperfusion injury, particularly the proximal events of innate immune activation during I/R, are also discussed.

WARM ISCHEMIA REPERFUSION INJURY

The process of warm I/R injury involves activation of immune pathways and is dominated by hepatocellular injury. There are 2 distinct phases that occur in warm I/R injury (**Fig. 1**). The initial phase defined as the period less than 2 hours after reperfusion and the late phase of injury, which occurs at 6 to 48 hours after reperfusion.[6–8] The early phase is marked by activation of immune cells and production of oxidant stress; the later injury is mediated by neutrophil accumulation and hepatocellular injury.[9] The events in I/R injury described here are laid out in as chronologically correct order as possible, but these events likely overlap or occur simultaneously in vivo. This description is an attempt to delineate and simplify the events involved in I/R injury, which in reality is a complex intersection of several different pathways.

Kupffer cells are the resident macrophages of the liver and are key cell types involved in the earliest stages of I/R injury. They were identified in the early 1980s as an early source of ROS production in ischemia to the liver.[10,11] Oxidative stress can damage cells through multiple mechanisms, including lipid peroxidation, DNA oxidation, and enzyme denaturation. However, ROS produced during oxidative stress can also serve as molecules that mediate intracellular signaling pathways.[12] Although damage from oxidant stress occurs during this early phase of injury, ROS can activate inflammatory pathways that lead to neutrophil accumulation in the liver. The recruitment and activation of other immune cells to the stressed liver ultimately contributes to a larger portion of the injury than the early oxidative stress itself.

In addition to oxidant-mediated damage, the production of cytokines and chemokines also plays a key role in the pathogenesis of I/R injury locally and systemically.

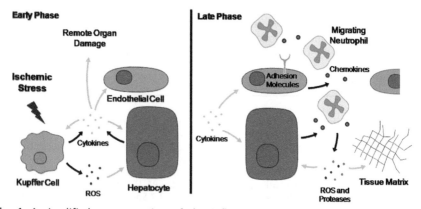

Fig. 1. A simplified representation of the inflammatory pathways in I/R injury. Initial ischemic stress results in release of cytokines and ROS, which leads to the expression of chemokines and adhesion molecules resulting in neutrophil migration to the site of injury. Subsequently, neutrophils release factors resulting in parenchymal damage and degradation of the tissue matrix.

Kupffer cells, in addition to their role in early production of ROS, also release these mediators.[13] Tumor necrosis factor-alpha (TNFα) and interleukin-1 (IL-1) are among the earliest cytokines to be systemically increased in I/R, with increased levels occurring within minutes of reperfusion of the liver.[13,14] Parenchymal cells of the liver (hepatocytes) may regulate the release of these cytokines during ischemic stress. Hepatocyte expression of interleukin-12 (IL-12) has been shown to be crucial to the production of TNFα and IL-1 at reperfusion.[15] The resultant increase in serum TNFα and IL-1 contribute significantly to the final pattern of I/R injury, contributing to local and remote organ injury.[16–18] In the local hepatic environment, TNFα and IL-1 mediate organ injury through multiple mechanisms. They promote additional release of inflammatory cytokines, creating a positive feedback loop that increases damage following I/R.[13,14] In addition, TNFα and IL-1 also up-regulate the production of chemokines and adhesion molecules that attract neutrophils to the liver, which ultimately are responsible for the later phases of injury.

The production of chemokines and adhesion molecules in the liver serves to recruit other immune cell types, such as neutrophils, to the site of injury.[19–21] Some of the chemokines that may contribute to the recruitment of neutrophils during I/R injury include interleukin-8, cytokine-induced neutrophil chemoattractant, macrophage inflammatory proteins, monocyte chemoattractants, and ENA-78, among others.[19,20,22–24] The release of these molecules occurs from multiple cell types (including Kupffer cells, endothelial cells, and hepatic parenchymal cells) and results in a proinflammatory state caused by the resultant infiltration of immune cells within the injured organ.[22,25] These molecules are also produced in remote organs, such as the lungs, in response to systemic levels of TNFα and contribute to injury at those sites by a similar mechanism.[19,26]

Although chemokines serve to attract neutrophils to ischemic areas of injury via a chemokine gradient within the liver tissue,[20] adhesion molecules are required for neutrophils to transmigrate from the bloodstream to the sites of injury. The initial interaction between neutrophils (and platelets) in the blood supply and the endothelial cells in the liver is mediated by a family of selectins, molecules on the endothelial cell surface that interact with these cells in the circulating blood.[27–31] The adhesion of platelets to endothelial cells via selectins ultimately contributes to platelet sequestration and hepatic injury.[29,31] However, neutrophils go on to more significant cell-cell interactions mediated by integrins (expressed on neutrophils and other leukocytes) and immunoglobulins (expressed on endothelial cells) that facilitate neutrophil arrest and extravasation into the hepatic parenchyma at the sites of ischemic injury.[32–36] This buildup of neutrophils in the liver marks the late phase of I/R injury.

Neutrophil-mediated injury in warm I/R occurs through oxidant- and protease-mediated mechanisms. The neutrophils release proteases and other cytotoxic enzymes through granule exocytosis.[37,38] These enzymes can degrade cellular membranes and matrix components. Inhibition of neutrophil elastase, one of the enzymes responsible for destruction of the extracellular matrix, results in decreased hepatic injury.[39] In addition, there is a significant release of ROS into the hepatic parenchyma from activated neutrophils that produce ROS through a largely nicotinamide adenine dinucleotide phosphate hydrogen (NADPH) oxidase–dependent pathway. The NADPH oxidase activation results largely in superoxide production, which is then converted into several other forms of reactive oxygen molecules.[9,33,40,41] These oxygen radicals serve to cause parenchymal damage and facilitate protease-mediated injury through deactivation of native antiproteases.

In contrast to the pathways described earlier that lead to liver injury during I/R, protective pathways are also activated during I/R to counteract and limit the inflammatory response. One such protective pathway is the heme oxygenase (HO) system that is activated during oxidative stress and leads to the controlled breakdown of heme following I/R injury. This HO-mediated heme breakdown leads to the release of 3 byproducts: a more neutral reduced iron, carbon monoxide (CO), and biliverdin, which can be converted to the endogenous antioxidant bilirubin.[42,43] The HO system expression is induced in hepatocytes following liver I/R.[44,45] To demonstrate its effectiveness in protecting against I/R, induction or overexpression of the HO system leads to decreased liver injury.[46] In addition to activation of the HO system to promote protection against liver I/R, the specific byproducts of HO-mediated heme breakdown have been shown to be protective. Bilirubin has been shown to act as an antioxidant[45] and exogenous administration of CO is protective against I/R injury.[47,48] Thus, the balance between activation of inflammatory and antiinflammatory pathways seems to modulate the inflammatory response, and extent of organ injury, following I/R.

COLD ISCHEMIA REPERFUSION INJURY

Cold I/R, in contrast to warm I/R, is dominated by damage to the sinusoidal endothelial cells and disruption of the microcirculation rather than damage to the hepatocytes. Cold storage occurs specifically in the setting of transplantation, in which a donor graft is harvested and perfused with a preservation solution before cold storage. While cold storage times that occur in human transplantation vary greatly, animal studies generally focus on storage times of up to 18 hours, although some extend cold storage to 24 hours or more. In addition to the issues involved in cold I/R injury, transplantation of livers involves additional factors such as immunologic tolerance and rejection.

One major difference between cold and warm I/R injury is that cold storage has specific effects on the various cellular subsets within the liver graft. Specifically, endothelial cells are more susceptible to cold storage. In studies using multiple cold storage solutions, endothelial cells demonstrate high cell death compared with hepatic parenchymal cells at the same time point.[2,49] This cold storage–induced injury seems to occur through apoptosis and coagulative necrosis.[50] The degree of endothelial damage has been correlated with functional impairment of the liver following reperfusion. The remaining viable endothelial cells contribute to I/R injury by expression of adhesion molecules as noted earlier. In addition, increasing cold storage times correlate with increasing Kupffer cell activation on reperfusion,[49] resulting in increased ROS and cytokine production as outlined earlier.

RECENT ADVANCEMENTS AND CURRENT RESEARCH
Nitric Oxide System

The nitric oxide (NO) system is an important component in liver I/R injury, although its involvement is complex and seems to have protective and injurious results.[51] Although the involvement of NO in liver I/R injury has long been established, its specific role is still a topic of current investigation. Nitric oxide is an important signaling molecule in the liver and is formed by the enzyme nitric oxide synthase (NOS) from the precursor amino acid arginine in the bloodstream. The isoforms of NOS that are responsible for physiologically important NO production during I/R injury are the inducible form (iNOS) and the endothelial form (eNOS). The eNOS form is constitutively expressed in endothelial cells of the liver and the iNOS form is induced during I/R injury[52] and regulated by many of the same cytokines (TNFα and IL-1 among others) that are discussed earlier and are involved in I/R injury.[53,54]

Several studies note the potential injurious role of NO during liver I/R. The production of NO during I/R injury seems to disturb the microcirculation of the liver and lead to mitochondrial dysfunction.[55] In addition, the use of a nonspecific NOS inhibitor has been reported to be protective.[56] In contrast, several studies report a protective effect of NO during I/R. In 1 recent study, compounds produced specifically to deliver NO to the liver were protective during I/R injury.[57] To support endogenous NO production, supplementation with an NO donor has been shown to be protective in warm and cold I/R injury.[58–61] In addition, inhibition of arginase, an enzyme competing with NOS for the substrate arginine, increases NOS activity and is protective in warm[62] and cold[63] models of I/R.

Some studies have attempted to determine individual roles for eNOS and iNOS during I/R, and it has been hypothesized that eNOS-derived NO may be protective and iNOS-derived NO is injurious.[64] A protective role of eNOS-derived NO has been demonstrated in warm[65] and cold[66] I/R injury. In addition, specific inhibition of iNOS has led to decreased injury in warm[67,68] and cold[69] I/R models. In contrast, adenoviral delivery for overexpression of iNOS in the donor graft has been protective in a cold storage I/R model,[70] and a protective role for Kupffer cell–derived iNOS in warm I/R has been shown.[71]

The role of nitric oxide in I/R injury remains a complex question with unclear answers. The specific source of NO, whether from eNOS or iNOS, may determine whether NO plays a protective or injurious role following I/R. Furthermore, its function may also include other factors, many of which have not been fully elucidated. The timing of the release of NO, the amount of NO released, or the downstream activation of NO-responsive elements may be additional determinants in NO's effects in liver I/R injury.

Immune System Activation: Danger Model of Injury

Much of the recent investigation in I/R injury is focused on the involvement of the immune system and specifically its mechanism of activation. The involvement of activated immune cells in I/R injury is clear as described above, though it still remains to be elucidated what activates the immune system during this injury process. Although the immune response to infection is well established, I/R injury occurs in the absence of pathogens. Therefore, much work has focused on the role of pattern recognition receptors known to be involved in immune processes and endogenous danger signaling as a mechanism for activation of the immune system leading to I/R injury.

Traditionally, innate immunity has referred to the initial proinflammatory response that occurs in response to an invading microorganism; however, clinicians have long recognized that sterile tissue injury can activate many of the same inflammatory pathways that are seen following microbial invasion. However, the mechanisms by which tissues notify the immune system of cell damage in the setting of noninfectious inflammation remains to be fully elucidated. In an effort to reconcile this apparent conundrum, Matzinger[72,73] hypothesized that the innate immune system is designed to recognize events that are of potential danger to the host. In this scenario, both pathogens and tissue damage represent threats to homeostasis that are capable of activating inflammatory cascades. The manner in which both microbial products (pathogen-associated molecular patterns [PAMPs]) and/or endogenous molecules (damage-associated molecular patterns [DAMPs]) are able to signal the presence of danger has recently been attributed to their ability to activate cellular receptors, referred to as pattern recognition receptors (PRRs).[74] Several endogenous DAMPs released during noninfectious inflammation, such as occurring following liver I/R, are able to activate the immune system through PRRs.[75–77] One particular DAMP, high mobility group box-1 (HMGB1), has received particular interest in I/R injury as it is a central mediator of the injury response.

HMGB1

HMGB1 is a nuclear protein that functions in stabilizing nucleosome formation, facilitating DNA bending, and enhancing transcription, replication, and repair. However, when released extracellularly, it can activate immune responses. Its proinflammatory properties were first described in 1999 in an endotoxemia animal model, in which it was found to be a late mediator of lethality.[77,78] HMGB1 can be released by active (secretion) and passive (necrosis) mechanisms.[79–81] The active mechanism is regulated by acetylation or phosphorylation and occurs in a variety of cell types including many of the immune cells involved in I/R injury as well as from hepatocytes themselves.[77,79,80,82–85] This active release is stimulated by many of the cytokines described earlier, such as TNFα, IL-1, and oxidative stress.[85–89] The release of HMGB1 subsequently results in a substantial proinflammatory response.

The release of HMGB1 into the extracellular milieu, whether during I/R or other states of injury, has a variety of effects, many of them proinflammatory in nature. HMGB1 stimulation of immune cells such as neutrophils and monocytes results in release of cytokines and increased cellular adhesion and migration.[90–93] HMGB1 stimulation of neutrophils results in cytokine production and NADPH oxidase–dependent production of ROS.[94–96] Most of these effects occur through interactions with PRRs, such as the receptor for advanced glycation end products (RAGE) and multiple members of the toll-like receptor (TLR) family.[91,96–98] Some of these receptors are discussed later in relation to their involvement in I/R injury.

HMGB1 has been found to be a central mediator of hepatic I/R injury. It is up-regulated in hepatic parenchyma as early as 1 hour after reperfusion and can be found to be increased in the serum following I/R.[85,99] HMGB1 is released in response to oxidative stress and antioxidants reduce HMGB1 release in in vitro and in vivo models.[85,99] Blocking the effects of HMGB1 using a neutralizing antibody or hemoperfusion through a HMGB1 absorptive column results in significantly decreased I/R injury,[99,100] a result that highlights its harmful role in this process. Many of these effects of HMGB1 in I/R injury have been tied to its interaction with specific PRRs, notably TLR4.

More recently, HMGB1 has been studied in human liver transplant recipient patients.[101] In this study, 20 patients were enrolled and HMGB1 as well as other cytokines and markers of liver damage were sampled. HMGB1 was systemically increased as early as 10 minutes following portal vein reperfusion but decreased to baseline levels by 8 hours after reperfusion. The source of HMGB1 appeared to be from graft hepatocytes, as demonstrated by comparing portal vein and hepatic vein levels as well as immunohistochemistry. Systemic levels correlated more with markers of overall graft damage such as alanine aminotransferase or graft steatosis than levels of individual cytokines such as TNFα or IL-6.

PRRs and TLRs

PRRs were originally noted for their ability to recognize PAMPs and initiate an immune response. These cellular receptors have since been shown to also recognize and respond to endogenous DAMPs. Although the category of PRRs is broad, the TLR family of receptors has gained particular interest in I/R injury. These receptors have many similarities but recognize different molecular signals and activate different inflammatory pathways.[102]

One of the most well-studied TLRs in hepatic I/R is TLR4. Although this receptor was first noted to respond to bacterial endotoxin (LPS), it is now known to be activated by multiple endogenous molecules.[103] TLR4 is activated during hepatic I/R as well as

I/R injury in multiple other organs.[103] Mice that have nonfunctional TLR4 mutations are protected against hepatic warm I/R, have reduced ROS, cytokine, and HMGB1 levels, and have increased protective HO-1 levels.[85,104,105] Several studies have demonstrated that functional TLR4 on bone marrow–derived (immune) cells rather than hepatocytes is important for injury in warm I/R.[106,107] However, a recent study suggests that TLR4 on bone marrow–derived cells and non–bone marrow–derived cells are important, although the protective mechanisms may be different.[108] The importance of TLR4 in I/R injury has been verified in the transplant model as well. Donor grafts with nonfunctional TLR4 have lower cytokine levels and less hepatocellular injury compared with grafts with functional TLR4, regardless of the TLR4 status of the recipient.[109]

In addition to TLR4, other members of the TLR family seem to be involved in liver I/R injury. The receptor TLR9 is known to recognize DNA, whether endogenous or bacterial. Blocking the TLR9 pathway, through inhibition or knockout strains of mice, results in protection from warm I/R injury and decreased levels of cytokines and ROS.[110] These findings also appeared to be mediated by TLR9 on neutrophils and other bone marrow–derived cells.[110] In addition, TLR2 has been linked to hepatic ischemia. Multiple studies have correlated increased expression of the TLR2 gene with increased liver injury following ischemia reperfusion, although specific TLR2 signaling has yet to be implicated.[111,112]

SUMMARY

The molecular mechanisms leading to injury during hepatic I/R are complex and involve multiple inflammatory pathways. These pathways are known to involve activation of the innate immune system and activation of Kupffer cells and neutrophils as well as other inflammatory cells. However, the early initiating events leading to the activation of the immune system are still not completely delineated, but are known to involve the release of endogenous molecules that are recognized by PRRs. Further research investigating how the immune system is activated following I/R injury is a topic of current research and may lead to novel protective strategies against I/R injury.

REFERENCES

1. Bilzer M, Gerbes AL. Preservation injury of the liver: mechanisms and novel therapeutic strategies. J Hepatol 2000;32(3):508–15.
2. Caldwell-Kenkel JC, Currin RT, Tanaka Y, et al. Reperfusion injury to endothelial cells following cold ischemic storage of rat livers. Hepatology 1989;10(3):292–9.
3. Fan C, Zwacka RM, Engelhardt JF. Therapeutic approaches for ischemia/reperfusion injury in the liver. J Mol Med 1999;77(8):577–92.
4. Lemasters JJ, Bunzendahl H, Thurman RG. Reperfusion injury to donor livers stored for transplantation. Liver Transpl Surg 1995;1(2):124–38.
5. McKeown CM, Edwards V, Phillips MJ, et al. Sinusoidal lining cell damage: the critical injury in cold preservation of liver allografts in the rat. Transplantation 1988;46(2):178–91.
6. Jaeschke H. Mechanisms of reperfusion injury after warm ischemia of the liver. J Hepatobiliary Pancreat Surg 1998;5(4):402–8.
7. Lentsch AB, Kato A, Yoshidome H, et al. Inflammatory mechanisms and therapeutic strategies for warm hepatic ischemia/reperfusion injury. Hepatology 2000;32(2):169–73.
8. Teoh NC, Farrell GC. Hepatic ischemia reperfusion injury: pathogenic mechanisms and basis for hepatoprotection. J Gastroenterol Hepatol 2003;18(8):891–902.

9. Jaeschke H, Farhood A, Smith CW. Neutrophils contribute to ischemia/reperfusion injury in rat liver in vivo. FASEB J 1990;4(15):3355–9.

10. Jaeschke H, Smith CV, Mitchell JR. Reactive oxygen species during ischemia-reflow injury in isolated perfused rat liver. J Clin Invest 1988;81(4):1240–6.

11. Jaeschke H, Smith CV, Mitchell JR. Hypoxic damage generates reactive oxygen species in isolated perfused rat liver. Biochem Biophys Res Commun 1988; 150(2):568–74.

12. Semenza GL. Cellular and molecular dissection of reperfusion injury: ROS within and without. Circ Res 2000;86(2):117–8.

13. Wanner GA, Ertel W, Muller P, et al. Liver ischemia and reperfusion induces a systemic inflammatory response through Kupffer cell activation. Shock 1996;5(1):34–40.

14. Shirasugi N, Wakabayashi G, Shimazu M, et al. Up-regulation of oxygen-derived free radicals by interleukin-1 in hepatic ischemia/reperfusion injury. Transplantation 1997;64(10):1398–403.

15. Lentsch AB, Yoshidome H, Kato A, et al. Requirement for interleukin-12 in the pathogenesis of warm hepatic ischemia/reperfusion injury in mice. Hepatology 1999;30(6):1448–53.

16. Colletti LM, Remick DG, Burtch GD, et al. Role of tumor necrosis factor-alpha in the pathophysiologic alterations after hepatic ischemia/reperfusion injury in the rat. J Clin Invest 1990;85(6):1936–43.

17. Colletti LM, Burtch GD, Remick DG, et al. The production of tumor necrosis factor alpha and the development of a pulmonary capillary injury following hepatic ischemia/reperfusion. Transplantation 1990;49(2):268–72.

18. Colletti LM, Cortis A, Lukacs N, et al. Tumor necrosis factor up-regulates intercellular adhesion molecule 1, which is important in the neutrophil-dependent lung and liver injury associated with hepatic ischemia and reperfusion in the rat. Shock 1998;10(3):182–91.

19. Colletti LM, Kunkel SL, Walz A, et al. Chemokine expression during hepatic ischemia/reperfusion-induced lung injury in the rat. The role of epithelial neutrophil activating protein. J Clin Invest 1995;95(1):134–41.

20. Lentsch AB, Yoshidome H, Cheadle WG, et al. Chemokine involvement in hepatic ischemia/reperfusion injury in mice: roles for macrophage inflammatory protein-2 and KC. Hepatology 1998;27(4):1172–7.

21. Luster AD. Chemokines–chemotactic cytokines that mediate inflammation. N Engl J Med 1998;338(7):436–45.

22. Colletti LM, Kunkel SL, Walz A, et al. The role of cytokine networks in the local liver injury following hepatic ischemia/reperfusion in the rat. Hepatology 1996; 23(3):506–14.

23. Lichtman SN, Lemasters JJ. Role of cytokines and cytokine-producing cells in reperfusion injury to the liver. Semin Liver Dis 1999;19(2):171–87.

24. Yoshimura T, Matsushima K, Oppenheim JJ, et al. Neutrophil chemotactic factor produced by lipopolysaccharide (LPS)-stimulated human blood mononuclear leukocytes: partial characterization and separation from interleukin 1 (IL 1) 1987. J Immunol 2005;175(9):5569–74.

25. Hisama N, Yamaguchi Y, Ishiko T, et al. Kupffer cell production of cytokine-induced neutrophil chemoattractant following ischemia/reperfusion injury in rats. Hepatology 1996;24(5):1193–8.

26. Yoshidome H, Lentsch AB, Cheadle WG, et al. Enhanced pulmonary expression of CXC chemokines during hepatic ischemia/reperfusion-induced lung injury in mice. J Surg Res 1999;81(1):33–7.

27. Burke J, Zibari GB, Brown MF, et al. Hepatic ischemia-reperfusion injury causes E-selectin upregulation. Transplant Proc 1998;30(5):2321–3.
28. Sawaya DE Jr, Zibari GB, Minardi A, et al. P-selectin contributes to the initial recruitment of rolling and adherent leukocytes in hepatic venules after ischemia/reperfusion. Shock 1999;12(3):227–32.
29. Singh I, Zibari GB, Brown MF, et al. Role of P-selectin expression in hepatic ischemia and reperfusion injury. Clin Transplant 1999;13(1 Pt 2):76–82.
30. Yadav SS, Howell DN, Gao W, et al. L-selectin and ICAM-1 mediate reperfusion injury and neutrophil adhesion in the warm ischemic mouse liver. Am J Physiol 1998;275(6 Pt 1):G1341–52.
31. Yadav SS, Howell DN, Steeber DA, et al. P-Selectin mediates reperfusion injury through neutrophil and platelet sequestration in the warm ischemic mouse liver. Hepatology 1999;29(5):1494–502.
32. Farhood A, McGuire GM, Manning AM, et al. Intercellular adhesion molecule 1 (ICAM-1) expression and its role in neutrophil-induced ischemia-reperfusion injury in rat liver. J Leukoc Biol 1995;57(3):368–74.
33. Jaeschke H, Farhood A, Bautista AP, et al. Functional inactivation of neutrophils with a Mac-1 (CD11b/CD18) monoclonal antibody protects against ischemia-reperfusion injury in rat liver. Hepatology 1993;17(5):915–23.
34. Kuzume M, Nakano H, Yamaguchi M, et al. A monoclonal antibody against ICAM-1 suppresses hepatic ischemia-reperfusion injury in rats. Eur Surg Res 1997;29(2):93–100.
35. Nakano H, Kuzume M, Namatame K, et al. Efficacy of intraportal injection of anti-ICAM-1 monoclonal antibody against liver cell injury following warm ischemia in the rat. Am J Surg 1995;170(1):64–6.
36. Vollmar B, Glasz J, Menger MD, et al. Leukocytes contribute to hepatic ischemia/reperfusion injury via intercellular adhesion molecule-1-mediated venular adherence. Surgery 1995;117(2):195–200.
37. Li XK, Matin AF, Suzuki H, et al. Effect of protease inhibitor on ischemia/reperfusion injury of the rat liver. Transplantation 1993;56(6):1331–6.
38. Mavier P, Preaux AM, Guigui B, et al. In vitro toxicity of polymorphonuclear neutrophils to rat hepatocytes: evidence for a proteinase-mediated mechanism. Hepatology 1988;8(2):254–8.
39. Uchida Y, Freitas MC, Zhao D, et al. The inhibition of neutrophil elastase ameliorates mouse liver damage due to ischemia and reperfusion. Liver Transpl 2009;15(8):939–47.
40. Jaeschke H. Reactive oxygen and ischemia/reperfusion injury of the liver. Chem Biol Interact 1991;79(2):115–36.
41. Ozaki M, Deshpande SS, Angkeow P, et al. Inhibition of the Rac1 GTPase protects against nonlethal ischemia/reperfusion-induced necrosis and apoptosis in vivo. FASEB J 2000;14(2):418–29.
42. Otterbein LE, Soares MP, Yamashita K, et al. Heme oxygenase-1: unleashing the protective properties of heme. Trends Immunol 2003;24(8):449–55.
43. Maines MD. The heme oxygenase system: a regulator of second messenger gases. Annu Rev Pharmacol Toxicol 1997;37:517–54.
44. Ito K, Ikeda S, Shibata T, et al. Immunohistochemical analysis of heme oxygenase-I in rat liver after ischemia. Biochem Mol Biol Int 1997;43(3):551–6.
45. Yamaguchi T, Terakado M, Horio F, et al. Role of bilirubin as an antioxidant in an ischemia-reperfusion of rat liver and induction of heme oxygenase. Biochem Biophys Res Commun 1996;223(1):129–35.

46. Kato H, Amersi F, Buelow R, et al. Heme oxygenase-1 overexpression protects rat livers from ischemia/reperfusion injury with extended cold preservation. Am J Transplant 2001;1(2):121–8.

47. Kaizu T, Nakao A, Tsung A, et al. Carbon monoxide inhalation ameliorates cold ischemia/reperfusion injury after rat liver transplantation. Surgery 2005;138(2):229–35.

48. Amersi F, Shen XD, Anselmo D, et al. Ex vivo exposure to carbon monoxide prevents hepatic ischemia/reperfusion injury through p38 MAP kinase pathway. Hepatology 2002;35(4):815–23.

49. Caldwell-Kenkel JC, Currin RT, Tanaka Y, et al. Kupffer cell activation and endothelial cell damage after storage of rat livers: effects of reperfusion. Hepatology 1991;13(1):83–95.

50. Gao W, Bentley RC, Madden JF, et al. Apoptosis of sinusoidal endothelial cells is a critical mechanism of preservation injury in rat liver transplantation. Hepatology 1998;27(6):1652–60.

51. Chen T, Zamora R, Zuckerbraun B, et al. Role of nitric oxide in liver injury. Curr Mol Med 2003;3(6):519–26.

52. Hur GM, Ryu YS, Yun HY, et al. Hepatic ischemia/reperfusion in rats induces iNOS gene transcription by activation of NF-kappaB. Biochem Biophys Res Commun 1999;261(3):917–22.

53. Geller DA, Nussler AK, Di SM, et al. Cytokines, endotoxin, and glucocorticoids regulate the expression of inducible nitric oxide synthase in hepatocytes. Proc Natl Acad Sci U S A 1993;90(2):522–6.

54. Nussler AK, Di SM, Billiar TR, et al. Stimulation of the nitric oxide synthase pathway in human hepatocytes by cytokines and endotoxin. J Exp Med 1992;176(1):261–4.

55. Glantzounis GK, Rocks SA, Sheth H, et al. Formation and role of plasma S-nitrosothiols in liver ischemia-reperfusion injury. Free Radic Biol Med 2007;42(6):882–92.

56. Lin HI, Wang D, Leu FJ, et al. Ischemia and reperfusion of liver induces eNOS and iNOS expression: effects of a NO donor and NOS inhibitor. Chin J Physiol 2004;47(3):121–7.

57. Katsumi H, Nishikawa M, Yasui H, et al. Prevention of ischemia/reperfusion injury by hepatic targeting of nitric oxide in mice. J Control Release 2009;140(1):12–7.

58. Geller DA, Chia SH, Takahashi Y, et al. Protective role of the L-arginine-nitric oxide synthase pathway on preservation injury after rat liver transplantation. JPEN J Parenter Enteral Nutr 2001;25(3):142–7.

59. Li SQ, Liang LJ. Protective mechanism of L-arginine against liver ischemic-reperfusion injury in rats. Hepatobiliary Pancreat Dis Int 2003;2(4):549–52.

60. Chattopadhyay P, Verma N, Verma A, et al. L-Arginine protects from pringle manoeuvere of ischemia-reperfusion induced liver injury. Biol Pharm Bull 2008;31(5):890–2.

61. Taha MO, Simoes MJ, Haddad MA, et al. L-Arginine supplementation protects against hepatic ischemia-reperfusion lesions in rabbits. Transplant Proc 2009;41(3):816–9.

62. Jeyabalan G, Klune JR, Nakao A, et al. Arginase blockade protects against hepatic damage in warm ischemia-reperfusion. Nitric Oxide 2008;19(1):29–35.

63. Reid KM, Tsung A, Kaizu T, et al. Liver I/R injury is improved by the arginase inhibitor, N (omega)-hydroxy-nor-L-arginine (nor-NOHA). Am J Physiol Gastrointest Liver Physiol 2007;292(2):G512–7.

64. Albrecht EW, Stegeman CA, Heeringa P, et al. Protective role of endothelial nitric oxide synthase. J Pathol 2003;199(1):8–17.
65. Duranski MR, Elrod JW, Calvert JW, et al. Genetic overexpression of eNOS attenuates hepatic ischemia-reperfusion injury. Am J Physiol Heart Circ Physiol 2006;291(6):H2980–6.
66. Theruvath TP, Zhong Z, Currin RT, et al. Endothelial nitric oxide synthase protects transplanted mouse livers against storage/reperfusion injury: role of vasodilatory and innate immunity pathways. Transplant Proc 2006;38(10): 3351–7.
67. Meguro M, Katsuramaki T, Nagayama M, et al. A novel inhibitor of inducible nitric oxide synthase (ONO-1714) prevents critical warm ischemia-reperfusion injury in the pig liver. Transplantation 2002;73(9):1439–46.
68. Takamatsu Y, Shimada K, Yamaguchi K, et al. Inhibition of inducible nitric oxide synthase prevents hepatic, but not pulmonary, injury following ischemia-reperfusion of rat liver. Dig Dis Sci 2006;51(3):571–9.
69. Tsuchihashi S, Kaldas F, Chida N, et al. FK330, a novel inducible nitric oxide synthase inhibitor, prevents ischemia and reperfusion injury in rat liver transplantation. Am J Transplant 2006;6(9):2013–22.
70. Kaizu T, Ikeda A, Nakao A, et al. Donor graft adenoviral iNOS gene transfer ameliorates rat liver transplant preservation injury and improves survival. Hepatology 2006;43(3):464–73.
71. Hsu CM, Wang JS, Liu CH, et al. Kupffer cells protect liver from ischemia-reperfusion injury by an inducible nitric oxide synthase-dependent mechanism. Shock 2002;17(4):280–5.
72. Matzinger P. Tolerance, danger, and the extended family. Annu Rev immunol 1994;12:991–1045.
73. Matzinger P. The danger model: a renewed sense of self. Science 2002; 296(5566):301–5.
74. Medzhitov R, Janeway CA Jr. Innate immunity: the virtues of a nonclonal system of recognition. Cell 1997;91(3):295–8.
75. Roth J, Vogl T, Sorg C, et al. Phagocyte-specific S100 proteins: a novel group of proinflammatory molecules. Trends Immunol 2003;24(4):155–8.
76. Scheibner KA, Lutz MA, Boodoo S, et al. Hyaluronan fragments act as an endogenous danger signal by engaging TLR2. J Immunol 2006;177(2): 1272–81.
77. Wang H, Bloom O, Zhang M, et al. HMG-1 as a late mediator of endotoxin lethality in mice. Science 1999;285(5425):248–51.
78. Bustin M. Regulation of DNA-dependent activities by the functional motifs of the high-mobility-group chromosomal proteins. Mol Cell Biol 1999;19(8):5237–46.
79. Abraham E, Arcaroli J, Carmody A, et al. HMG-1 as a mediator of acute lung inflammation. J Immunol 2000;165(6):2950–4.
80. Lotze MT, Tracey KJ. High-mobility group box 1 protein (HMGB1): nuclear weapon in the immune arsenal. Nat Rev Immunol 2005;5(4):331–42.
81. Scaffidi P, Misteli T, Bianchi ME. Release of chromatin protein HMGB1 by necrotic cells triggers inflammation. Nature 2002;418(6894):191–5.
82. Bonaldi T, Talamo F, Scaffidi P, et al. Monocytic cells hyperacetylate chromatin protein HMGB1 to redirect it towards secretion. EMBO J 2003;22(20):5551–60.
83. Nickel W. The mystery of nonclassical protein secretion. A current view on cargo proteins and potential export routes. Eur J Biochem 2003;270(10):2109–19.
84. Youn JH, Shin JS. Nucleocytoplasmic shuttling of HMGB1 is regulated by phosphorylation that redirects it toward secretion. J Immunol 2006;177(11):7889–97.

85. Tsung A, Klune JR, Zhang X, et al. HMGB1 release induced by liver ischemia involves Tolllike receptor 4 dependent reactive oxygen species production and calcium-mediated signaling. J Exp Med 2007;204(12):2913–23.

86. Rendon-Mitchell B, Ochani M, Li J, et al. IFN-gamma induces high mobility group box 1 protein release partly through a TNF-dependent mechanism. J Immunol 2003;170(7):3890–7.

87. Rouhiainen A, Kuja-Panula J, Wilkman E, et al. Regulation of monocyte migration by amphoterin (HMGB1). Blood 2004;104(4):1174–82.

88. Tang D, Shi Y, Kang R, et al. Hydrogen peroxide stimulates macrophages and monocytes to actively release HMGB1. J Leukoc Biol 2007;81(3):741–7.

89. Wahamaa H, Vallerskog T, Qin S, et al. HMGB1-secreting capacity of multiple cell lineages revealed by a novel HMGB1 ELISPOT assay. J Leukoc Biol 2007;81(1):129–36.

90. Andersson U, Wang H, Palmblad K, et al. High mobility group 1 protein (HMG-1) stimulates proinflammatory cytokine synthesis in human monocytes. J Exp Med 2000;192(4):565–70.

91. Kokkola R, Andersson A, Mullins G, et al. RAGE is the major receptor for the proinflammatory activity of HMGB1 in rodent macrophages. Scand J Immunol 2005;61(1):1–9.

92. Orlova VV, Choi EY, Xie C, et al. A novel pathway of HMGB1-mediated inflammatory cell recruitment that requires Mac-1-integrin. EMBO J 2007;26(4):1129–39.

93. Rouhiainen A, Tumova S, Valmu L, et al. Pivotal advance: analysis of proinflammatory activity of highly purified eukaryotic recombinant HMGB1 (amphoterin). J Leukoc Biol 2007;81(1):49–58.

94. Fan J, Li Y, Levy RM, et al. Hemorrhagic shock induces NAD(P)H oxidase activation in neutrophils: role of HMGB1–TLR4 signaling. J Immunol 2007;178(10):6573–80.

95. Park JS, Arcaroli J, Yum HK, et al. Activation of gene expression in human neutrophils by high mobility group box 1 protein. Am J Physiol Cell Physiol 2003;284(4):C870–9.

96. Park JS, Svetkauskaite D, He Q, et al. Involvement of toll-like receptors 2 and 4 in cellular activation by high mobility group box 1 protein. J Biol Chem 2004;279(9):7370–7.

97. Hori O, Brett J, Slattery T, et al. The receptor for advanced glycation end products (RAGE) is a cellular binding site for amphoterin. Mediation of neurite outgrowth and co-expression of rage and amphoterin in the developing nervous system. J Biol Chem 1995;270(43):25752–61.

98. Park JS, Gamboni-Robertson F, He Q, et al. High mobility group box 1 protein interacts with multiple Toll-like receptors. Am J Physiol Cell Physiol 2006;290(3):C917–24.

99. Tsung A, Sahai R, Tanaka H, et al. The nuclear factor HMGB1 mediates hepatic injury after murine liver ischemia-reperfusion. J Exp Med 2005;201(7):1135–43.

100. Yamamoto T, Ono T, Ito T, et al. Hemoperfusion with a high-mobility group box 1 adsorption column can prevent the occurrence of hepatic ischemia-reperfusion injury in rats. Crit Care Med 2010;38(3):879–85.

101. Ilmakunnas M, Tukiainen EM, Rouhiainen A, et al. High mobility group box 1 protein as a marker of hepatocellular injury in human liver transplantation. Liver Transpl 2008;14(10):1517–25.

102. Kumar H, Kawai T, Akira S. Toll-like receptors and innate immunity. Biochem Biophys Res Commun 2009;388(4):621–5.

103. Kaczorowski DJ, Tsung A, Billiar TR. Innate immune mechanisms in ischemia/reperfusion. Front Biosci (Elite Ed) 2009;1:91–8.
104. Shen XD, Ke B, Zhai Y, et al. Toll-like receptor and heme oxygenase-1 signaling in hepatic ischemia/reperfusion injury. Am J Transplant 2005;5(8):1793–800.
105. Wu HS, Zhang JX, Wang L, et al. Toll-like receptor 4 involvement in hepatic ischemia/reperfusion injury in mice. Hepatobiliary Pancreat Dis Int 2004;3(2): 250–3.
106. Tsung A, Hoffman RA, Izuishi K, et al. Hepatic ischemia/reperfusion injury involves functional TLR4 signaling in nonparenchymal cells. J Immunol 2005; 175(11):7661–8.
107. Tsung A, Zheng N, Jeyabalan G, et al. Increasing numbers of hepatic dendritic cells promote HMGB1-mediated ischemia-reperfusion injury. J Leukoc Biol 2007;81(1):119–28.
108. Hui W, Jinxiang Z, Heshui W, et al. Bone marrow and non-bone marrow TLR4 regulates hepatic ischemia/reperfusion injury. Biochem Biophys Res Commun 2009;389(2):328–32.
109. Shen XD, Ke B, Zhai Y, et al. Absence of toll-like receptor 4 (TLR4) signaling in the donor organ reduces ischemia and reperfusion injury in a murine liver transplantation model. Liver Transpl 2007;13(10):1435–43.
110. Bamboat ZM, Balachandran VP, Ocuin LM, et al. Toll-like receptor 9 inhibition confers protection from liver ischemia-reperfusion injury. Hepatology 2010; 51(2):621–32.
111. Jin X, Wang L, Wu HS, et al. N-Acetylcysteine inhibits activation of toll-like receptor 2 and 4 gene expression in the liver and lung after partial hepatic ischemia-reperfusion injury in mice. Hepatobiliary Pancreat Dis Int 2007;6(3): 284–9.
112. Zhang JX, Wu HS, Wang H, et al. Protection against hepatic ischemia/reperfusion injury via downregulation of toll-like receptor 2 expression by inhibition of Kupffer cell function. World J Gastroenterol 2005;11(28):4423–6.

Hepatic Cysts and Liver Abscess

Kaye M. Reid-Lombardo, MD*, Saboor Khan, MBBS, PhD, FRCS,
Guido Sclabas, MD, MS

KEYWORDS

- Hepatic cysts • Polycystic liver disease • Hepatic abscess
- Caroli's disease • Hydatid cyst • Hepatic parasites

LIVER CYSTS

Hepatic cysts were considered to be a rare entity until 30 years ago when a Mayo Clinic report showed an incidence of 17 per 10,000 operations.[1] With the evolution of modern imaging techniques, reports of the prevalence of simple cysts has increased with rates of 3% to 5% on ultrasonography[2,3] to as high as 18% on CT.[4] The differential diagnosis of hepatic cysts is extensive, with varying causes, prevalence, manifestations, and severity. Cystic lesions may represent a congenital disorder, which may be inherited, a cystic malformation of intrahepatic bile ducts, or an infectious process.

PRIMARY HEPATIC AND BILIARY CYSTS
Simple Cysts

Epidemiology
Simple hepatic cysts are typically thin-walled masses that are uncommon before the 40 years of age. Large cysts tend to occur more frequently in women older than 50 years. They are often found incidentally and for the most part are commonly asymptomatic. The female to male ratio is 4:1, and the prevalence is approximately 3%.[5] The radiographic presentation varies from solitary to multiple and from small to large. The average size reported is 3 cm.[6] Simple cysts are believed to be the result of excluded hyperplastic bile duct rests. Microscopically, the cysts are bordered by a single layer

Dr Reid Lombardo was funded by Grant Number 1 UL1 RR024150 from the National Center for Research Resources (NCRR), a component of the National Institutes of Health (NIH), and the NIH Roadmap for Medical Research. Its contents are solely the responsibility of the authors and do not necessarily represent the official view of NCRR or NIH. Information on NCRR is available at http://www.ncrr.nih.gov/. Information on Reengineering the Clinical Research Enterprise can be obtained from http://nihroadmap.nih.gov.
Division of Gastroenterologic and General Surgery, Mayo Clinic, 200 First Street South West, Rochester, MN 55905, USA
* Corresponding author.
E-mail address: reidlombardo.kaye@mayo.edu

of cuboid or columnar epithelium (resembling biliary epithelium); cyst fluid is produced by this epithelium lining the cyst. The cyst fluid may be serous, turbid, or frankly bilious.

Rarely, the presence of a dominant cyst may cause pain because of its enlarging size, pressure, or bleeding into the cyst wall. The symptoms may include abdominal pain, early satiety, and epigastric fullness. Symptoms should only be attributed to the cyst when clinically the cyst is large and all other likely clinical diagnoses have been eliminated. Although complications such as bleeding and rupture have been described, they are exceedingly rare.

Diagnosis

Although diagnosed typically as an incidental finding, an initial evaluation with ultrasound will show characteristic anechoic lesions with sharp, smooth borders, and strong posterior wall echoes.[7] A CT may be used to confirm the water density associated typically with a simple cyst, and to screen for other likely pathologies causing symptoms.

Management

Asymptomatic cysts are best managed with observation alone. For symptomatic liver cysts, a wide therapeutic range extends from no intervention (minimal symptoms) to ultrasound-guided aspiration (which may be used to confirm symptom resolution), and finally to operative resection. However, although aspiration is a viable tool to help diagnose the cysts as a source of symptoms, it is insufficient as a definitive treatment in most patients because of the high recurrence rate.[8] Aspiration of cyst fluid followed by sclerotherapy is reasonable, because it may provide respite from symptoms in up to 80% of patients.[9]

More definitive treatment options, including cyst fenestration (laparoscopic or open), which mandates resection of the cyst roof or, rarely, hepatic resection (depending on the size and location of cyst), provide long-term relief in up to 90% of patients.[10–12] Over the past decade, laparoscopic cyst deroofing/fenestration has produced acceptable long-term results and should be considered the preferred treatment.[13] Finally, the cyst wall should be subjected to pathologic assessment to ensure that a cystadenoma is not missed. If a cystadenoma is diagnosed unexpectedly, the patient should undergo a formal hepatic resection to excise the cyst in its entirety.

Polycystic Liver Disease

Etiology

Adult polycystic liver disease (AD-PCLD) occurs as an autosomal dominant disease and is associated with polycystic kidney disease (PKD). Those afflicted are found to have mutations of PKD1 (40%–75%), and approximately 75% have mutations of the *PKD2* gene.[14] This condition is responsible for the formation of a large number of hepatic cysts. Rarely, this disease presents in the absence of renal disease; this patient subgroup has been identified as having a mutation in the protein kinase C substrate 80 K–H (PRKCSH).[15]

Epidemiology

In contradistinction to simple hepatic cysts, AD-PCLD is usually extensive with numerous hepatic cysts. These cysts are similar to simple cysts, but the distinguishing features include their number, size, bilobar distribution, and presence of numerous microcysts. The prevalence and number of hepatic cysts tend to be greater in women and increase with advancing age, severity of renal cystic disease, and renal dysfunction. At 60 years of age, approximately 80% of patients with autosomal dominant AD-PCLD will have hepatic cysts, with women having more and larger cysts.

Pregnancy and female hormones tend to increase the risk for severe hepatic cystic disease.

Presentation

Patients with AD-PCLD will lack symptoms until cystic size/number increase to a critical level (cyst to parenchyma volume ratio of >1). The symptoms may include abdominal pain, bloating, postprandial fullness, and shortness of breath depending on which lobe is enlarged. The first presentation is likely secondary to a complication such as infection,[16] intracystic bleeding, extrinsic compression of the biliary or digestive tract, traumatic rupture, or even Budd-Chiari syndrome. Despite the enlarging hepatic cysts, patients rarely develop hepatic-related pathologies, such as hepatic failure/portal hypertension (eg, jaundice, ascites, encephalopathy, variceal bleeding). In contrast, those with concomitant renal disease are prone to progressive renal failure, which in turn can worsen the hepatic disease. An association with cerebral artery aneurysm[17] and valvular heart disease[18] has been described.

Imaging

Initial evaluation may include an ultrasound that will show multiple fluid-filled round or oval cysts, with distinct margins in the liver or kidneys (**Fig. 1**). Imaging with CT is, however, the preferred modality, and may also show other complicating pathologies associated with AD-PCLD (eg, cerebral aneurysm, diverticulosis, inguinal hernia). Patients with polycystic livers will have cysts that are hyperintense on transverse (T2)-weighted MRI and hypointense on longitudinal (T1)-weighted MRI, except when they are complicated by hemorrhage.

Management

Management of the symptomatic patient with AD-PCLD presents challenges that are best managed in experienced hepatobiliary units. No medical therapies are available to either reduce the cyst size or prevent further increase in size or number. Symptoms are related mainly to the volume of the liver rather than to a specific cyst; therefore, the aim is to decompress the liver as a whole or remove as many cysts as feasible. Selected patients with massive hepatomegaly from AD-PCLD experience benefit from operative intervention. The type of operation performed must be tailored to individual presentation, distribution of the cysts, coincident sectoral vascular patency, parenchymal preservation, and hepatic reserve. Hepatic resection can be performed

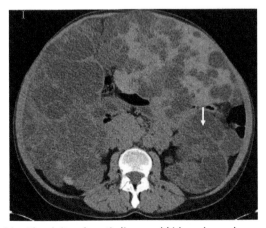

Fig. 1. A 47-year-old with adult polycystic liver and kidney (*arrow*).

with acceptable morbidity and mortality,[19] prompt and durable relief of symptoms, and maintenance of liver function.

More recently, the laparoscopic approach was used to treat 45 patients with AD-PCLD with excellent short- and intermediate-term results.[12] The laparoscopic approach for AD-PCLD was historically more limited to deroofing of the dominant hepatic cyst, rather than used for surgical resection with good outcome.[11] Although, immediate symptom relief from AD-PCLD after laparoscopic fenestration may be adequate, in the long-term most patients experience recurrence of symptoms.[20] Whether PCLD will have a broader laparoscopic use in the future remains to be seen. Cyst fenestration (laparoscopic or open)[9] and liver transplantation, although effective in selected patients, are less broadly applicable.[18,21] Simultaneous renal and hepatic transplantation may be appropriate for patients with coexistent renal failure.[22,23]

Hepatic Cystadenoma/Cystadenocarcinoma

Epidemiology

Cystadenoma is a rare benign cystic neoplasm of the liver that tends to affect women older than 40 years. The usual presentation is abdominal pain, anorexia, nausea, and abdominal swelling. Jaundice is a possibility secondary to fistulation into the biliary tree or from formation of mucinous plugs.[7,24]

Morphologically, it is characterized by large, multiple loculi filled with mucinous or mucin-like material (**Fig. 2**). The lining epithelium is cuboidal or columnar and thin-walled. In places, the epithelium forms papillary projections that are thick, compact, and cellular, resembling ovarian stroma;[25,26] these neoplasms are reminiscent of mucinous cystic neoplasms of the pancreas. Because of the risk for malignancy or malignant transformation giving rise to cystadenocarcinoma,[27,28] the cyst wall must be carefully assessed at surgical resection.

Evaluation

Diagnosis is based on imaging. Ultrasonography shows single, large, anechoic, fluid-filled ovoid or globular area.[29] Internal echoes are seen corresponding to the septations forming multiple loculi secondary to papillary growths originating from the lining. CT shows comparable abnormalities with septation, mural nodules, and calcification. In some, the fluid shows a greater density than water. On MRI, the tumor is strongly hyperintense on T2-weighted images, although it also may be hyperintense or heterogeneous because of mucinous content.[30] Although carbohydrate antigen 19-9 (CA 19-9) levels in the fluid may be increased, this measure alone is not diagnostic.[31] Nevertheless, a diagnostic algorithm has been suggested based on cyst fluid analysis

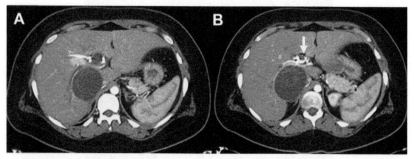

Fig. 2. A 25-year-old woman with cystadenoma arising from the right posterior lobe of the liver. Enucleation showed low-grade dysplasia. Note stent in the common hepatic duct (*white arrow*) to treat biliary obstruction (*A, B*).

for CA 19-9 and carcinoembryonic antigen (CEA), which have been found to be increased in patients with cystadenoma,[32] similar to pancreatic mucinous cystic neoplasms (**Table 1**). Patients with increased tumor markers require histopathologic assessment of the cyst wall.[32] Serologic tests for hydatid disease must be performed in all cases.

Management
Cystadenoma of the liver even in asymptomatic patients should be treated with complete excision. Partial excision exposes patients to the risk for recurrence and malignancy (cystadenocarcinoma). Complete excision is the only option for cure.[33] A diagnosis of cystadenocarcinoma mandates a formal surgical resection along the same lines as other hepatic malignancies.[33] Aggressive resection of cystadenocarcinoma may provide a chance for long-term survival; however, for most patients, the risk for postresection recurrence and death is high.[34]

Unfortunately, a risk exists for misdiagnosing a cystadenoma as a simple cyst on imaging. Hence, if a postoperative histopathologic report after a laparoscopic fenestration/partial resection shows cystadenoma, the preoperative imaging should be reviewed to reassess the extent of the disease. Further cross-sectional imaging should also be performed to plan a complete excision of the cystadenoma. The risk for malignancy mandates a full resection of this entity. When a complete laparoscopic enucleation of the cyst may be assured, a strict clinical, biochemical, and radiologic follow-up could be considered the definitive treatment, demanding operative intervention only in the presence of recurrence or a high suspicion for malignancy.[35] The timeframe of progression from cystadenoma to cystadenocarcinoma has previously been difficult to predict. Reassuringly, cystadenocarcinoma remains a rare tumor,[33] prompting speculation that malignancy arises as a late manifestation.

Diagnosis
Mucinous fluid on needle aspiration indicates an underlying cystadenoma. However, in the presence of cystadenocarcinoma, biopsy or aspiration could potentially disseminate the malignancy. Therefore, preoperative needle biopsy is not recommended to focus the differential. A mixed solid and cystic component on imaging or constitutional symptoms (eg, weight loss, pain) indicates malignant transformation.

Bile Duct Cysts (Caroli's Disease)

Etiology
Caroli's disease is a congenital malformation characterized by multifocal dilation of segmental bile ducts, the main consequence of which is recurrent bacterial cholangitis. Development of these biliary cystic dilations is believed to result from the arrest of

Table 1
Distinctive characteristics of cystadenoma and simple hepatic cyst

	Cystadenoma	Simple Cyst
Number of cysts	1	>1
Septations	Present	Absent
Papillary projections	Present	Absent
Cyst fluid	Mucinous	Serous
Cyst fluid CA19-9	Likely elevated	Not elevated
Partial excision	Causes recurrence	Recurrence unlikely
Malignancy	Possible (adenocarcinoma)	Unlikely

or a derangement in the normal embryologic remodeling of ducts. If the large intrahepatic bile ducts are affected, the result is Caroli's disease; however, congenital hepatic fibrosis may result if smaller biliary radicles are involved. These two disorders may also coexist. Caroli's disease (or syndrome) is associated with an autosomal recessive trait;[36] the mutated gene remains unknown.

Presentation

Caroli's disease usually presents between ages 5 and 20 years, although it is likely to be present at birth. It may remain unrecognized unless imaging is performed for another indication.[37] Attacks of cholangitis occur typically without any apparent precipitating cause.[36,38] Unfortunately, in some instances, biliary infection is secondary to ill-advised therapeutic interventions, such as operative T-tube placement or endoscopic retrograde cholangiopancreatography. The main symptom is fever without pain or jaundice, and therefore the underlying pathology may not be apparent.

Congenital hepatic fibrosis may also present as portal hypertension and hepatic failure when these two disorders coexist. The course of the disease is complicated by recurrent cholangitis; some patients may experience 10 to 20 episodes per year. The bile is saturated with cholesterol crystals, which predispose patients to the formation of intrahepatic stones. The primary intrahepatic bile duct stones may migrate and cause obstructive jaundice and pancreatitis. Unless calcified, these may not be visible on CT. Another consequence of the disease is the increased risk for malignancy, which may be challenging to diagnose.[39]

The main characteristic of these bile duct cysts is their communication with the biliary tree. The condition may also manifest with signs of biliary gas or intrahepatic stones. Caroli's disease is important to differentiate from PCLD, dilated bile ducts secondary to biliary obstruction, and duct ectasia (primary sclerosing cholangitis). The important distinction is that with Caroli's disease, ultrasound or CT will show cysts of varying sizes with a clear biliary communication.[40] MRI has replaced direct cholangiography as a diagnostic modality (**Fig. 3**).[41,42]

Management

Treatment of cholangitis associated with Caroli's disease is with appropriate antibiotics. The prevention of recurrent cholangitis is difficult. Although long-term antibiotics

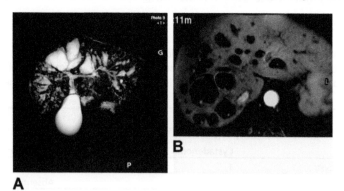

Fig. 3. MRI showing Caroli's disease in its diffuse form, associated with hepatic fibrosis. (A) MRI reconstruction showing the segmental dilation of the intrahepatic bile ducts. (B) After injection of contrast medium, tiny dots corresponding to protal branches and hepatic arteries protruding into the lumen of the cysts can be seen. (*Reproduced from* Blumgart L, editor. Surgery of the liver, biliary tract, and pancreas, vol. 2. 4th edition. Philadelphia: Saunders; 2007. p. 1017; with permission.)

are not always efficacious, they should be considered. Ursodiol should be offered to all patients to prevent lithiasis and treat stones.[41] Operative or endoscopic drainage procedures are beset with a heightened infection rate and should be used with caution. In the localized form of Caroli's disease (often involving just the left liver), partial hepatectomy is indicated and is associated with improvement of symptoms and a decrease in the risk for malignant transformation.[37] In the diffuse form with recurrent bacterial cholangitis (with or without hepatic fibrosis), hepatic transplantation may be the only option.[43] Patients with Caroli's disease are at an increased risk for cholangiocarcinoma, and therefore screening is mandatory.

HEPATIC AND BILIARY CONDITIONS SECONDARY TO INFECTIONS
Pyogenic Liver Abscess

Liver abscesses were uniformly fatal until the first half of the last century when operative drainage was found to be associated with recovery and cure.[44] Results were further improved with the advent of antibiotics, enhanced imaging techniques, and percutaneous and minimally invasive techniques. With these developments, the spectrum of causation shifted from portal pyemia to preexisting hepatobiliary disease or its treatment.[45]

Etiology

Pyogenic liver abscess (PLA) secondary to appendicitis, diverticulitis (**Fig. 4**), or other intra-abdominal infective processes has decreased dramatically because of improvements in the treatment of the primary condition, which typically includes source control and early initiation of antibiotics.[46] Nonetheless, these diagnoses may still be relevant in patients with delayed treatment or those residing in the underdeveloped world. Biliary obstruction (benign or malignant), stenting, or instrumentation is now a more common cause for PLA. Hematogenous spread from other sources, such as bacterial endocarditis and intravenous drug abuse, are other classic examples of why PLA might develop. Patients who are immunocompromised or diabetic are especially prone to develop PLA; those who are diabetic have a 3.6-fold increased risk for developing PLA compared with population controls.[47–51]

Modern treatments for hepatic neoplasms with radiofrequency or microwave ablation and chemoembolization may be complicated by PLA.[52] Hepatic trauma, especially if associated with necrosis, intrahepatic hematoma, or bile leak, may become secondarily infected and lead to PLA. Vascular thrombosis complicating hepatic transplantation is a serious event, with the parenchyma becoming secondarily predisposed to infection with bacteria and fungi. Direct extension of infection into the liver from contiguous visceral (gall bladder, stomach/duodenum) infection can also be

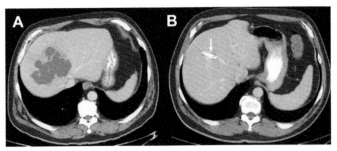

Fig. 4. (*A*) Pyogenic abscess secondary to diverticulitis. (*B*) Resolution of abscess after treatment with CT-guided drainage catheter and intravenous antibiotics. Drainage catheter in residual abscess cavity (*white arrow*).

a cause of PLA. Despite these numerous possible origins, in a small portion of patients no identifiable cause is found, leasing to the entity termed *cryptogenic PLA*, which is reported to account for 15% to 53% of all PLAs currently.[53]

Clinical presentation
Typically, early symptoms of PLA are insidious, nonspecific, and evolve over days to several weeks. Symptoms may include malaise, headache, loss of appetite, myalgia, and arthralgia. More specific symptoms of fever, chills, or abdominal pain (which may not be localized to the right upper quadrant) are late features. If adjacent to the diaphragm, pleuritic pain, cough, and dyspnea may occur. Septic shock may ensue in patients in the setting of biliary obstruction and delayed diagnosis. Predisposing conditions (**Box 1**) may cause symptoms/complications separate from the liver abscess.

Diagnosis
Laboratory investigations may show an increased white cell count with shift and C-reactive protein. Liver function derangement is common but may be associated with sepsis rather than biliary obstruction. Hyperglycemia may be the first indication in a patient with diabetes.[50]

Box 1
Frequent causes of pyogenic liver abscess

Cryptogenic

Hepatobiliary

    Biliary enteric anastomoses

    Biliary procedures: endoscopic or percutaneous

    Gall stones

    Malignancy involving common bile duct, gall bladder, pancreas, and ampullary

Portal

    Appendicitis

    Chronic inflammatory bowel disease

    Diverticulitis

    Gastrointestinal malignancy

    Pancreatitis

    Pelvic and anorectal sepsis

    Postoperative

Arterial

    Dental infections

    Endocarditis

    Ear, nose, or throat sepsis

    Vascular sepsis

Traumatic

    Abdominal trauma

    Ablation: radiofrequency or ethanol

    Chemoembolization

Plain abdominal and chest radiography is usually nonspecific, unless a coexistent pleural effusion/collapse of lung or elevation of diaphragm is present. Gas-forming organisms may cause an air/fluid level within the dilated biliary tree. Appearance on ultrasound varies according to disease stage. Initially, the abscess may be hyperechoic and indistinct; but with maturation and pus formation, it becomes hyperechoic with a distinct margin. Thick pus or multiple small lesions might be confused with solid lesions. Evaluating an abscess on the dome of the liver may have some limitations. Ultrasonography may highlight biliary tract pathology (gallstones, ductal dilation, or solid lesions) and has a sensitivity of 75% to 95%.[54]

CT is more accurate (sensitivity, 95%), especially with contrast enhancement.[55,56] Peripheral enhancement of the abscess wall is virtually diagnostic of PLA in the appropriate clinical setting; moreover, by allowing imaging of the abdomen, the CT may also show the likely cause of noncryptogenic PLA in approximately 70% of the cases.[57] MRI does not seem to have any specific advantage over CT; however, it may further delineate previously unsuspected liver lesions or intraductal pathology, while investigating the biliary tract noninvasively.

Liver abscesses may be single or multiple. Cryptogenic abscesses are more likely to be single (70% on the right side), whereas multiple small abscesses tend to be secondary to an underlying biliary pathology or from metastatic seeding (eg, bacterial endocarditis, intravenous drug abuse). A PLA of less than 2 cm in diameter is described as a microabscess. Multiple microabscesses have been reported as having two distinct imaging characteristics: the first, *diffuse miliary*, is associated with staphylococcal infection, and the second, *cluster*, which seems to coalesce, is more likely to be secondary to infections from coliform organisms.[58]

Microbiology

Blood cultures should be performed on patients suspected of having PLA (**Box 2**). Blood cultures are more likely to be positive in noncryptogenic PLA and polymicrobial (*Escherichia coli*, Klebsiella,[59] Bacteroides) infections. Klebsiella infections are more likely to form single-site infections, which may metastasize, and seem to occur more commonly in the Asian population.[60,61] There is increasing evidence implicating Klebsiella and testifying to its virulence.[62–64] Nonhematogenous spread from a nongastrointestinal source is likely to be monomicrobial and either *Staphylococcus aureus* or *Streptococcus*. *Staphylococcus* PLA is most common and occurs in the setting of chronic granulomatous disease, disorders of granulocyte function, and hematologic malignancy. In contrast, PLA caused by the *Streptococcus milleri* group of organisms exhibits stellate necrosis with abscess;[65,66] the pus is often inspissated and too thick to be aspirated effectively.

Treatment

The principles of management include drainage of pus, parenteral antibiotics, and treatment of the underlying condition (if one can be found). Advances in imaging have allowed earlier diagnosis and a shift in management away from open drainage to percutaneous aspiration or tube (catheter) drainage.[67]

Broad-spectrum antibiotics should to be started before blood culture results are available. Antibiotics should be directed at all gram-positive and -negative aerobes and anaerobes. The exact choice should be dictated by the suspected pathogens based on history, presentation, and, potentially, hospital flora. Parenteral antibiotics should be administered for up to 2 weeks, followed by appropriate oral therapy for another 4 to 6 weeks. Biliary obstruction should be relieved, if present.

Box 2
Microbiology of liver abscess

Pyogenic
  Gram-negative aerobes
    Escherichia coli
    Klebsiella pneumoniae
    Proteus spp
    Enterobacter cloacae
    Citrobacter freundii
    Others
  Gram-positive aerobes
    Streptococcus milleri
    Staphylococcus aureus
    Enterococcus spp
    Others
  Gram-negative anaerobes
    Bacteroides spp
    Fusobacterium spp
  Gram-positive anaerobes
    Clostridium spp
    Peptostreptococcus spp
Other
  Fungal
    Candida
    Aspergillus
    Actinomycosis
    Yersinia
  Parasites
    Entameba histolytica
    Fasciola hepatica
    Clonorchis sinensis
    Ascariasis

Percutaneous drainage is performed under ultrasound or CT guidance. Aspiration of the PLA should confirm the diagnosis while obtaining pus for culture. Whether a drain is placed after an initially successful aspiration has been the subject of some debate. Several studies have shown reasonable results with repeat aspirations;[68] in contrast, a randomized controlled trial showed catheter drainage to be more effective than percutaneous needle aspiration in the management of liver abscess.[69] A second, randomized, controlled trial supports the use of percutaneous needle aspiration as a valid alternative for simple abscesses 50 mm in diameter or smaller.[69,70] In contrast, a unilocular abscess less than 5 cm in diameter is most likely to respond to aspiration, but the treatment is prone to failure if the pus is thick and difficult to aspirate or drain. Large multiloculated cavities with thick pus may require several catheter/tube drains. The catheters should to be irrigated daily to prevent blockage. Even though catheter treatment may be necessary, long-term placement is prone to complications, such as bleeding.[71]

Failure of nonoperative measures mandates early surgical intervention, whether secondary to viscous pus, an enlarging cavity, inability to treat the contributing condition, or progressive sepsis.[72] Traditionally, an open approach has several steps: ultrasound localization, division of loculations, loosening of debris from the wall abscess, and placement of dependent drains. Postoperative irrigation may be used and can occasionally be advantageous.

Certain patients may require treatment with liver resection, including those with liver atrophy, multiple PLAs causing near-complete hepatic disruption, and longstanding obstruction. In addition, patients tend to experience dense, septate staphylococcal abscesses. Aggressive operative intervention is advocated.[73] Patients with advanced sepsis have also been shown to have reasonable outcome after aggressive liver resection.[74] More recently, a laparoscopic approach has been used effectively in this setting.[56,75]

The risk factors associated with mortality include septic shock, jaundice, coagulopathy, diabetes leukocytosis, hypoalbuminemia, intraperitoneal rupture, and malignancy.[76-78] A high initial "Acute Physiology, Age, and Chronic Health Evaluation (APACHE II)" score has also been linked to an increased risk for mortality.[79]

PARASITIC HEPATIC CYSTS
Hydatid Cyst

Epidemiology
Hydatid cysts are caused by the zoonotic parasites, *Echinococcus granulosus* or *E multilocularis*. The lifecycle of the echinococcus parasite requires a definitive host, which is often a dog, and an intermediate host, which is commonly a sheep. Humans become accidental intermediate hosts when they get infected from dogs. The disease occurs principally in sheep-grazing areas of the world and is endemic in many Mediterranean countries, the Middle and Far East, South America, Australia, and East Africa. The incidence in these areas depends on the level of health care and veterinary control. In the Western hemisphere, immigrants from endemic areas have a greater incidence of hydatid diagnosis.

Pathogenesis
If the parasite survives and reaches the liver parenchyma, it develops into a cyst, which is visible after 3 weeks and may measure up to 3 cm in diameter after 3 months. The mature cyst consists of a layer of living tissue, which includes a germinal layer surrounding the fluid-filled central hydatid cavity and a laminated layer. These two layers form the endocyst. The germinal membrane has absorptive function for nutrition and also produces daughter cysts. The compressive force of the host's tissue around the endocyst produces a fibrous layer called *ectocyst* or *pericyst*. The cyst fluid is typically colorless, unless there is communication with a bile duct, it becomes infected, or it is degenerating. Hydatid fluid pressure can reach high levels, which explains the risk for rupture after trauma or operative manipulation.

Presentation
Small (<5 cm) cysts are usually asymptomatic and are sometimes detected incidentally. The expansion of larger cysts or the inflammatory reaction around the cyst can

irritate the surrounding parietal peritoneum and cause moderate right upper-quadrant pain. Acute pain indicates a purulent cyst or rupture. When the antigenic cyst fluid is released into circulation it can cause an acute intense allergic manifestation. Extrusion into the biliary tree may cause jaundice, cholangitis, or, rarely, acute pancreatitis. Bronchobiliary fistula resulting from hepatobronchial fistula and ascites, or acute hepatic failure resulting from Budd-Chiari syndrome (caused by pressure on hepatic veins or inferior vena cava) are other rare but possible complications.

Diagnosis

The diagnosis of hydatid cyst is based on history and likelihood of past exposure but requires imaging and serology. Parasitology of cyst contents confirms the diagnosis. Routine blood tests are usually not helpful, derangement of liver function is unusual, and eosinophilia is only seen in 25% to 40% of patients. Serologic testing for *E granulosis* includes immunoelectrophoresis, enzyme-linked immunosorbent assay, and Western blotting.[80-82] The sensitivity and specificity of the various tests vary between 60% and 95%. These tests may be used for diagnosis, posttreatment follow-up, and epidemiologic studies.

The World Health Organization (WHO) developed a classification system based on ultrasound appearance to improve uniformity of reporting and judge the effect of different treatment modalities.[83] Although ultrasound is the first imaging study that should be performed, CT gives more precise information on the morphology of the cyst (**Fig. 5**). The cyst may have a low signal intensity rim on T2-weighted MRI, which is a characteristic sign of hydatid disease.[84]

Management

The treatment for hydatid cystic disease of the liver depends on the size, symptoms, location, and experience of the clinical team treating the patient.[85] Treatment modalities include operative (conservative vs resection) strategies, percutaneous drainage, and chemotherapy. Conservative operative treatment has the goal of preventing spillage of cyst contents, inactivating the daughter cysts, obliterating the biliary communications (if present), and management of residual cyst cavity. This treatment strategy has a recurrence rate of approximately 10%.[86] The more aggressive operative approaches of either pericystectomy or a formal hepatic resection should be reserved for experienced centers.[86,87] Cystectomy is associated with a high risk for

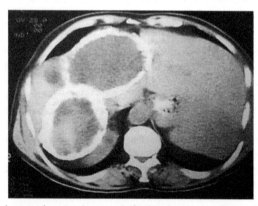

Fig. 5. CT of the abdomen, showing large, calcified hydatid cysts. (*Reproduced from* Cameron JL, editor. Current surgical therapy. 17th edition. St Louis (MO): Mosby Inc; 2001. p. 344; with permission.)

bile leak/fistula, but has a lower recurrence rate.[88,89] Laparoscopic resection techniques can help treat hydatid cysts.[90]

Various methods of percutaneous-based treatments include, broadly, image-guided aspiration of cyst fluid, injection of a protoscolicidal, or reaspiration.[91] These treatments have a small associated risk for allergic reaction. More recently, techniques of radiofrequency ablation have also been used with good success.[92–95] Chemotherapy includes the use of antihelminthic drugs, such as benzimidazole carbamates (mebendazole and albendazole), that kill the parasite through impairing glucose uptake. These pharmacologic approaches are used as an adjunct to other modalities in extended treatment courses aimed at eradication.[96] Response to treatment is nearly dependent on cyst morphology. Success rates up to 80% are possible for a univesicular cyst if treatment is continued for 3 to 6 months.[97]

Amebiasis-Related Liver Abscess

The protozoan *Entameba histolytica* is the causative organism for amebic colitis and hepatic abscess, affecting chiefly individuals living in or visiting tropical and temperate climates. As a causative agent of hepatic abscesses, it boroughs through the intestinal mucosal barrier and enters the portal, eventually forming an abscess in the liver. Direct extension or lymphatic spread is not believed to occur. Hepatic involvement is typically silent, and parenchymal necrosis ensues, resulting in the typical "anchovy sauce" appearance. Typically, the lesions are single, large, and loculated. Amebae are also known to lyse neutrophils.[98–100]

Epidemiology

Typically, this disease affects young men, and symptoms last approximately 10 days. Travelers from nonendemic areas may develop the disease between 2 and 5 months after becoming infected. Usually, abrupt abdominal pain and fever occurs. Active colitis and liver abscess occur rarely together. Occasionally, diarrhea may be present. Complications may include secondary bacterial infection, rupture into the peritoneal or thoracic cavity, and pericardial involvement.[101]

Laboratory investigations show leukocytosis without eosinophilia. Liver function tests show moderate increases in alkaline phosphatase, and the prothrombin time is typically elevated. Affected individuals will almost always have positive serum anti-amebic antibodies, which can be confirmed with various serologic tests (eg, indirect hemagglutination). Ultrasonography has a diagnostic accuracy of 90%. CT may not add to the diagnostic accuracy but delineates the morphologic characteristics.

The treatment of uncomplicated abscess is metronidazole, emetine hydrochloride, chloroquine phosphate, or diloxanide furoate.[102,103] Patients with inconclusive serology, pregnancy, failure of symptom resolution, and imminent rupture should be considered for percutaneous aspiration and drainage if aspiration alone is unsuccessful.

Parasites Affecting the Liver

Clonorchis sinensis

Clonorchis sinensis is a flat trematode worm measuring 10 to 25 mm, endemic in East Asia and transmitted through the consumption of raw, freshwater fish. Clinical manifestations may occur up to 20 years after infection and involve recurrent pyogenic cholangitis, itself a risk factor for the development of cholangiocarcinoma. Praziquantel is the preferred drug treatment.

Ascaris lumbricoides

Ascaris lumbricoides infects a quarter of the world's population and is common in Asia, Africa, and Central America. Hepatic disease tends to occur with a heavy worm load and often involves the biliary system (eg, biliary ascariasis, acute suppurative cholangitis, acute pancreatitis). Stool microscopy is diagnostic. Treatment with albendazole is usually sufficient, with endoscopic intervention needed rarely.

Fungal Hepatic Infections

Hepatic abscesses complicated by fungi are being recognized with increasing frequency in immunocompromised patients[104] and those with malignant diseases. Risk factors and treatment of patients with pure fungal, mixed fungal, and pyogenic abscesses (see **Box 2**) have not been well described. *Candida* is likely to affect children. In patients with mixed fungal/pyogenic hepatic abscesses who fail to improve after drainage and broad-spectrum antibiotics, early antimycotic therapy should be considered before the onset of fungemia.

RARE CONDITIONS
Congenital Hepatic Fibrosis

Congenital hepatic fibrosis is a recessive inherited disease that belongs to the family of malformations in the hepatic ductal plate. This disorder consists of markedly increased portal spaces because of abundant connective tissue, with numerous bile ductules that are ectatic and communicating with the biliary tree. Bile ductular proliferation (cluster of small cysts) is an essential component. Typically, patients (aged 5–20 years) present with variceal bleeding secondary to portal hypertension. Liver failure is rare. No treatment options are available, and the management is based on surveillance to detect secondary complications, such as gastroesophageal varices and hepatopulmonary syndrome. Afflicted patients are encouraged seek genetic counseling and avoid situations that may impair hepatic function, such as hepatotoxic medications, alcohol consumption, obesity, and infections with hepatitis A or B and HIV. Diagnosed patients should be vaccinated for hepatitis A and B.

Ciliated Foregut Cysts

This cyst is likely related to developmental anomaly of the anterior foregut, leading to a detached outpouching of the hepatic diverticulum or enteric foregut. The cysts are typically small, solitary, uniloculated, and run a benign course.

Degenerative, Trauma, and Masquerading Cysts

Hepatic cysts are seen increasingly after ablative procedures (radiofrequency and microwave) because of coagulative necrosis of the parenchyma. The tumor causes a pseudocyst to form. If infection ensues, it should be treated as a hepatic abscess. Posttraumatic cysts are rare and form usually after incomplete resolution of subcapsular or intrahepatic hematomas, usually single with a thick, pseudocyst wall. Rarely, cystic conditions of neighboring viscera, especially if these protrude into hepatic parenchyma, have been mislabeled as hepatic cysts.

REFERENCES

1. Sanfelippo PM, Beahrs OH, Weiland LH. Cystic disease of the liver. Ann Surg 1974;179(6):922–5.
2. Caremani M, Vincenti A, Benci A, et al. Echographic epidemiology of non-parasitic hepatic cysts. J Clin Ultrasound 1993;21(2):115–8.
3. Rungsinaporn K, Phaisakamas T. Frequency of abnormalities detected by upper abdominal ultrasound. J Med Assoc Thai 2008;91(7):1072–5.

4. Carrim ZI, Murchison JT. The prevalence of simple renal and hepatic cysts detected by spiral computed tomography. Clin Radiol 2003;58(8):626–9.

5. Charlesworth P, Ade-Ajayi N, Davenport M. Natural history and long-term follow-up of antenatally detected liver cysts. J Pediatr Surg 2007;42(3):494–9.

6. Bae KT, Zhu F, Chapman AB, et al. Magnetic resonance imaging evaluation of hepatic cysts in early autosomal-dominant polycystic kidney disease: the consortium for radiologic imaging studies of polycystic kidney disease cohort. Clin J Am Soc Nephrol 2006;1(1):64–9.

7. Liang P, Cao B, Wang Y, et al. Differential diagnosis of hepatic cystic lesions with gray-scale and color Doppler sonography. J Clin Ultrasound 2005;33(3):100–5.

8. Saini S, Mueller PR, Ferrucci JT Jr, et al. Percutaneous aspiration of hepatic cysts does not provide definitive therapy. AJR Am J Roentgenol 1983; 141(3):559–60.

9. Erdogan D, van Delden OM, Rauws EA, et al. Results of percutaneous sclerotherapy and surgical treatment in patients with symptomatic simple liver cysts and polycystic liver disease. World J Gastroenterol 2007;13(22):3095–100.

10. Cruz N, Vazquez Quintana E. Surgical management of hepatic cysts. Bol Asoc Med P R 1979;71(12):455–8.

11. Gall T, Oniscu G, Madhavan K, et al. Surgical management and longterm follow-up of non-parasitic hepatic cysts. HPB (Oxford) 2009;11(3):235–41.

12. Gamblin TC, Holloway SE, Heckman JT, et al. Laparoscopic resection of benign hepatic cysts: a new standard. J Am Coll Surg 2008;207(5):731–6.

13. Palanivelu C, Jani K, Malladi V. Laparoscopic management of benign nonparasitic hepatic cysts: a prospective nonrandomized study. South Med J 2006; 99(10):1063–7.

14. Juran BD, Lazaridis KN. Genetics of hepatobiliary diseases. Clin Gastroenterol Hepatol 2006;4(5):548–57.

15. Drenth JP, te Morsche RH, Smink R, et al. Germline mutations in PRKCSH are associated with autosomal dominant polycystic liver disease. Nat Genet 2003; 33(3):345–7.

16. Sallee M, Rafat C, Zahar J-R, et al. Cyst infections in patients with autosomal dominant polycystic kidney disease. Clin J Am Soc Nephrol 2009;4(7):1183–9.

17. Rossetti S, Chauveau D, Kubly V, et al. Association of mutation position in polycystic kidney disease 1 (pkd1) gene and development of a vascular phenotype. Lancet 2003;361(9376):2196–201.

18. Schnelldorfer T, Torres VE, Zakaria S, et al. Polycystic liver disease: a critical appraisal of hepatic resection, cyst fenestration, and liver transplantation. Ann Surg 2009;250(1):112–8.

19. Que F, Nagorney DM, Gross JB Jr, et al. Liver resection and cyst fenestration in the treatment of severe polycystic liver disease. Gastroenterology 1995;108(2): 487–94.

20. Robinson TN, Stiegmann GV, Everson GT. Laparoscopic palliation of polycystic liver disease. Surg Endosc 2005;19(1):130–2.

21. Russell RT, Pinson CW. Surgical management of polycystic liver disease. World J Gastroenterol 2007;13(38):5052–9.

22. Barahona-Garrido J, Camacho-Escobedo J, Cerda-Contreras E, et al. Factors that influence outcome in non-invasive and invasive treatment in polycystic liver disease patients. World J Gastroenterol 2008;14(20):3195–200.

23. Morgan DE, Lockhart ME, Canon CL, et al. Polycystic liver disease: multimodality imaging for complications and transplant evaluation. Radiographics 2006; 26(6):1655–68 [quiz: 55].

24. Gonzalez M, Majno P, Terraz S, et al. Biliary cystadenoma revealed by obstructive jaundice. Dig Liver Dis 2009;41(7):e11–3.
25. Lam MM, Swanson PE, Upton MP, et al. Ovarian-type stroma in hepatobiliary cystadenomas and pancreatic mucinous cystic neoplasms: an immunohistochemical study. Am J Clin Pathol 2008;129(2):211–8.
26. Lee JH, Chen DR, Pang SC, et al. Mucinous biliary cystadenoma with mesenchymal stroma: expressions of ca 19–9 and carcinoembryonic antigen in serum and cystic fluid. J Gastroenterol 1996;31(5):732–6.
27. Buetow PC, Buck JL, Pantongrag-Brown L, et al. Biliary cystadenoma and cystadenocarcinoma: clinical-imaging-pathologic correlations with emphasis on the importance of ovarian stroma. Radiology 1995;196(3):805–10.
28. Teoh AY, Ng SS, Lee KF, et al. Biliary cystadenoma and other complicated cystic lesions of the liver: diagnostic and therapeutic challenges. World J Surg 2006; 30(8):1560–6.
29. Gaines PA, Sampson MA. The prevalence and characterization of simple hepatic cysts by ultrasound examination. Br J Radiol 1989;62(736):335–7.
30. Williams DM, Vitellas KM, Sheafor D. Biliary cystadenocarcinoma: seven year follow-up and the role of MRI and MRCP. Magn Reson Imaging 2001;19(9):1203–8.
31. Park KH, Kim JS, Lee JH, et al. [significances of serum level and immunohistochemical stain of ca19–9 in simple hepatic cysts and intrahepatic biliary cystic neoplasms]. Korean J Gastroenterol 2006;47(1):52–8 [in Korean].
32. Koffron A, Rao S, Ferrario M, et al. Intrahepatic biliary cystadenoma: role of cyst fluid analysis and surgical management in the laparoscopic era. Surgery 2004; 136(4):926–36.
33. Vogt DP, Henderson JM, Chmielewski E. Cystadenoma and cystadenocarcinoma of the liver: a single center experience. J Am Coll Surg 2005; 200(5):727–33.
34. Lee JH, Lee KG, Park HK, et al. Biliary cystadenoma and cystadenocarcinoma of the liver: 10 cases of a single center experience. Hepatogastroenterology 2009;56(91–92):844–9.
35. Fiamingo P, Veroux M, Cillo U, et al. Incidental cystadenoma after laparoscopic treatment of hepatic cysts: which strategy? Surg Laparosc Endosc Percutan Tech 2004;14(5):282–4.
36. Taylor AC, Palmer KR. Caroli's disease [comment]. Eur J Gastroenterol Hepatol 1998;10(2):105–8.
37. Yonem O, Bayraktar Y. Clinical characteristics of Caroli's syndrome. World J Gastroenterol 2007;13(13):1934–7.
38. Mercadier M, Chigot JP, Clot JP, et al. Caroli's disease. World J Surg 1984;8(1): 22–9.
39. Chapman RW. Risk factors for biliary tract carcinogenesis. Ann Oncol 1999; 10(Suppl 4):308–11.
40. Brancatelli G, Federle MP, Vilgrain V, et al. Fibropolycystic liver disease: CT and MR imaging findings. Radiographics 2005;25(3):659–70.
41. Ananthakrishnan AN, Saeian K. Caroli's disease: identification and treatment strategy. Curr Gastroenterol Rep 2007;9(2):151–5.
42. Mortele KJ, Ros PR. Cystic focal liver lesions in the adult: differential CT and MR imaging features. Radiographics 2001;21(4):895–910.
43. Ammori BJ, Jenkins BL, Lim PC, et al. Surgical strategy for cystic diseases of the liver in a western hepatobiliary center. World J Surg 2002;26(4):462–9.
44. Larson LM, Rosenow JH. Solitary pyogenic liver abscess; review of literature and report of case. Minn Med 1950;33(6):588–92 passim.

45. Land MA, Moinuddin M, Bisno AL. Pyogenic liver abscess: changing epidemiology and prognosis. South Med J 1985;78(12):1426–30.
46. Branum GD, Tyson GS, Branum MA, et al. Hepatic abscess. Changes in etiology, diagnosis, and management. Ann Surg 1990;212(6):655–62.
47. Thomsen RW, Jepsen P, Sorensen HT. Diabetes mellitus and pyogenic liver abscess: risk and prognosis. Clin Infect Dis 2007;44(9):1194–201.
48. Wiwanitkit V. Causative agents of liver abscess in HIV-seropositive patients: a 10-year case series in Thai hospitalized patients. Trop Doct 2005;35(2):115–7.
49. Hansen PS, Schonheyder HC. Pyogenic hepatic abscess. A 10-year population-based retrospective study. APMIS 1998;106(3):396–402.
50. Kaplan GG, Gregson DB, Laupland KB. Population-based study of the epidemiology of and the risk factors for pyogenic liver abscess. Clin Gastroenterol Hepatol 2004;2(11):1032–8.
51. Tsai FC, Huang YT, Chang LY, et al. Pyogenic liver abscess as endemic disease, Taiwan. Emerg Infect Dis 2008;14(10):1592–600.
52. Poggi G, Riccardi A, Quaretti P, et al. Complications of percutaneous radiofrequency thermal ablation of primary and secondary lesions of the liver. Anticancer Res 2007;27(4C):2911–6.
53. Lok KH, Li KF, Li KK, et al. Pyogenic liver abscess: clinical profile, microbiological characteristics, and management in a Hong Kong hospital. J Microbiol Immunol Infect 2008;41(6):483–90.
54. Lin AC, Yeh DY, Hsu YH, et al. Diagnosis of pyogenic liver abscess by abdominal ultrasonography in the emergency department. Emerg Med J 2009;26(4):273–5.
55. Barreda R, Ros PR. Diagnostic imaging of liver abscess. Crit Rev Diagn Imaging 1992;33(1–2):29–58.
56. Wang CL, Guo XJ, Qiu SB, et al. Diagnosis of bacterial hepatic abscess by CT. Hepatobiliary Pancreat Dis Int 2007;6(3):271–5.
57. Auh YH, Lim JH, Kim KW, et al. Loculated fluid collections in hepatic fissures and recesses: CT appearance and potential pitfalls. Radiographics 1994; 14(3):529–40.
58. Ralls PW. Inflammatory disease of the liver. Clin Liver Dis 2002;6(1):203–25.
59. Golia P, Sadler M. Pyogenic liver abscess: klebsiella as an emerging pathogen. Emerg Radiol 2006;13(2):87–8.
60. Pastagia M, Arumugam V. Klebsiella pneumoniae liver abscesses in a public hospital in queens, New York. Travel Med Infect Dis 2008;6(4):228–33.
61. Sng CC, Jap A, Chan YH, et al. Risk factors for endogenous klebsiella endophthalmitis in patients with klebsiella bacteraemia: a case-control study. Br J Ophthalmol 2008;92(5):673–7.
62. Lee SS, Chen YS, Tsai HC, et al. Predictors of septic metastatic infection and mortality among patients with klebsiella pneumoniae liver abscess. Clin Infect Dis 2008;47(5):642–50.
63. Moffie BG, Wijbenga JA. Liver abscess due to klebsiella pneumoniae showing the mucoid phenotype. J Infect 2008;57(4):353–4.
64. Yu VL, Hansen DS, Ko WC, et al. Virulence characteristics of klebsiella and clinical manifestations of k. Pneumoniae bloodstream infections. Emerg Infect Dis 2007;13(7):986–93.
65. Allison HF, Immelman EJ, Forder AA. Pyogenic liver abscess caused by streptococcus milleri. Case reports. S Afr Med J 1984;65(11):432–5.
66. Corredoira J, Casariego E, Moreno C, et al. Prospective study of streptococcus milleri hepatic abscess. Eur J Clin Microbiol Infect Dis 1998;17(8):556–60.

67. Jepsen P, Vilstrup H, Schonheyder HC, et al. A nationwide study of the incidence and 30-day mortality rate of pyogenic liver abscess in Denmark, 1977–2002. Aliment Pharmacol Ther 2005;21(10):1185–8.
68. Chung YF, Tan YM, Lui HF, et al. Management of pyogenic liver abscesses—percutaneous or open drainage? Singapore Med J 2007;48(12):1158–65 [quiz: 65].
69. Zerem E, Hadzic A. Sonographically guided percutaneous catheter drainage versus needle aspiration in the management of pyogenic liver abscess. AJR Am J Roentgenol 2007;189(3):W138–42.
70. Yu SC, Ho SS, Lau WY, et al. Treatment of pyogenic liver abscess: prospective randomized comparison of catheter drainage and needle aspiration. Hepatology 2004;39(4):932–8.
71. Pearce N, Knight R, Irving H, et al. Non-operative management of pyogenic liver abscess. HPB (Oxford) 2003;5(2):91–5.
72. Hope WW, Vrochides DV, Newcomb WL, et al. Optimal treatment of hepatic abscess. Am Surg 2008;74(2):178–82.
73. Kobayashi S, Murayama S, Takanashi S, et al. Clinical features and prognoses of 23 patients with chronic granulomatous disease followed for 21 years by a single hospital in japan. Eur J Pediatr 2008;167(12):1389–94.
74. Hsieh HF, Chen TW, Yu CY, et al. Aggressive hepatic resection for patients with pyogenic liver abscess and apache ii score > or = 15. Am J Surg 2008;196(3):346–50.
75. Siu WT, Chan WC, Hou SM, et al. Laparoscopic management of ruptured pyogenic liver abscess. Surg Laparosc Endosc 1997;7(5):426–8.
76. Chen SC, Tsai SJ, Chen CH, et al. Predictors of mortality in patients with pyogenic liver abscess. Neth J Med 2008;66(5):196–203.
77. Chung YF. Pyogenic liver abscess–predicting failure to improve outcome. Neth J Med 2008;66(5):183–4.
78. Ruiz-Hernandez JJ, Leon-Mazorra M, Conde-Martel A, et al. Pyogenic liver abscesses: mortality-related factors. Eur J Gastroenterol Hepatol 2007; 19(10):853–8.
79. Alvarez Perez JA, Gonzalez JJ, Baldonedo RF, et al. Clinical course, treatment, and multivariate analysis of risk factors for pyogenic liver abscess. Am J Surg 2001;181(2):177–86.
80. Biava MF, Dao A, Fortier B. Laboratory diagnosis of cystic hydatic disease. World J Surg 2001;25(1):10–4.
81. Ito A, Nakao M, Sako Y. Echinococcosis: serological detection of patients and molecular identification of parasites. Future Microbiol 2007;2:439–49.
82. Parija SC. A review of some simple immunoassays in the serodiagnosis of cystic hydatid disease. Acta Trop 1998;70(1):17–24.
83. Group WHOIW. International classification of ultrasound images in cystic echinococcosis for application in clinical and field epidemiological settings. Acta Trop 2003;85(2):253–61.
84. von Sinner WN. New diagnostic signs in hydatid disease; radiography, ultrasound, CT and MRI correlated to pathology. Eur J Radiol 1991;12(2):150–9.
85. Voros D, Katsarelias D, Polymeneas G, et al. Treatment of hydatid liver disease. Surg Infect (Larchmt) 2007;8(6):621–7.
86. Yagci G, Ustunsoz B, Kaymakcioglu N, et al. Results of surgical, laparoscopic, and percutaneous treatment for hydatid disease of the liver: 10 years experience with 355 patients. World J Surg 2005;29(12):1670–9.

87. Daradkeh S, El-Muhtaseb H, Farah G, et al. Predictors of morbidity and mortality in the surgical management of hydatid cyst of the liver. Langenbecks Arch Surg 2007;392(1):35–9.

88. Agarwal S, Sikora SS, Kumar A, et al. Bile leaks following surgery for hepatic hydatid disease. Indian J Gastroenterol 2005;24(2):55–8.

89. Kayaalp C, Bzeizi K, Demirbag AE, et al. Biliary complications after hydatid liver surgery: incidence and risk factors. J Gastrointest Surg 2002;6(5):706–12.

90. Palanivelu C, Jani K, Malladi V, et al. Laparoscopic management of hepatic hydatid disease. JSLS 2006;10(1):56–62.

91. Nasseri Moghaddam S, Abrishami A, Malekzadeh R. Percutaneous needle aspiration, injection, and reaspiration with or without benzimidazole coverage for uncomplicated hepatic hydatid cysts. Cochrane Database Syst Rev 2006;(2): CD003623.

92. Brunetti E, Filice C. Radiofrequency thermal ablation of echinococcal liver cysts. Lancet 2001;358(9291):1464.

93. Papaconstantinou I, Kontos M, Prassas E, et al. Radio frequency ablation (RFA)-assisted pericystectomy for hepatic echinococcosis: an alternative technique. Surg Laparosc Endosc Percutan Tech 2006;16(5):338–41.

94. Sahin M, Kartal A, Haykir R, et al. RF-assisted cystectomy and pericystectomy: a new technique in the treatment of liver hydatid disease. Eur Surg Res 2006; 38(2):90–3.

95. Zacharoulis D, Poultsidis A, Roundas C, et al. Liver hydatid disease: radiofrequency-assisted pericystectomy. Ann R Coll Surg Engl 2006;88(5):499–500.

96. Arif SH, Shams Ul B, Wani NA, et al. Albendazole as an adjuvant to the standard surgical management of hydatid cyst liver. Int J Surg 2008;6(6):448–51.

97. Ayles HM, Corbett EL, Taylor I, et al. A combined medical and surgical approach to hydatid disease: 12 years' experience at the hospital for tropical diseases, London. Ann R Coll Surg Engl 2002;84(2):100–5.

98. Jarumilinta R, Kradolfer F. The toxic effect of entamoeba histolytica on leucocytes. Ann Trop Med Parasitol 1964;58:375–81.

99. Guerrant RL, Brush J, Ravdin JI, et al. Interaction between entamoeba histolytica and human polymorphonuclear neutrophils. J Infect Dis 1981;143(1):83–93.

100. Stanley SL Jr. Amoebiasis. Lancet 2003;361(9362):1025–34.

101. Rao S, Solaymani-Mohammadi S, Petri WA Jr, et al. Hepatic amebiasis: a reminder of the complications. Curr Opin Pediatr 2009;21(1):145–9.

102. Chavez-Tapia NC, Hernandez-Calleros J, Tellez-Avila FI, et al. Image-guided percutaneous procedure plus metronidazole versus metronidazole alone for uncomplicated amoebic liver abscess. Cochrane Database Syst Rev 2009; 1:CD004886.

103. Ralls PW, Barnes PF, Johnson MB, et al. Medical treatment of hepatic amebic abscess: rare need for percutaneous drainage. Radiology 1987;165(3):805–7.

104. van den Berg JM, van Koppen E, Ahlin A, et al. Chronic granulomatous disease: the European experience. PLoS ONE 2009;4(4):e5234.

Management of an Incidental Liver Mass

Cherif Boutros, MD, MSc, Steven C. Katz, MD,
N. Joseph Espat, MD, MS*

KEYWORDS

- Incidental liver mass • Benign liver tumors • Liver metastases
- Hepatocellular carcinoma

The wide availability and use of advanced imaging modalities, including ultrasonography (US), CT, MRI, and positron emission tomography (PET), have led to increased identification of incidental liver masses (ILMs). The discovery of an ILM typically occurs during the course of an evaluation for an unrelated suspected or existing clinical problem. ILMs have also been detected during whole-body cross-sectional imaging offered on a proprietary basis for screening purposes.[1] On detection of ILM, it is incumbent on caring physicians to balance the potential risks posed by a lesion with the costs of further evaluation or treatment. Real harm can result from failure to diagnose a malignancy or inappropriate work-up of a harmless lesion. Through careful consideration of patient factors and imaging characteristics of ILMs, clinicians can recommend a safe, effective, and efficient course of action.

This article begins by considering the clinical factors that should be incorporated into the risk assessment of ILMs. Subsequently, the radiologic features of ILMs are reviewed, which are used in conjunction with clinical circumstances to define the risk of malignancy and the need for further evaluation and management. Specific indications for biopsy or therapeutic intervention are discussed. The article concludes with consideration of the specific pathologic entities accounting for the majority of ILMs. An algorithmic approach is outlined as a conceptual framework to assist with the development of an individualized assessment and management strategy for each patient confronted with an ILM (**Fig. 1**).

CLINICAL FACTORS RELATED TO INCIDENTAL LIVER MASS RISK

Although most of this discussion focuses on the radiographic or physical characteristics of ILMs, placing incidental imaging findings in the appropriate clinical context is of the utmost importance. Factors, including patient age, gender, history of malignancy,

Department of Hepatobiliary and Surgical Oncology, Roger Williams Medical Center, 825 Chalkstone Avenue, Prior 4, Providence, RI 02908, USA
* Corresponding author.
E-mail address: jespat@hepatisurgery.com

Surg Clin N Am 90 (2010) 699–718
doi:10.1016/j.suc.2010.04.005
0039-6109/10/$ – see front matter © 2010 Pubished by Elsevier Inc.

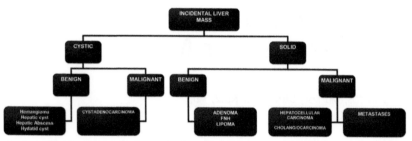

Fig. 1. An algorithmic approach to the hepatic mass. Hepatic masses can be grouped by architectural composition (solid or cystic), further subcategorized as benign or malignant, and if a malignant process is suspected or confirmed, then the mass is primary or metastatic in origin.

medication usage, and general medical history, in large part define the appropriate level of concern clinicians should assume for ILMs. By considering each patient's unique clinical circumstances in association with key radiographic features, clinicians can arrive at an appropriate plan of action.

History of Malignancy

The liver is a frequent site of metastatic disease and several factors account for the predilection of blood-borne neoplastic cells to establish secondary tumors within the intrahepatic milieu. The liver receives direct portal venous drainage from the gastrointestinal tract and is thus the first potential visceral site for metastases from numerous intra-abdominal tumor sites. It has been estimated that 40% to 50% of breast cancer patients develop liver metastases at some point in their disease.[2,3] Similarly, 35% to 50% of patients with colorectal cancer develop liver metastases.[4–6] Nearly two-thirds of patients with metastatic gastrointestinal stromal tumor have hepatic involvement.[7] The unique anatomic and biologic properties of the liver sinusoids and sinusoidal endothelial cells may also promote the development of metastases.[8,9] Therefore, in patients with a history of malignancy, in particular the tumor types discussed previously, a high degree of suspicion is warranted when ILMs are detected.

Medication Usage and Environmental Exposure

An association between steroid usage and liver neoplasia has been described.[10] Originally considered a risk factor for hepatic adenoma (HA), steroid administration has also been associated with focal nodular hyperplasia (FNH) and hepatocellular carcinoma (HCC).[11] An association between oral contraceptive use and hepatic tumors has been reported.[12–14] Growth of hepatic tumors during pregnancy or in the immediate postoperative period suggests an association with heightened endogenous estrogen levels.[15,16] Neoplastic liver lesions have been linked to anabolic steroid use, with reported cases of death from rupture.[17,18]

Exposure to vinyl chloride is a risk factor for the development of liver angiosarcoma.[19] Cohort studies have demonstrated a strong relationship between cumulative vinyl chloride exposure and risk of malignancy.[20] As with other anatomic sites, exposure to radiation is associated with the development of hepatic lymphoma. The liver is radiosensitive, with parenchymal toxicity occurring at 30 to 35 Gy.[21] Accidental exposure to radiation or whole-body radiation with bone marrow transplant may result in hepatotoxicity and increased risk of radiation-associated tumors.[21]

Age and Gender

Women are more likely to be diagnosed with certain benign liver tumors, including HA. HCC, however, is more common in men.[22] The reason for male predominance in HCC is unclear. Although male predominance was initially thought related to a higher rate of smoking and alcohol abuse, animal studies have implicated hormonal factors.[23] Specifically, women may be protected by the inhibitory effect of estrogen on interleukin-6. Although HCC is typically found in individuals beyond their fifth or sixth decade, fibrolamellar HCC tends to occur in younger individuals.[24] Hepatoblastoma is a malignant hepatic tumor that occurs almost exclusively in the pediatric populations. Therefore, consideration of patient age provides some guidance in assessing the cause of an ILM.

Medical Conditions

In addition to a history of malignant disease, other medical conditions may bear relevance to ILMs. The presence of cirrhosis, as a consequence of viral or alcoholic hepatitis, may lead to the presence of ILMs, including HCC and regenerative nodules. Documentation of the underlying cause of chronic hepatitis or cirrhosis is important, because the biologic features of malignant ILMs vary according the inciting factor.[25] Hepatitis C virus–related HCC has a greater tendency for multifocality and intrahepatic recurrence, whereas hepatitis B virus–related tumors are more likely to be solitary and large.[26–28] As discussed previously, the fibrolamellar type of HCC occurs most commonly in young patients with no history of hepatitis or cirrhosis, and these patients generally have normal α-fetoprotein (AFP) levels.[24]

Patients with primary sclerosing cholangitis (PSC) are at elevated risk for cholangiocarcinoma, which may present as an intrahepatic mass. Therefore, an ILM detected in a patient with a history of PSC or the associated condition, ulcerative colitis, warrants a high degree of suspicion. The only effective treatment for advanced PSC is orthotopic liver transplantation, which, in the absence of cholangiocarcinoma, is associated with a 5-year survival rate of 89%.[29] In cases of primary biliary cirrhosis (PBC), HCC is may develop several years after the onset of fibrotic changes in up to 40% of patients.[30] Patients with hemochromatosis are at elevated risk for HCC,[31] as are those suffering from autoimmune hepatitis[32] or Wilson disease.[33] The presence of any of these conditions warrants a heightened degree of suspicion when evaluating ILMs.

RADIOGRAPHIC FEATURES OF INCIDENTAL LIVER MASSES

At autopsy, ILMs may be identified in more than 50% of cases.[34] As imaging technology continues to improve, clinicians and patients will be faced with an increasing incidence of ILMs. Previous studies reported the frequency of clinically apparent ILMs as ranging from 10% to 33%.[35–37] The range in frequency of ILMs can be accounted for by variability in patient characteristics, imaging technique, and imaging interpretation. An appreciation of the tissue properties each imaging technique depends on can provide clinicians with clues to the cause of an ILM. Likewise, recognizing the limitations of imaging tests is helpful when attempting to define the risk posed by an ILM. This section focuses on the imaging tests that most commonly result in ILMs coming to clinical attention.

Ultrasonography

US is inexpensive and used for a wide range of indications. The liver is often imaged as part of examinations performed for biliary or urinary tract symptoms. Its ultimate usefulness as a diagnostic tool is operator dependent. US defines masses based on differential acoustic impedance relative to the surrounding tissues. For this reason, US is an excellent modality for defining a lesion as solid or cystic, based on the degree of echogenicity, shadowing characteristics, and through transmission.[38] As discussed later, establishing whether or not a lesion is solid or cystic is an important step in defining the risk of malignancy for ILM. The flow characteristics of ILMs, as detected with Doppler imaging, may provide additional information.[39]

CT Scans

Identification of a liver mass by CT scan depends on differential attenuation between the lesion and surrounding parenchyma in addition to its intravenous contrast uptake and washout characteristics. On unenhanced images, the attenuation of normal liver is typically brighter relative to neoplastic masses, which are hypoattenuating due to higher water content.[40]

Primary and metastatic liver tumors derive their blood supply primarily from the hepatic arterial circulation when they reach a size permitting detection on CT scans.[41] Intense arterial enhancement is characteristic of HCC and neuroendocrine tumors, whereas colorectal cancer liver metastases tend to be less vascular.[42] The pattern or timing of enhancement is important in certain instances as well. Although FNH lesions fill from the central scar region, hemangiomas demonstrate centripetal, globular peripheral enhancement.[43]

MRI

MRI machines emit short radio wave bursts, which align hydrogen protons that emit signals when the radio waves cease and the protons assume their native alignment.[44,45] The intensity of radio wave emission by tissue depends on the number of protons and hence water content. T1-weighted MRI demonstrates tissue, such as fat, as bright, whereas water-dense lesions, such as cysts, have high signal intensity on T2-weighted imaging. There are many other MRI techniques, the discussion of which is beyond the scope of this article. Although some liver lesions can be easily diagnosed on the basis of T1/T2 principles, the use of intravenous contrast material can add additional information.[46] For example, as for CT scans, early peripheral globular enhancement is essentially diagnostic of a hemangioma.[43] The most widely used MRI contrast agent is gadolinium,[47] and iron oxide may be useful to the detection of smaller intrahepatic tumors.[48]

Nuclear Medicine Imaging Techniques

Detection of ILM by scintigraphy is infrequent and the liver is usually first imaged with US, CT, or MRI. Rarely, a radiolabeled erythrocyte scan may demonstrate a hemangioma or a hepatobiliary iminodiacetic acid (HIDA) scan may reveal FNH.[46] PET scans are performed with increasing frequency to stage and monitor treatment response in cancer patients. In patients undergoing PET for cancer staging, a second malignancy is detected in 4% to 6% of cases.[49,50] Fluorodeoxyglucose (FDG)-PET depends on tissue glucose uptake and metabolism. Therefore, FDG-avid ILMs are, by definition, metabolically active relative to surrounding tissue. FDG-avid incidental lesions were previously termed, *PET-associated incidental neoplasms*.[51]

FURTHER IMAGING FOR INCIDENTAL LIVER MASSES

Determining the need for additional imaging after detection of ILM is of paramount importance. In some cases, the imaging test with which the lesion was detected provides sufficient information to permit confident diagnosis. Additional imaging is often beneficial, particularly when the incremental information is more specific or provides complementary data about the ILM physical properties. Understanding the features and limitations of each imaging technique facilitates safe and effective evaluation. Avoiding unnecessary tests is important to minimize delays in definitive management and risk of harm to patients.

Ultrasonography

US is inexpensive and poses no direct significant health risk to patients. Furthermore, US is accurate, is noninvasive, and can detect lesions as small as 1 cm within the liver. US readily distinguishes between solid and cystic lesions. Doppler US has made it possible to assess the presence of vascular flow, which may help define the nature of an ILM. US is also useful for serial interval imaging if observation is determined the appropriate course of action. US has been reported as 80% accurate for the detection of liver metastases.[52]

The development and use of microbubble contrast agents allows for dynamic sonographic images, which may be recorded in the arterial and venous phases.[53] Furthermore, the ability to calculate the transit time of contrast from the hepatic artery to hepatic veins can help define the degree of hepatic parenchymal injury in patients with hepatitis or cirrhosis.[54] As discussed previously, an appreciation of conditions affecting the liver parenchyma may allow for more accurate ILM risk assessment. Many studies have been performed to define the role of contrast-enhanced US for the characterization of liver lesions. HCC nodules show a high degree of vascularity when viewed with contrast-enhanced US.[55] Contrast-enhanced US may be superior compared with unenhanced US for the detection of intrahepatic metastases.[56]

CT Scans

Although modern CT scanners are accurate, liver lesions less than 1 cm in size may not be detected or adequately characterized.[57] CT has a reported sensitivity of 65% to 93% and specificity of 75% to 90% for detecting primary and metastatic tumors.[58–60] Modern helical CT scanners provide exquisitely detailed hepatic anatomic information as well, which is useful before resection or biopsy. CT scans performed with intravenous contrast and multiphase acquisitions allow determining the relationship of liver masses to critical vascular and biliary structures. The appearance of a lesion on CT is dependent on several features, including vascular density and pattern of enhancement with intravenous contrast. HCC lesions enhance on arterial phase and display washout of contrast material during the portal phase. Hepatic colorectal metastases have low attenuation compared with the surrounding parenchyma during portal phase scanning. Hypervascular neuroendocrine or renal metastases may be obscured in the portal phase but are hyperintense in the arterial phase.[61]

MRI

Sensitivity of MRI for HCC or liver metastases ranges from 93% to 97%.[62] In another study that included 80 malignant hepatic tumors identified by intraoperative US, the sensitivity and specificity of iron oxide–enhanced MRI were 87% and 97%, respectively.[63] Because MRI depends in large part on hydrogen proton density and, hence, water composition, the nature of tissue can be defined (ie, fat, fluid, or blood).[64] As with CT, MRI reveals lesion architecture (solid or cystic), the degree of lesion heterogeneity, and the relationship of a mass to vascular or biliary structures. Magnetic resonance angiography and magnetic resonance cholangiopancreatography are useful in circumstances in which ILMs lie in proximity to or communicate with critical structures. Accurate definition of lesion proximity to biliary and vascular structures is critical for planning safe and effective image-guided biopsies or surgical resection.

Nuclear Medicine Studies

Scintigrams performed with radiolabeled tracers are occasionally useful for defining the biologic properties of ILMs. For example, technetium Tc 99m sulfur colloid may assist in the diagnosis of FNH because the tracer identifies Kupffer cells within these lesions.[65] Technetium Tc 99m–labeled red blood scintigraphy can secure the diagnosis of hemangioma.[66] Although scintigraphy may detect hemangiomas as small as 1.5 cm,[67,68] CT and MRI can are sufficient in the majority of cases.

An incidental lesion detected by US, CT, or MRI may be further characterized by PET. Under certain circumstances, a PET scan may not only help detect metastatic disease but also define the biologic aggressiveness of tumors.[51] The incremental value of PET over routine imaging, clinical assessment, and tissue acquisition for the evaluation of ILMs, however, remains to be defined.[69,70] FDG-PET has demonstrated a sensitivity of 94% and a specificity of 91% in the detection of hepatic metastases from colorectal cancer[71–73] and may change management in up to 40% of patients.[73,74] An important limitation of traditional FDG-PET imaging is the inability to provide detailed anatomic information. This often requires that PET imaging is complemented by CT or MRI.[75] For HCC, PET is less reliable because approximately half of HCCs are not FDG avid.[76] PET, however, may alter management in up to 30% of patients with HCC by focusing the biopsy on the metabolically active site, identifying distant metastases, or detecting local recurrence.[77] Furthermore, whole-body FDG-PET imaging may demonstrate an index primary cancer or additional intra- or extrahepatic metastases in cases of malignant ILMs.[78]

INDICATIONS FOR BIOPSY AND RESECTION

In selected cases, the most appropriate imaging test after detection of an ILM is performed with a pathologist's microscope after a percutaneous biopsy or surgical resection. The decision of whether or not to pursue a tissue diagnosis rests largely on the clinical context in addition to the imaging characteristics of the ILM. A history of malignancy raises the level of suspicion when an ILM is detected. If the clinical factors and imaging characteristics are not definitive, a tissue diagnosis may be necessary before pursuing a therapeutic option.

Image-Guided Biopsy

US or CT may be used to guide percutaneous liver biopsy of an ILM. Tissue may be acquired by fine-needle aspiration (FNA) or a core needle biopsy. FNA provides cytologic information in the absence of tissue architecture.[79] Despite the fact that more tissue is retrieved by core needle biopsy, the diagnostic rates are not significantly different from FNA and the two may be complementary, with a combined sensitivity of 90%.[80,81] FNA, however, limited by the inability to provide tissue architecture, may underdiagnose well-differentiated HCC. In such cases, a core biopsy may be required.[82,83]

Complications of percutaneous biopsy include intraperitoneal hemorrhage, hemobilia, pneumothorax, infection, and bile leak. The risk of parenchymal bleeding is less than 1% and is usually self-limited.[84] Pericardial tamponade has also been reported.[85] The risk of needle track seedling is reported to be less than 1% with an average latency of 24 months.[86] Percutaneous biopsies should only be performed when the information gained alters the management of an ILM. For example, a hypervascular tumor in a cirrhotic patient with a markedly elevated AFP level can securely be diagnosed as an HCC without tissue confirmation. Although percutaneous biopsies are safe, even a small level of risk is difficult to justify if the cytologic or histologic information does not affect the diagnosis or treatment.

Surgical Biopsy

With the advent of safe and effective image-guided percutaneous liver biopsies, the need to excise a mass for purely diagnostic purposes is limited. In cases when a percutaneous biopsy is nondiagnostic, open or laparoscopic liver biopsy may be appropriate. Laparoscopy has emerged as an important adjunct to the staging of several abdominal malignancies. Direct imaging with the laparoscope and the use of intraoperative US may help define the nature of an ILM and facilitate safe excision. Intraoperative US may reveal liver masses not detected by cross-sectional imaging in 27% of cases.[57]

ILMs may also be detected during the course of an operation performed for an unrelated indication. As with ILMs detected by imaging, those found during laparotomy or laparoscopy must be considered in the overall clinical context. A common scenario during which an ILM is found intraoperatively is during a colectomy for carcinoma. Surgical excision of such lesions may be warranted for diagnostic or therapeutic purposes, depending on the number of tumors and their location in the liver.[87] Intraoperatively detected ILMs may also be addressed with ablative techniques or regional therapeutic strategies.[88]

SPECIFIC CAUSES

Clinical and radiographic features of ILMs are reported in **Table 1**.

Hepatic Hemangioma

Hepatic hemangiomas (HHs) are congenital vascular malformations and are the most common benign hepatic tumor. In a series of 115 patients, nearly 50% of patients were asymptomatic at the time of diagnosis.[89] Although US, CT, and scintigraphy can be used to diagnose HH, MRI with contrast is currently the most accurate with reported sensitivity and specificity of 85% to 95%.[90,91] The approach to diagnosing HH, however, in a given patient depends on several factors, including clinical history, the preference of the patient and referring physician, and the imaging technique available.[92]

On CT scan, HHs are sharply defined masses that are usually hypoattenuating compared with the adjacent hepatic parenchyma on unenhanced images. On enhanced images, the vascular components of HHs have the same attenuation value as normal blood vessels.[93] As discussed previously, HHs demonstrate characteristic sequential contrast opacification, beginning at the periphery of the lesion and proceeding toward the center (**Fig. 2**).[94] On MRI, HHs have low signal intensity on T1-weighted images and are heterogenously intense on T2-weighted images. HHs demonstrate a relative increase in signal in heavily T2-weighted images compared with moderate T2-weighted images, unlike other ILMs with the exception of hepatic cysts.[92] After administration of gadolinium, HHs demonstrate peripheral nodular enhancement on T1-weighted images (**Fig. 3**). Needle or core biopsy for a suspected HH is discouraged because the diagnostic yield is poor[89] and can lead to hemorrhage.[95] The indications for surgical resection of HH are symptoms or the inability to rule out malignancy.[89] Resection of HH due to concern for a malignant process has been associated with the lack of MRI.[96]

Table 1
Clinical and radiographic features of incidental liver masses

Pathology	Pertinent History	Pertinent Laboratory Studies	Radiologic Studies
Hepatic adenoma	Young adult women History of oral contraceptive use May present acutely with severe pain due to hemorrhage	None	US: solid lesion, without biliary structures CT: solid lesion, contrast enhancement due to vascularity MRI: solid, enhancing mass
Focal nodular hyperplasia	Usually asymptomatic	None	US: solid homogeneous lesion CT/MRI: solid lesion with central scar, large feeding artery May be difficult to differentiate from HA
Lipoma	Usually asymptomatic	None	US: identified as a homogenous lesion MRI: bright on T1 sequence (**Fig. 8**)
Hemangioma	Usually asymptomatic	Thrombocytopenia in rare cases	CT and MRI: peripheral, centripetal enhancing pattern
Simple hepatic cyst	RUQ pain or fullness if large May occur in association with polycystic kidney disease	Leukocytosis if infected	US: cystic structure with no vascular flow CT or MRI: fluid-filled homogenous lesion Septations or nodules may indicate neoplasia
Hydatid cyst	Suspect if patient from endemic areas	Serologic test for *E granulosus*	US: heterogeneous, multilocculated CT/MRI: heterogeneous with internal layer and daughter cysts
Hepatocellular carcinoma	Suspect if cirrhosis or chronic viral hepatitis are present Other risk factors include PSC, PBC, or hemochromatosis	Viral serology Elevated AFP	US: peritumoral arterial flow on Doppler interrogation CT/MRI: intense in arterial phase, with washout in portal phase
Cholangiocarcinoma	Jaundice if biliary obstruction is present	Possible evidence of cholestasis	US: dilations of the biliary tree if hilar. CT/MRI: hypoattenuating mass
Metastases	History of extrahepatic malignancy	Elevated CEA if colorectal Elevated chromogranin or urinary 5-HIAA if neuroendocrine	CT: hypoattenuating mass MRI: may be more sensitive than CT to identify the number of lesions

Abbreviations: CEA, carcinoembryonic antigen; 5-HIAA, 5-hydroxyindoleacetic acid; RUQ, right upper quadrant.

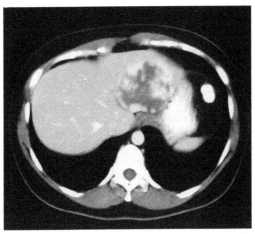

Fig. 2. A CT scan with contrast in the arterial phase demonstrating early, peripheral enhancements of a hemangioma of the liver.

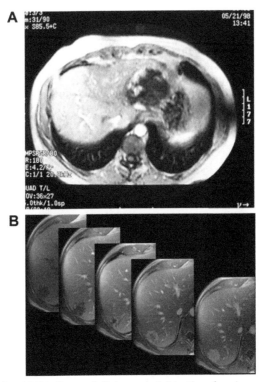

Fig. 3. (*A*) T1-weighted MRI after gadolinium administration showing peripheral enhancement of a hemangioma. (*B*) Serial picture of MRI with gadolinium showing the typical centripetal vascular filling pattern of a hemangioma over time.

Focal Nodular Hyperplasia

As the name implies, FNH is a nodular hyperplasia of hepatocytes associated with Kupffer cells. A central scar is highly characteristic but present in less than 50% of cases.[97] FNH accounts for 8% of benign hepatic tumors, usually is an incidental finding, and is associated with a female predominance.[97] Because the management of FNH is nonsurgical in asymptomatic cases, it is important to make the diagnosis radiologically. Because FNH is composed primarily of hepatocytes, the density of FNH is similar to the normal hepatic parenchyma. This manifests as an isoechoic lesion on US or isodense mass on a CT scan. A triple-phase CT scan or MRI with contrast may show enhancement or high signal intensity in the arterial phase, allowing a lesion to be distinguished from the surrounding parenchyma. A central artery is visualized in 20% to 30% of cases on CT scan or MRI (**Fig. 4**). The central scar is characteristically opacified in late phases on CT scan and hyperintense on T2.[98] MRI is the preferred modality for confirming diagnosis of FNH (**Fig. 5**).[99,100] Scintigraphy using technetium Tc 99m sulfur colloid or HIDA scan may aid in the confirmation of FNH, but false-positive tests have been reported in cases of adenoma and hepatoblastoma.[101,102] In the extraordinarily rare cases when FNH cannot be confirmed by radiologic studies, liver biopsy is indicated to rule out malignancy and to avoid unnecessary resection. Histologic evaluation of FNH may reveal fibrous septae, a dystrophic artery, ductal proliferation, sinusoidal dilatation, and perisinusoidal fibrosis.[103] Immunohistochemical studies can help differentiate FNH from other entities in select cases.[104]

Hepatic Adenoma

HAs are benign tumors of normal hepatocytes and sinusoidal endothelial cells, with no portal triads. HAs are more common in women than in men (9:1) and have been associated with the use of oral contraceptives.[12–14] Other risk factors include anabolic steroids and history of Budd-Chiari syndrome.[105] Radiologically, HAs are differentiated from FNH by a regular smooth border and internal heterogeneity. CT scans with intravenous contrast reveal the hypervascular nature of HA and have largely replaced arteriography (**Fig. 6**).

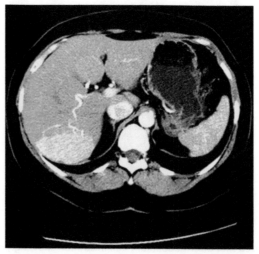

Fig. 4. CT scan with intravenous contrast illustrating a dominant central artery supplying FNH.

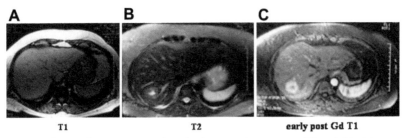

| T1 | T2 | early post Gd T1 |

Fig. 5. MRI of FNH demonstrating the classic central scar on a T1-weighted image (*A*), T2-weighted image (*B*), and T1 image after gadolinium (Gd) administration (*C*).

Although HA can be incidentally discovered, patients may present with abdominal pain related to hemorrhage within the adenoma or intraperitoneal rupture. In approximately 50% of cases, multiple adenomas may be found.[106] Surgical resection was traditionally recommended on the basis of symptoms or size greater than 5 cm given the risk of malignant transformation and hemorrhage.[107] Therefore, particularly during pregnancy all ILMs definitely diagnosed as HA should be resected if patients are appropriate surgical candidates. With the application of minimally invasive liver resection techniques, the indications for liver resection may be expanding, particularly with indeterminate ILMs.[108] Ultimately, the decision to perform a liver resection should be based on a careful assessment of the risks of observation relative to the risks of surgical intervention.

Cystic Lesions

Hepatic cysts are most commonly benign, simple cysts and may be found in up to 2.5% of the population on US.[109] Cysts are solitary in 70% and asymptomatic in the majority of patients. In patients with multiple hepatic and renal cysts, a hereditary syndrome should be considered, because the liver is the most frequent extrarenal site of involvement.[110] The diagnosis is typically made by US, which reveals a hypoechoic spherical or oval lesion with clear borders and no acoustic shadow. When these typical findings are present, US is sufficient. The presence of internal septations or

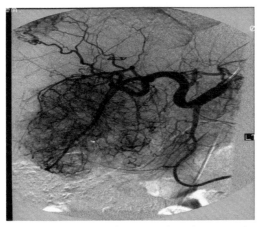

Fig. 6. Angiogram showing a hypervascular HA with a characteristic network-like filling pattern.

mural nodularity, cystadenoma or cystadenocarcinoma, however, should be suspected and further evaluation is warranted. On CT, hepatic cysts are round, hypodense, and the walls do not enhance with contrast. On MRI, hepatic lesions demonstrate high intensity on T2 sequences given their high water content (**Fig. 7**). Mural nodules may enhance with intravenous contrast on CT or MRI. In cases when a neoplastic cyst cannot be excluded, FNA with cytology and CEA concentration determination may be useful.[111] Even large hepatic cysts do not require treatment, unless symptomatic. Treatment options include percutaneous sclerosis, cyst marsupialization, or cystectomy. If a cyst demonstrates suspicious features, such as mural nodularity, it is imperative to generously sample the cyst wall to exclude malignancy.

Hydatid Cysts

Hydatid cysts are frequent causes of ILMs in geographic regions endemic for *Echinococcus granulosus*. Typical imaging features vary by stage and include an anechoic cyst with a thick wall, a detached internal layer, multiple daughter cysts, and dense calcifications.[112] These features are discernable on US or CT. MRI may detect

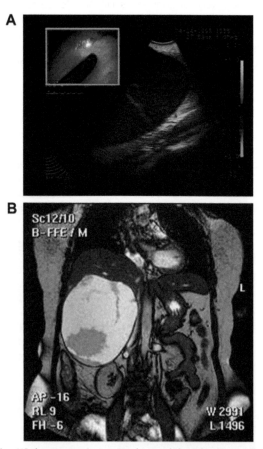

Fig. 7. Intraoperative US demonstrating a simple cyst (*A*) and a T2-weighted MRI of cytadenoma (*B*). Note the hyperintense character and intacystic trabeculae of the cystadenoma on the T2-weighted images.

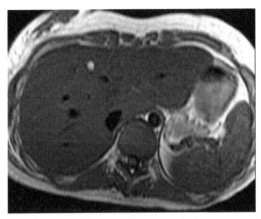

Fig. 8. MRI of a hepatic lipoma. This central, anterior lesion appears bright lesion on T1 similar to subcutaneous fat.

communication with the biliary tree. When hydatid disease is suspected, serologic testing is warranted to secure the diagnosis.

Biliary Hamartomas

Biliary hamartomas are benign congenital liver lesions characterized by the presence of a fibrous stroma. These lesions are peripherally distributed, hypodense, and range from 1 mm to 3 cm in size. On MRI, biliary hamartomas are hypointense on T1 sequences and strongly hyperintense in T2 sequences.

Malignant Incidental Liver Masses

As discussed previously, indications for surgical management of benign liver masses include uncertain diagnosis, severe or progressive symptoms, hemorrhage, or rupture.[113] The key determination when an ILM is found is whether or not a mass is benign or malignant. In a retrospective analysis of patients undergoing liver resection for suspected malignancy, lesion size less than 4 cm, discrepant radiology findings, and stability over time were correlates of a benign pathologic diagnosis.[114] This underscores the need to review prior imaging when it is available.

On CT and MRI, malignant ILMs may demonstrate an enhancing rim or diffuse heterogeneous enhancement. A hypoattenuatting or hypointense halo surrounding the mass also is highly suggestive of malignancy, although can be seen with adenomas.[92] Peripheral washout on delayed images can be found in cholangiocarcinoma and hepatic metastases[115] but is seen more frequently in hypervascular tumors, such as HCC and metastases from neuroendocrine or renal cell primaries.[116] Demonstration of vascular invasion to the portal or hepatic veins is consistent with a malignancy and is seen more commonly with HCC than metastases.[92]

As emphasized throughout this article, clinical factors are important for determining the likelihood of malignancy when an ILM is noted. A history of prior malignancy, particularly one with a predilection for liver metastases, is an obvious risk factor for malignant ILMs. In general, the likelihood of malignancy increases with advancing age and larger tumor size.[117] When the diagnosis of a malignant ILM is not secure or a patient is not an ideal operative candidate, then percutaneous tissue sampling or observation may be appropriate. For example, biopsy to prove HCC may be needed for small lesions in the 1- to 2-cm range if other supporting clinical features are not present.[118]

SUMMARY

As use of more sensitive imaging techniques increases , the rate of ILM detection will continue to increase. It is imperative to accurately assess the risk of malignancy and probability of hemorrhage and determine if symptoms are likely due to the ILM and not an unrelated condition. By carefully considering patient history and specific imaging features, the caring physician can arrive at a safe, efficient, and appropriate plan for diagnosis and, when indicated, definitive management.

REFERENCES

1. Furtado CD, Aguirre DA, Sirlin CB, et al. Whole-body CT screening: spectrum of findings and recommendations in 1192 patients. Radiology 2005;237(2): 385–94.
2. Hoe AL, Royle GT, Taylor I. Breast liver metastases—incidence, diagnosis and outcome. J R Soc Med 1991;84(12):714–6.
3. Zinser JW, Hortobagyi GN, Buzdar AU, et al. Clinical course of breast cancer patients with liver metastases. J Clin Oncol 1987;5(5):773–82.
4. Power DG, Healey-Bird BR, Kemeny NE. Regional chemotherapy for liver-limited metastatic colorectal cancer. Clin Colorectal Cancer 2008;7(4):247–59.
5. Khatri VP, Chee KG, Petrelli NJ. Modern multimodality approach to hepatic colorectal metastases: solutions and controversies. Surg Oncol 2007;16(1): 71–83.
6. Pawlik TM, Choti MA. Surgical therapy for colorectal metastases to the liver. J Gastrointest Surg 2007;11(8):1057–77.
7. DeMatteo RP, Lewis JJ, Leung D, et al. Two hundred gastrointestinal stromal tumors: recurrence patterns and prognostic factors for survival. Ann Surg 2000;231(1):51–8.
8. Katz SC, Pillarisetty VG, Bleier JI, et al. Liver sinusoidal endothelial cells are insufficient to activate T cells. J Immunol 2004;173(1):230–5.
9. Tang L, Yang J, Liu W, et al. Liver sinusoidal endothelial cell lectin, LSECtin, negatively regulates hepatic T-cell immune response. Gastroenterology 2009; 137(4):1498–508, e1–5.
10. Baum JK, Bookstein JJ, Holtz F, et al. Possible association between benign hepatomas and oral contraceptives. Lancet 1973;2(7835):926–9.
11. Klatskin G. Hepatic tumors: possible relationship to use of oral contraceptives. Gastroenterology 1977;73(2):386–94.
12. Edmondson HA, Henderson B, Benton B. Liver-cell adenomas associated with use of oral contraceptives. N Engl J Med 1976;294(9):470–2.
13. Rooks JB, Ory HW, Ishak KG, et al. Epidemiology of hepatocellular adenoma. The role of oral contraceptive use. JAMA 1979;242(7):644–8.
14. Christopherson WM, Mays ET, Barrows G. Hepatocellular carcinoma in young women on oral contraceptives. Lancet 1978;2(8079):38–9.
15. Malt RA, Hershberg RA, Miller WL. Experience with benign tumors of the liver. Surg Gynecol Obstet 1970;130(2):285–91.
16. Motsay GJ, Gamble WG. Clinical experience with hepatic adenomas. Surg Gynecol Obstet 1972;134(3):415–8.
17. Wilson JD. Androgen abuse by athletes. Endocr Rev 1988;9(2):181–99.
18. Creagh TM, Rubin A, Evans DJ. Hepatic tumours induced by anabolic steroids in an athlete. J Clin Pathol 1988;41(4):441–3.
19. Blair A, Kazerouni N. Reactive chemicals and cancer. Cancer Causes Control 1997;8(3):473–90.

20. Simonato L, L'Abbe KA, Andersen A, et al. A collaborative study of cancer incidence and mortality among vinyl chloride workers. Scand J Work Environ Health
1991;17(3):159–69.
21. Lawrence TS, Robertson JM, Anscher MS, et al. Hepatic toxicity resulting from
cancer treatment. Int J Radiat Oncol Biol Phys 1995;31(5):1237–48.
22. Wands J. Hepatocellular carcinoma and sex. N Engl J Med 2007;357(19):
1974–6.
23. Nakatani T, Roy G, Fujimoto N, et al. Sex hormone dependency of
diethylnitrosamine-induced liver tumors in mice and chemoprevention by
leuprorelin. Jpn J Cancer Res 2001;92(3):249–56.
24. Stipa F, Yoon SS, Liau KH, et al. Outcome of patients with fibrolamellar hepatocellular carcinoma. Cancer 2006;106(6):1331–8.
25. Roayaie S, Haim MB, Emre S, et al. Comparison of surgical outcomes for hepatocellular carcinoma in patients with hepatitis B versus hepatitis C: a western
experience. Ann Surg Oncol 2000;7(10):764–70.
26. Yamanaka N, Tanaka T, Tanaka W, et al. Correlation of hepatitis virus serologic
status with clinicopathologic features in patients undergoing hepatectomy for
hepatocellular carcinoma. Cancer 1997;79(8):1509–15.
27. Schwartz M. Liver transplantation: the preferred treatment for early hepatocellular carcinoma in the setting of cirrhosis? Ann Surg Oncol 2007;14(2):
548–52.
28. Shah SA, Greig PD, Gallinger S, et al. Factors associated with early recurrence
after resection for hepatocellular carcinoma and outcomes. J Am Coll Surg
2006;202(2):275–83.
29. Harrison PM. Prevention of bile duct cancer in primary sclerosing cholangitis.
Ann Oncol 1999;10(Suppl 4):208–11.
30. Jones DE, Metcalf JV, Collier JD, et al. Hepatocellular carcinoma in primary
biliary cirrhosis and its impact on outcomes. Hepatology 1997;26(5):
1138–42.
31. Deugnier YM, Guyader D, Crantock L, et al. Primary liver cancer in genetic
hemochromatosis: a clinical, pathological, and pathogenetic study of 54 cases.
Gastroenterology 1993;104(1):228–34.
32. Ryder SD, Koskinas J, Rizzi PM, et al. Hepatocellular carcinoma complicating
autoimmune hepatitis: role of hepatitis C virus. Hepatology 1995;22(3):718–22.
33. Kumagi T, Horiike N, Abe M, et al. Small hepatocellular carcinoma associated
with Wilson's disease. Intern Med 2005;44(5):439–43.
34. Karhunen PJ. Benign hepatic tumours and tumour like conditions in men. J Clin
Pathol 1986;39(2):183–8.
35. Volk M, Strotzer M, Lenhart M, et al. Frequency of benign hepatic lesions incidentally detected with contrast-enhanced thin-section portal venous phase
spiral CT. Acta Radiol 2001;42(2):172–5.
36. Schwartz LH, Gandras EJ, Colangelo SM, et al. Prevalence and importance of
small hepatic lesions found at CT in patients with cancer. Radiology 1999;
210(1):71–4.
37. Kuszyk BS, Bluemke DA, Urban BA, et al. Portal-phase contrast-enhanced
helical CT for the detection of malignant hepatic tumors: sensitivity based on
comparison with intraoperative and pathologic findings. AJR Am J Roentgenol
1996;166(1):91–5.
38. Eberhardt SC, Choi PH, Bach AM, et al. Utility of sonography for small hepatic
lesions found on computed tomography in patients with cancer. J Ultrasound
Med 2003;22(4):335–43 [quiz: 345–6].

39. Ohto M, Kato H, Tsujii H, et al. Vascular flow patterns of hepatic tumors in contrast-enhanced 3-dimensional fusion ultrasonography using plane shift and opacity control modes. J Ultrasound Med 2005;24(1):49–57.
40. Tidebrant G, Asztely M, Lukes P, et al. Comparison of non-enhanced, bolus enhanced, and delayed scanning techniques in computed tomography of hepatic tumours. Acta Radiol 1990;31(2):161–6.
41. Honda H, Matsuura Y, Onitsuka H, et al. Differential diagnosis of hepatic tumors (hepatoma, hemangioma, and metastasis) with CT: value of two-phase incremental imaging. AJR Am J Roentgenol 1992;159(4):735–40.
42. Foley WD. Liver: surgical planning. Eur Radiol 2005;15(Suppl 4):D89–95.
43. Valette PJ, Pilleul F, Crombe-Ternamian A. MDCT of benign liver tumors and metastases. Eur Radiol 2003;13(Suppl 5):M31–41.
44. Scherzinger AL, Hendee WR. Basic principles of magnetic resonance imaging—an update. West J Med 1985;143(6):782–92.
45. Turner DA. Nuclear magnetic resonance in oncology. Semin Nucl Med 1985; 15(2):210–23.
46. Braga L, Guller U, Semelka RC. Modern hepatic imaging. Surg Clin North Am 2004;84(2):375–400.
47. Semelka RC, Helmberger TK. Contrast agents for MR imaging of the liver. Radiology 2001;218(1):27–38.
48. Schultz JF, Bell JD, Goldstein RM, et al. Hepatic tumor imaging using iron oxide MRI: comparison with computed tomography, clinical impact, and cost analysis. Ann Surg Oncol 1999;6(7):691–8.
49. Choi JY, Lee KS, Kwon OJ, et al. Improved detection of second primary cancer using integrated [18F] fluorodeoxyglucose positron emission tomography and computed tomography for initial tumor staging. J Clin Oncol 2005;23(30): 7654–9.
50. Kojima S, Zhou B, Teramukai S, et al. Cancer screening of healthy volunteers using whole-body 18F-FDG-PET scans: the Nishidai clinic study. Eur J Cancer 2007;43(12):1842–8.
51. Katz SC, Shaha A. PET-associated incidental neoplasms of the thyroid. J Am Coll Surg 2008;207(2):259–64.
52. Smith TJ, Kemeny MM, Sugarbaker PH, et al. A prospective study of hepatic imaging in the detection of metastatic disease. Ann Surg 1982;195(4):486–91.
53. Cosgrove D. The advances are significant improvements in both the microbubbles used as contrast agents and in the software that allows their selective detection. Eur Radiol 2004;14(Suppl 8):1–3.
54. Albrecht T, Blomley MJ, Cosgrove DO, et al. Non-invasive diagnosis of hepatic cirrhosis by transit-time analysis of an ultrasound contrast agent. Lancet 1999; 353(9164):1579–83.
55. Choi BI, Kim AY, Lee JY, et al. Hepatocellular carcinoma: contrast enhancement with Levovist. J Ultrasound Med 2002;21(1):77–84.
56. Skjoldbye B, Pedersen MH, Struckmann J, et al. Improved detection and biopsy of solid liver lesions using pulse-inversion ultrasound scanning and contrast agent infusion. Ultrasound Med Biol 2002;28(4):439–44.
57. Scaife CL, Ng CS, Ellis LM, et al. Accuracy of preoperative imaging of hepatic tumors with helical computed tomography. Ann Surg Oncol 2006;13(4):542–6.
58. Matsuo M, Kanematsu M, Inaba Y, et al. Pre-operative detection of malignant hepatic tumours: value of combined helical CT during arterial portography and biphasic CT during hepatic arteriography. Clin Radiol 2001;56(2): 138–45.

59. Kehagias D, Metafa A, Hatziioannou A, et al. Comparison of CT, MRI and CT during arterial portography in the detection of malignant hepatic lesions. Hepatogastroenterology 2000;47(35):1399–403.
60. Schmidt J, Strotzer M, Fraunhofer S, et al. Intraoperative ultrasonography versus helical computed tomography and computed tomography with arterioportography in diagnosing colorectal liver metastases: lesion-by-lesion analysis. World J Surg 2000;24(1):43–7 [discussion: 48].
61. Mahfouz AE, Hamm B, Mathieu D. Imaging of metastases to the liver. Eur Radiol 1996;6(5):607–14.
62. Kim YK, Kwak HS, Kim CS, et al. Detection and characterization of focal hepatic tumors: a comparison of T2-weighted MR images before and after the administration of gadoxetic acid. J Magn Reson Imaging 2009;30(2):437–43.
63. Vogl TJ, Schwarz W, Blume S, et al. Preoperative evaluation of malignant liver tumors: comparison of unenhanced and SPIO (Resovist)-enhanced MR imaging with biphasic CTAP and intraoperative US. Eur Radiol 2003;13(2):262–72.
64. Biagini C. [Role of magnetic resonance imaging in the tissue characterization of tumors]. Radiol Med 1986;72(6):379–92 [in Italian].
65. Buetow PC, Pantongrag-Brown L, Buck JL, et al. Focal nodular hyperplasia of the liver: radiologic-pathologic correlation. Radiographics 1996;16(2):369–88.
66. Royal HD, Israel O, Parker JA, et al. Scintigraphy of hepatic hemangiomas: the value of Tc-99m-labeled red blood cells: concise communication. J Nucl Med 1981;22(8):684–7.
67. Krausz Y, Levy M, Antebi E, et al. Liver hemangioma. A perioperative Tc-99m RBC SPECT correlation. Clin Nucl Med 1997;22(1):35–7.
68. Guze BH, Hawkins RA. Utility of the SPECT Tc-99m labeled RBC blood pool scan in the detection of hepatic hemangiomas. Clin Nucl Med 1989;14(11):817–8.
69. Yapar Z, Kibar M, Yapar AF, et al. The value of 18F-fluorodeoxyglucose positron emission tomography/computed tomography in carcinoma of an unknown primary: diagnosis and follow-up. Nucl Med Commun 2010;31(1):59–66.
70. Pace L, Nicolai E, Klain M, et al. Diagnostic value of FDG PET/CT imaging. Q J Nucl Med Mol Imaging 2009;53(5):503–12.
71. Orlacchio A, Schillaci O, Fusco N, et al. Role of PET/CT in the detection of liver metastases from colorectal cancer. Radiol Med 2009;114(4):571–85.
72. Kinkel K, Lu Y, Both M, et al. Detection of hepatic metastases from cancers of the gastrointestinal tract by using noninvasive imaging methods (US, CT, MR imaging, PET): a meta-analysis. Radiology 2002;224(3):748–56.
73. Desai DC, Zervos EE, Arnold MW, et al. Positron emission tomography affects surgical management in recurrent colorectal cancer patients. Ann Surg Oncol 2003;10(1):59–64.
74. Rydzewski B, Dehdashti F, Gordon BA, et al. Usefulness of intraoperative sonography for revealing hepatic metastases from colorectal cancer in patients selected for surgery after undergoing FDG PET. AJR Am J Roentgenol 2002;178(2):353–8.
75. Ruers TJ, Langenhoff BS, Neeleman N, et al. Value of positron emission tomography with [F-18]fluorodeoxyglucose in patients with colorectal liver metastases: a prospective study. J Clin Oncol 2002;20(2):388–95.
76. Salem N, MacLennan GT, Kuang Y, et al. Quantitative evaluation of 2-deoxy-2[F-18]fluoro-D-glucose-positron emission tomography imaging on the woodchuck model of hepatocellular carcinoma with histological correlation. Mol Imaging Biol 2007;9(3):135–43.

77. Delbeke D, Pinson CW. 11C-acetate: a new tracer for the evaluation of hepato-cellular carcinoma. J Nucl Med 2003;44(2):222–3.

78. MacManus MP, Hicks RJ, Matthews JP, et al. High rate of detection of unsus-pected distant metastases by pet in apparent stage III non-small-cell lung cancer: implications for radical radiation therapy. Int J Radiat Oncol Biol Phys 2001;50(2):287–93.

79. Nasuti JF, Gupta PK, Baloch ZW. Diagnostic value and cost-effectiveness of on-site evaluation of fine-needle aspiration specimens: review of 5,688 cases. Diagn Cytopathol 2002;27(1):1–4.

80. Stewart CJ, Coldewey J, Stewart IS. Comparison of fine needle aspiration cytology and needle core biopsy in the diagnosis of radiologically detected abdominal lesions. J Clin Pathol 2002;55(2):93–7.

81. Ohlsson B, Nilsson J, Stenram U, et al. Percutaneous fine-needle aspiration cytology in the diagnosis and management of liver tumours. Br J Surg 2002; 89(6):757–62.

82. Kulesza P, Torbenson M, Sheth S, et al. Cytopathologic grading of hepatocel-lular carcinoma on fine-needle aspiration. Cancer 2004;102(4):247–58.

83. Kuo FY, Chen WJ, Lu SN, et al. Fine needle aspiration cytodiagnosis of liver tumors. Acta Cytol 2004;48(2):142–8.

84. Riemann B, Menzel J, Schiemann U, et al. Ultrasound-guided biopsies of abdominal organs with an automatic biopsy system. A retrospective analysis of the quality of biopsies and of hemorrhagic complications. Scand J Gastroen-terol 2000;35(1):102–7.

85. Kucharczyk W, Weisbrod GL, Cooper JD, et al. Cardiac tamponade as a compli-cation of thin-needle aspiration lung biopsy. Chest 1982;82(1):120–1.

86. Kosugi C, Furuse J, Ishii H, et al. Needle tract implantation of hepatocellular carcinoma and pancreatic carcinoma after ultrasound-guided percutaneous puncture: clinical and pathologic characteristics and the treatment of needle tract implantation. World J Surg 2004;28(1):29–32.

87. Wanebo HJ, Semoglou C, Attiyeh F, et al. Surgical management of patients with primary operable colorectal cancer and synchronous liver metastases. Am J Surg 1978;135(1):81–5.

88. Fahy BN, D'Angelica M, DeMatteo RP, et al. Synchronous hepatic metastases from colon cancer: changing treatment strategies and results of surgical inter-vention. Ann Surg Oncol 2009;16(2):361–70.

89. Yoon SS, Charny CK, Fong Y, et al. Diagnosis, management, and outcomes of 115 patients with hepatic hemangioma. J Am Coll Surg 2003;197(3):392–402.

90. Unal O, Sakarya ME, Arslan H, et al. Hepatic cavernous hemangiomas: patterns of contrast enhancement on MR fluoroscopy imaging. Clin Imaging 2002;26(1):39–42.

91. Olcott EW, Li KC, Wright GA, et al. Differentiation of hepatic malignancies from hemangiomas and cysts by T2 relaxation times: early experience with multiply refocused four-echo imaging at 1.5 T. J Magn Reson Imaging 1999;9(1):81–6.

92. Heiken JP. Distinguishing benign from malignant liver tumours. Cancer Imaging 2007;7(Spec No A):S1–14.

93. Whitehouse RW. Computed tomography attenuation measurements for the char-acterization of hepatic haemangiomas. Br J Radiol 1991;64(767):1019–22.

94. Quinn SF, Benjamin GG. Hepatic cavernous hemangiomas: simple diagnostic sign with dynamic bolus CT. Radiology 1992;182(2):545–8.

95. Jenkins RL, Johnson LB, Lewis WD. Surgical approach to benign liver tumors. Semin Liver Dis 1994;14(2):178–89.

96. Mitchell DG, Saini S, Weinreb J, et al. Hepatic metastases and cavernous hemangiomas: distinction with standard- and triple-dose gadoteridol-enhanced MR imaging. Radiology 1994;193(1):49–57.

97. Bioulac-Sage P, Balabaud C, Wanless IR. Diagnosis of focal nodular hyperplasia: not so easy. Am J Surg Pathol 2001;25(10):1322–5.

98. Mortele KJ, Praet M, Van Vlierberghe H, et al. CT and MR imaging findings in focal nodular hyperplasia of the liver: radiologic-pathologic correlation. AJR Am J Roentgenol 2000;175(3):687–92.

99. Cherqui D, Rahmouni A, Charlotte F, et al. Management of focal nodular hyperplasia and hepatocellular adenoma in young women: a series of 41 patients with clinical, radiological, and pathological correlations. Hepatology 1995;22(6): 1674–81.

100. Kehagias D, Moulopoulos L, Antoniou A, et al. Focal nodular hyperplasia: imaging findings. Eur Radiol 2001;11(2):202–12.

101. Diament MJ, Parvey LS, Tonkin IL, et al. Hepatoblastoma: technetium sulfur colloid uptake simulating focal nodular hyperplasia. AJR Am J Roentgenol 1982;139(1):168–71.

102. Tanasescu DE, Waxman AD, Hurvitz C. Scintigraphic findings mimicking focal nodular hyperplasia in a case of hepatoblastoma. Clin Nucl Med 1991;16(4): 236–8.

103. Fabre A, Audet P, Vilgrain V, et al. Histologic scoring of liver biopsy in focal nodular hyperplasia with atypical presentation. Hepatology 2002;35(2): 414–20.

104. Makhlouf HR, Abdul-Al HM, Goodman ZD. Diagnosis of focal nodular hyperplasia of the liver by needle biopsy. Hum Pathol 2005;36(11):1210–6.

105. Vilgrain V, Lewin M, Vons C, et al. Hepatic nodules in Budd-Chiari syndrome: imaging features. Radiology 1999;210(2):443–50.

106. Dokmak S, Paradis V, Vilgrain V, et al. A single-center surgical experience of 122 patients with single and multiple hepatocellular adenomas. Gastroenterology 2009;137(5):1698–705.

107. Ribeiro A, Burgart LJ, Nagorney DM, et al. Management of liver adenomatosis: results with a conservative surgical approach. Liver Transpl Surg 1998;4(5): 388–98.

108. Koffron A, Geller D, Gamblin TC, et al. Laparoscopic liver surgery: shifting the management of liver tumors. Hepatology 2006;44(6):1694–700.

109. Gaines PA, Sampson MA. The prevalence and characterization of simple hepatic cysts by ultrasound examination. Br J Radiol 1989;62(736):335–7.

110. Chauveau D, Fakhouri F, Grunfeld JP. Liver involvement in autosomal-dominant polycystic kidney disease: therapeutic dilemma. J Am Soc Nephrol 2000;11(9): 1767–75.

111. Pinto MM, Kaye AD. Fine needle aspiration of cystic liver lesions. Cytologic examination and carcinoembryonic antigen assay of cyst contents. Acta Cytol 1989;33(6):852–6.

112. Gharbi HA, Hassine W, Abdesselem K. [Abdominal hydatidosis in echography. Reflections and characteristic aspects (Echinococcus granulosus)]. Ann Radiol (Paris) 1985;28(1):31–4 [in French].

113. Charny CK, Jarnagin WR, Schwartz LH, et al. Management of 155 patients with benign liver tumours. Br J Surg 2001;88(6):808–13.

114. Shimizu S, Takayama T, Kosuge T, et al. Benign tumors of the liver resected because of a diagnosis of malignancy. Surg Gynecol Obstet 1992;174(5): 403–7.

115. Mahfouz AE, Hamm B, Wolf KJ. Peripheral washout: a sign of malignancy on dynamic gadolinium-enhanced MR images of focal liver lesions. Radiology 1994;190(1):49–52.
116. Danet IM, Semelka RC, Leonardou P, et al. Spectrum of MRI appearances of untreated metastases of the liver. AJR Am J Roentgenol 2003;181(3):809–17.
117. Liu CL, Fan ST, Lo CM, et al. Hepatic resection for incidentaloma. J Gastrointest Surg 2004;8(7):785–93.
118. Bruix J, Sherman M. Practice Guidelines Committee AAftSoLD. Management of hepatocellular carcinoma. Hepatology 2005;42(5):1208–36.

Management of Benign Hepatic Tumors

Joseph F. Buell, MD[a],*, Hadrien Tranchart, MD[b],
Robert Cannon, MD[a], Ibrahim Dagher, MD[b]

KEYWORDS

- Benign • Liver tumor • Adenoma • Hemangioma
- Focal nodular hyperplasia

Traditionally the management of benign hepatic tumors has been conservative. This conservative approach to benign tumors can be attributed to the morbidity and mortality rates associated with surgery experienced in the late 1970s and early 1980s.[1–4] However, the last two decades have seen a plethora of new and more sensitive imaging modalities used in patients not previously imaged. With this increased utilization of diagnostic imaging studies and improvement in their resolution, there has been a dramatic rise in the detection of liver lesions. Multiple population studies have estimated that up to 20% of the population will have a benign tumor of the liver at autopsy.[5–7] Currently in the United States, approximately 250,000 patients are diagnosed with either a primary or metastatic tumor of the liver each year. Dramatic rises in hepatitis C and nonalcoholic steatosis have led to a rise in cirrhosis with an associated risk for hepatocellular cancer (HCC). These patients result in another diagnostic dilemma of HCC versus benign lesion.[8–11] These facts in conjunction with an improved imaging resolution have increased the number of evaluable patients. CT and MRI scanning have improved from centimeters to millimeters. Despite accuracy levels of 88% to 94%, this still leaves a significant proportion of patients with nondiagnostic imaging studies.[10–13]

Currently, there is a controversy with the choice of observation versus resection for incidental hepatic lesions. Aside from the challenge of incidental lesions, surgical doctrine for the management of benign tumors has been dogmatic: (1) symptomatic lesions or (2) asymptomatic adenomas greater than 5 cm.[14,15] These recommendations were based on an experiential doctrine that was evolved from decades of open hepatic

a Department of Surgery, Tulane Abdominal Transplant Institute, Tulane University, New Orleans, LA 70112, USA
b Department of General Surgery, Paris-Sud School of Medicine, Antoine Beclere Hospital, Clamart, France
* Corresponding author.
E-mail address: jbuell1@tulane.edu

Surg Clin N Am 90 (2010) 719–735
doi:10.1016/j.suc.2010.04.006
0039-6109/10/$ – see front matter © 2010 Elsevier Inc. All rights reserved.

resection, and reflect the low percentage of complications or observed incidence of malignant degeneration and the morbidity and mortality associated with open hepatic resections. Recent advances in laparoscopic hepatic resection, imaging techniques, and histological analysis may further impact the evolution of surgical dogma for the management of benign hepatic tumors.[16–20]

EVALUATION OF UNDIAGNOSED HEPATIC MASSES

The majority of hepatic masses are diagnosed incidentally during some form of radiologic evaluation. Benign tumors of the liver often lead to a diagnostic challenge, because many lesions have overlapping radiographic features. Routine laboratories, serologic evaluation of hepatitis, and tumor markers are often reliable for the diagnosis of benign hepatic tumors. Diagnosis of benign hepatic tumors is then left to a broad spectrum of diagnostic studies.

Ultrasound

Ultrasound is clearly the most simple and inexpensive modality to evaluate new hepatic lesions, it can easily determine a solid from cystic lesion but lacks the sensitivity to diagnose the type of solid mass. Benign tumors of the liver are solid and present as hypoechoic, isoechoic, or even hyperechoic.[21–23] Further diagnosis of a new hepatic lesion often requires additional imaging studies. Ultrasound has also been used to screen patients for the development of primary or metastatic disease in at-risk patients. Recently published hepatology guidelines advocate the screening of patients with chronic hepatitis B and C to undergo biyearly liver ultrasounds.[24–26] These recommendations reflect the simplicity, safety, and minimal expense of ultrasound. CT requires exposure to medical radiation with multiple exposures carrying an inherent risk for malignancy. Unfortunately, despite the simplicity of ultrasonography it does have limited sensitivity. This limitation most commonly arises from alterations in the background liver, including steatosis, fibrosis, and cirrhosis.

In early 2000, several contrast agents were developed to increase the sensitivity of ultrasound for the screening of at-risk livers for new hepatic lesions.[27–31] With these early agents, contrast enhanced ultrasound (CEUS) was felt to be complimentary rather than equivalent to other imaging modalities, such as triphasic CT or MRI. Recently, a second generation of CEUS agents has been described.[29–31] Improved imaging characteristics have been identified, particularly those of peri-tumor vasculature. These new agents, in combination with pulse inversion color flow Doppler ultrasound, appear to be comparable to standard advanced imaging technology. In a 1290-subject prospective trial, tumor differentiation was concordant with CEUS in 90 cases and discordant in 19 cases. In this trial, contrast-enhanced ultrasound compared with contrast-enhanced spiral CT demonstrated a sensitivity of 94.0/90.7%; a specificity of 83.0/81.5%, with a positive predictive value of 91.6/91.5% and a negative predictive value of 87.5/80.0%; and accuracy of 90.3/87.8%.[28] CEUS can be employed before CT is performed for the differentiation of liver tumors, because radiation exposure and invasive biopsies can be avoided in veritable numbers of cases.

Triphasic CT

CT has been widely used since the 1980s to evaluate everything from abdominal pain to liver masses. The majority of benign hepatic tumors now presenting for evaluation are discovered incidentally or during the evaluation of vague pain. Multiple generations of CT have been developed. The most diagnostic CT examination for hepatic tumors is performed using a multidetector helical scanner.[32–35] The examination is performed with intravenous iodinated contrast material injected into patients with three distinct scanning intervals commonly described as a triple-phase CT scan. The three components to the triple phase are: (1) early phase arterial dominant phase, (2) portal venous enhancement phase, and a (3) delayed hepatic phase. Evaluation of hepatic lesions in the context of an abnormal hepatic background, including steatosis, fibrosis, or cirrhosis, can be challenging. Imaging in a cirrhotic liver is significantly more challenging demonstrated by several prospective. Liver transplant recipients undergoing abdominal CT scan at least 1 month prior to liver explantation identified only 68% to 75% of lesions detected on explant specimens.[34,35]

MRI

MRI has become an important diagnostic technique in the detection of focal liver lesions. The large variations in tissue characteristics, such as relaxation times and proton density in liver tumors, necessitate the use of multiple pulse sequences to maximize lesion detection. For the detection of specific histologies, several ratios provide potential diagnostic criteria. These diagnostic criteria include elevated contrast-to-noise ratios, arterial-to-portal enhancement, and lesion-to-liver signal-intensity ratios. Despite the potentially diagnostic insights of these ratios, the combination of T1- and T2-weighted spin-echo and T2-weighted phase-contrast images have the advantage of distinguishing benign from malignant tumors.[36–40] Gadolinium is the standard material used for contrast-enhanced MRI, whereas ferumoxide, a second contrast agent, can be utilized in a double-contrast MR scan with a higher sensitivity for detection of dysplastic nodules and HCC greater than 1 cm.[39,40]

Sulfur Colloid Scan

Technetium 99 is utilized in the Sulfur Colloid scan. The contrast agent is rapidly taken up in the liver, spleen, and bone marrow by Kupffer cells of the liver. All hepatic tumors are cold except for focal nodular hyperplasia.[41]

Percutaneous Biopsy

In the instance where diagnostic imaging fails to elucidate a particular hepatic mass, tumor sampling may be considered. However, percutaneous biopsy of hepatic tumors continues to be controversial. Modern imaging has been estimated to be 90% to 98% diagnostic.[42–44] Percutaneous biopsy carries with it several technical complications, including pneumothorax, hemorrhage, and biopsy tract tumor seeding, even if those complications remain rare.[42–44]

SYMPTOMATOLOGY FROM LIVER MASSES

The liver is innervated by the vagus nerve and is surrounded by a visceral capsule known as the Glisson capsule. Masses arising in the liver can produce pain or discomfort through capsular distention or external compression of the diaphragm or stomach. The site of abdominal pain is variable, being reported as shoulder pain, back pain, right upper quadrant pain, nausea, or early satiety. Hepatic tumors can also lead to intrinsic compression of the biliary tree and jaundice. Other rare complications of benign tumor include malignant degeneration, Kasabach-Merritt syndrome, and spontaneous rupture. Malignant degeneration has been described in hepatocellular adenomas larger than 5 cm in diameter. Kasabach-Merritt syndrome can be seen in association with large hemangiomas, resulting in disseminated intravascular coagulation and thrombocytopenia. Bleeding or rupture can lead to acute pain or even peritonitis.

Large hemangiomas are prone to outgrow their blood supply and thrombose. Spontaneous hemorrhage and rupture has been described with hepatocellular adenomas and focal nodular hyperplasia. Hemorrhage can occur after histologic sampling, which can sometimes be conservatively managed. Spontaneous rupture is best served with emergent resection.

TUMOR TYPES
Hemangiomas

Hemangioma is the most common benign lesion of the liver, with an estimated prevalence of 5% to 20%.[45] Hemangiomas are frequently encountered in patients between the third and fifth decades of life with a female preponderance (sex ratio 6:1).[46] Multiple hemangiomas account for 10% of these patients.[47] Few hemangiomas are symptomatic, however when they are large (>4 cm); abdominal discomfort or pain caused by capsular stretch, rupture spontaneously or traumatically was reported, consumptive coagulopathy with low platelet count and hypofibrinogenaemia (Kasabach-Merritt syndrome). Hemangiomas have no malignant potential.

Imaging

The usual ultrasonographic appearance is hyperechoic and sharply marginated mass. Color Doppler shows filling vessels in the periphery of the lesion. The sensitivity of ultrasound ranges from 60% to 70% and specificity from 60% to 90%.[47] At CT scan, hemangiomas are seen as a well-circumscribed, hypodense mass with lobular margins, with a characteristic peripheral nodular enhancement following intravenous injection of contrast that progresses towards the center of the lesion (**Fig. 1**). Large hemangiomas may show fibrotic scars. The overall sensitivity of dynamic CT scans ranges from 75% to 85% and specificity from 75% to 100%.[47] At MRI, hemangiomas are hypointense on T1-weighted images and hyperintense on T2-weighted images.[48,49] Peripheral, nodular enhancement progressing centripetally to uniform

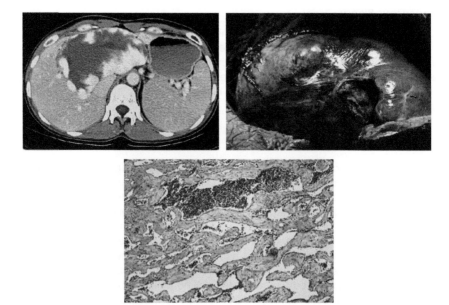

Fig. 1. Liver hemangioma.

filling is seen in typical hemangiomas. Accuracy of MRI has been reported to be the highest of all imaging modalities with a sensitivity up to 95%[50,51] and specificity up to 100%. Small lesions can show immediate and complete gadolinium enhancement.

Focal Nodular Hyperplasia

Focal nodular hyperplasia (FNH) has a reported frequency of 3% in adults.[52] It is typically discovered incidentally in women during their reproductive years (female/male ratios up to 8:1).[49] There are different theories regarding the pathogenesis of FNH: a congenital vascular malformation as telangiectasia and arteriovenous malformations, a vascular injury as the underlying mechanism for a hyperplastic response of liver parenchyma, or a proliferative lesion with a clonal nature.[53–55] FNH is asymptomatic in approximately 80% of cases with rare predisposition to hemorrhage and rupture and no incidence of malignant transformation.[55] Nevertheless, large lesions may be responsible for abdominal complaints.

Imaging

On ultrasound examination, FNH appears as a well-demarcated, homogeneous, isoechoic mass relative to the liver parenchyma with a hyperechoic central scar.[56] The sensitivity of ultrasound for FNH is low.[54] The evaluation in contrast-enhanced sonography of early arterial phase imaging contributes most to the differentiation of FNH and adenoma by showing the arterial phase filling direction and arterial morphology.[57] On CT scan, there is a transient, intense hyperdensity of the lesion on the arterial phase. The central scar becomes hyper dense on delayed imaging (**Fig. 2**). On MRI, FNH is isointense to mildly hypointense on T1-weighted images and is isointense to mildly hyperintense on T2-weighted images. The lesion shows homogeneous-intense arterial phase enhancement and isointensity on the venous and delayed-phase images. The scar characteristics and lack of capsule enhancement help to distinguish FNH from other arterial-phase enhancing tumors, such as HCC, adenoma, and fibrolamellar HCC. On T2-weighted images with iron particles, FNH shows decreased signal. MRI with superparamagnetic iron-oxide uptake with improved conspicuity of the central scar and septa facilitates comprehensive evaluation of FNH.[58] Accurate differentiation of FNH from hepatic adenoma is achievable on delayed T1-weighted gradient-echo sequences images after administration of gadobenate dimeglumine. The sensitivity and specificity of FNH from adenoma reach 97% and 100%, respectively.[59]

Hepatocellular Adenoma

Hepatocellular adenoma is an uncommon benign lesion of the liver that occurs more frequently in women in their third and fourth decades. The female/male ratio is up to 11:1.[45] Hepatic adenoma has been strongly associated with the use of oral contraception.[60,61] This incidence, however, has fallen since the introduction of pills containing smaller amounts of estrogens.[62] In men, they may be associated with the use of anabolic steroids.[63] Hepatic adenomas may be single or multiple, and they may occasionally reach a size larger than 20 cm, thus the clinical presentation varies widely. Pain in the right upper quadrant or epigastric region is common, occurring in 25% to 50% of patients. Especially large hepatocellular adenomas (>5 cm) have the potential to rupture and bleed spontaneously.[64] Spontaneous rupture occurs more often in men, especially steroid users.[65] Adenomas are noncancerous lesions, however, they can rarely become malignant. In a recent series an increased risk for complicated disease was reported in subjects with telangiectasia, adenomas greater than 5 cm, and men.[64]

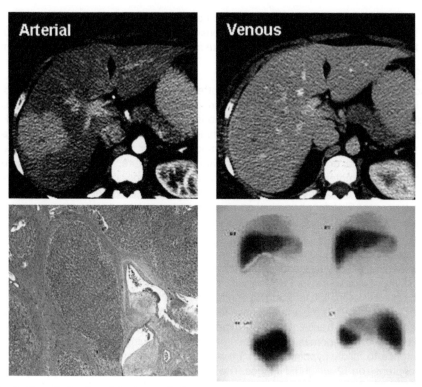

Fig. 2. Hepatic focal nodular hyperplasia.

Imaging

The ultrasonographic appearance of hepatocellular adenomas may be hypo-, iso-, or hyperechoic. Hepatic adenomas lack predictable diagnostic features on ultrasonography, which has a sensitivity of about 30%.[66] On CT scan, adenomas are seen typically as a discrete, hypodense lesion that shows arterial-phase enhancement and may become iso-attenuating on the delayed images.[67] Hepatic adenomas may show intralesional hypo or hyperdensities, depending on the presence or absence of necrosis or hemorrhage (**Fig. 3**). On MRI, adenomas are hypointense to hyperintense on T1-weighted images. On T2-weighted images the lesions are isointense to slightly hyperintense. Gadolinium enhancement is maximal during the arterial phase with rapid fading in the venous phase. A characteristic feature is that of decreased signal intensity on out-of-phase T1-weighted (or fat-suppressed) images because of their fat content.[48]

Adenomatosis

Liver adenomatosis is a rare clinical entity where arbitrarily greater than 10 adenomas are identified in a patient's liver without the background of glycogen storage disease. Patients with adenomatosis are often asymptomatic. Often these patients will present with a mixture of adenomas and focal nodular hyperplasias (**Fig. 4**), which has led some investigators to postulate that the central disturbance in hepatic adenomatosis is an abnormal hepatic vasculature that leads to hyperplasia and weakened vessel walls. These patients, like adenoma patients, are at risk for spontaneous hemorrhage

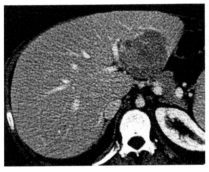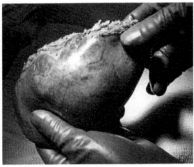

Fig. 3. Hepatic adenoma.

and malignant degeneration. Observed proliferation of hepatocytes and sinusoids, in combination with weakened connective tissue, possibly predispose these lesions to hemorrhage. Tumor diameter appears to be correlated with the occurrence of malignant degeneration, hence resection of dominant lesions has been advocated.

OTHER HYPERVASCULAR LESIONS
Regenerative Nodules

Nodular regenerative hyperplasia (NRH) is defined as multiple regenerative lesions which involve most of the liver and occur in the absence of fibrous septa. NRH is associated with a disturbance of hepatic blood flow leading to a nodular regeneration of hepatocytes. These nodules may compress the sinusoids, resulting in portal hypertension. In contrast to the regenerative nodules of cirrhosis, there is no surrounding fibrosis. The diagnosis requires liver biopsy. Radiologically, multiple nodules or apparently normal liver are visible. They are often hypodense on CT without significant enhancement. Treatment of NRH is usually focused on eliminating causative drugs and managing portal hypertension, although some patients with NRH have been treated with liver transplantation.[68,69] Large regenerative nodules (LRN) measuring between 5 mm and 5 cm in diameter have been reported with cirrhosis, certain forms of congenital heart disease, and with Budd-Chiari syndrome.[70–74] LRN do not require treatment, therapy is directed at the underlying liver disease. However, LRN have the potential to be misdiagnosed as hepatocellular carcinoma on imaging, because they appear as hypervascular masses within a chronically diseased liver.

Angiomyolipoma

Angiomyolipoma of the liver is a rare, benign mesenchymal tumor.[75] Grossly, angiomyolipomas are circumscribed, soft masses. Their histologic composition, which is

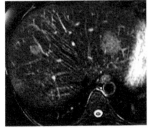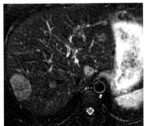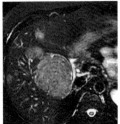

Fig. 4. Hepatic adenomatosis.

characterized by an admixture of mature fat cells, blood vessels and smooth muscle cells, largely determines their radiological appearance. Ultrasonographic examination of the lesion usually shows a hyperechoic mass.[76] On CT scan the lesion commonly appears as a well-defined, heterogeneous, hypoattenuating mass. A marked early and prolonged enhancement is usually seen after contrast.[76,77] On MRI, angiomyolipomas often show high signal intensity on T1- and T2-weighted images, and low signal intensity on fat-suppressed images, reflecting their high fat content.[48] Only three cases of malignant counterparts of this tumor have been reported, therefore a conservative approach is sufficient if the diagnosis of angiomyolipoma is established.[78–80]

Inflammatory Pseudotumor

Inflammatory pseudotumors are rare, benign lesions of unknown origin, but may be difficult to differentiate from malignant lesions. Recent studies have suggested a genetic basis, although precise etiology remains unknown.[81] The most common presentation of liver pseudotumors is of an incidental mass mimicking a malignancy, and the main pathological feature is the presence of myofibroblastic spindle cells without cellular atypia. They can be classified into two types: fibrohistiocytic and lymphoplasmacytic. CT scan shows a liver mass occasionally mimicking hepatocellular carcinoma or abscess.[82] Contrast-enhanced ultrasound with microbubbles and MRI scanning with the use of mangafodipir trisodium can be helpful as scintigraphy with Tc-99 m or Ga-67.[83–86] Management of this lesion is controversial. There is a possibility of recurrence or metastases of these lesions and a malignant conversion was reported.[87–89] Investigations to exclude malignancy should be undertaken, but if doubt remains, resection of the lesion should be considered.

SPECIAL CONSIDERATIONS WITH BENIGN LIVER TUMORS
Oral Contraceptives

The liver is morphologically and biochemically altered by sex hormones, including estrogens and androgenic steroids. In vitro and in vivo data indicate estrogens stimulate hepatocyte proliferation; whereas antiestrogens, such as tamoxifen, inhibit hepatocyte proliferation. In the case of androgens, patients with HCC have been shown to have significant upregulation of androgen receptors in particular testosterone. Extrinsic estrogens are most commonly administered in the form of oral birth control, whereas androgen exposure occurs in the form of anabolic steroids. No clear relationship between hemangiomas and sex hormones has been identified. Focal nodular hyperplasia occurs more commonly in young adult females with an 8:1 ratio to adult males.[90–94] An initial study by Scalori and colleagues[94] from Italy indicated there was a clear trend between oral contraception usage and the incidence of focal nodular hyperplasia. However, this data was controverted by a study by Mathieu and colleagues[95] who examined five separate forms of oral contraceptives varying from high-dose estrogens to pure progesterone therapy. This study found no correlation between extrinsic estrogens and focal nodular hyperplasia. A confounding variable to this question has subsequently been corrected with the reclassification of atypical focal nodular hyperplasia. In the last few years atypical FNH, or telangiectatic FNH, has been reclassified as an adenoma based on pathology and biologic behavior.

Hepatocellular adenomas have a clear association with the use of oral contraceptives.[93] The first suggestion of an association between oral contraceptives and adenomas was reported by Baum and colleagues[96] in 1973. Since this initial report, several series have confirmed this relationship. Current estimates have calculated that about 320 new cases of adenoma diagnosed in the United States can be attributed to oral contraceptive use. A case-controlled study by Heinemann and colleagues[63] identified an odds ratio of 1.25 for developing hepatic adenomas among oral contraceptive users. The incidence of hepatocellular adenomas has fallen since the introduction of low-dose estrogen oral contraception. Under the increasing estrogen exposure of pregnancy or during rapid growth, hepatic adenomas are at risk for hemorrhage or spontaneous rupture. The rate of rupture or simple hemorrhage has been reported to be between 25% and 42%, with the majority of these cases occurring in tumors greater than 5 cm in diameter.[92] Discontinuation of oral contraceptives can result in tumor shrinkage, but this is not universally observed. Ruptured or hemorrhagic adenomas should be resected. Several centers advocate a period of estrogen discontinuation prior to surgical resection, but operative intervention after hemorrhage or rupture is mandatory, which leaves management of asymptomatic adenomas to be considered. Two approaches to this problem have been adopted: (1) discontinuation of sex hormone therapy, caution over conception, and observation with or without biopsy for lesions less than 5 cm; or (2) resection of adenomas in females of child bearing age regardless of size.

Pregnancy and Hepatocellular Adenomas

Pregnancy causes significant physiologic and biochemical changes in a woman. Increased levels of estrogen and progesterone are observed, with an increased risk for gestational diabetes and fatty liver infiltrate. Pregnancy is associated with the physiologic change of hypervolemia. Aside from the physiologic changes secondary to hypervolemia, pregnant women can develop pregnancy-induced hypertension (PIH), previously known as preeclampsia or toxemia. An estimated 6% to 8% of first-time pregnancies are complicated by PIH. PIH is thought to be an immunologic event, where the body attempts to reject the fetus as foreign material.[97] The mother's kidneys are more prone to damage where there is significant vasoconstriction resulting in hypertension and protein spillage. The mother may exhibit proteinuria, hyperreflexia, visual disturbances, and ultimately seizure activity from brain edema. The women most at risk for PIH include first-time gestations, multiple fetuses, teenage mothers, women older than 40 years, familial history of PIH, or prior renal problems.

In 2% to 12% of pregnancies complicated by PIH, HEELP syndrome can also occur. HEELP syndrome is a constellation of symptoms, including hemolysis, elevated liver enzymes caused by hepatic tissue ischemia, and low platelets.[97–99] Secondarily, disseminated intravascular coagulation can develop leading to severe bleeding or hemorrhage. Placental abruption has also been described with this syndrome. Unfortunately, it has been the authors' experience to manage six women with adenomas discovered during pregnancy with four developing HEELP syndrome and ruptured adenomas. On occasion a pregnant woman may present with a new liver lesion during ultrasound examination. If hemorrhage or exponential growth is observed, surgical resection is safest for the fetus in the second trimester. As with the management of any patient with PIH or HEELP, expeditious delivery of a viable fetus will allow regression of the hypervolemic and exogenous estrogen state.

Malignant Degeneration of Adenomas

The most dire sequelae of hepatocellular adenomas is malignant degeneration into HCC.[100] Recent review of the literature identified the incidence of malignant degeneration varies from 5% to 11%, occurring almost exclusively in tumors greater than 5 cm in diameter, and often more than 10 cm in diameter.[101] Aside from hepatocellular adenomas, malignant degeneration can occur in the telangiectatic variant of focal nodular hyperplasia, recently reclassified as adenoma. This variant can most often be differentiated from typical focal nodular hyperplasia by the presence of glycogenated nuclei arising in nonalcoholic steatohepatitis. Identification of genetic mutations has become diagnostic for adenomas at risk for the development of malignant degeneration. The TCF1 gene mutation is rarely involved in cytologic atypia or malignant changes, whereas the β-catenin mutation is more prone to cytologic atypia and to the development of hepatocellular carcinoma (**Fig. 5**).[100]

It is well accepted that HCC can develop within a hepatic adenoma. Multiple series have documented the rate of malignant degeneration observed within adenomas. Micchelli and colleagues[100] performed a review of these series and determined the average incidence of malignancy with 165 adenomas was 9%. Improved imaging modalities have increased their diagnostic sensitivity, whereas tumor sampling of a HCC foci within an adenoma may be challenging. In addition, there was a 6% incidence of dysplastic lesions present in adenomas in this series. Dysplastic adenomas are considered a premalignant lesion. The literature has previously supported a 5 cm diameter for recommending resection of hepatic adenomas. However, Micchelli and colleagues reported that a 1-cm HCC arose in a 4-cm adenoma. Often small HCC are indolent in nature until they reach 2 cm, however, identification of a cancer within a 4-cm adenoma would suggest the 5 cm size may be arbitrary.

Iatrogenic and Traumatic Rupture of Hemangiomas

One of the most controversial areas of hepatic surgery has been the resection of hemangiomas. The lure of a laparoscopic procedure should not become an indication for resection of patients who are asymptomatic. With that clearly stated, several authors have advocated the resection of extensive hemangiomas in patients who are asymptomatic that perform dangerous tasks far from medical attention. This is only an opinion that has been advanced by other surgeons. However, the authors have had extensive experience with resection of hemangiomas after iatrogenic injury and blunt automobile trauma. Unfortunately, these cases are not managed at all hepatobiliary centers because of the lack of a level one trauma facility. One must take this experience with patients who are exsanguinated, coagulaopathic, and hypothermic to heart. Clinical experience with a trauma center sub population may in fact lend credence to a more aggresive philosophy to resect large hemangiomas in at-risk patients.

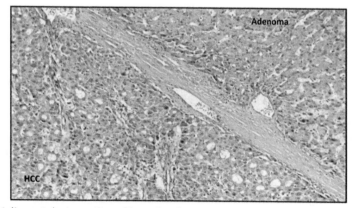

Fig. 5. Malignant degeneration of hepatic adenoma to HCC.

INTERNATIONAL APPROACHES TO THE MANAGEMENT OF BENIGN TUMORS

The traditional approach to the management of benign hepatic tumors of the liver has been established over decades of experience with open hepatic resection. This surgical dictum should be considered in the setting of open resections that carry a higher incidence of complications and mortality. Today, modern hepatic surgery carries a mortality rate of less than 1%, whereas the long-term impact of laparoscopic hepatic surgery has not been observed. Symptomatic, benign, hepatic tumors are an indication for resection. However, the degree of symptomatology indicating resection is unclear. To better evaluate this question, we should examine the current recommendations for benign hepatic tumors by individual histologies. Symptomatic hemangiomas often tend to be large, varying from 5 to 20 cm in diameter. These large lesions can cause significant pain, chronic vague pain, or stomach compression early satiety. Another indication for resection has been a consumptive coagulopathy, or Kasabach-Merritt syndrome. These lesions are often of significant size, greater than 15 cm. Resection of focal nodular hyperplasia is only indicated for significant symptoms. Hepatocellular adenoma is a lesion with multiple indications for resection aside from significant symptoms, which include risk for hemorrhage and malignant degeneration. Multiple studies have demonstrated increasing size correlates with the incidence of these complications. Traditional surgical dictum has reserved 5 cm as an indication for surgical management.

IMPACT OF LAPAROSCOPIC LIVER SURGERY

In recent years, laparoscopic hepatic surgery has become a principle mode of resection for benign hepatic tumors at large hepatobiliary centers.[17–21] Laparoscopic liver resection has been used equivalently in all hepatic tumors, including hemangiomas, focal nodular hyperplasia, and hepatocellular adenomas. Laparoscopic liver resection has also been employed in patients who are cirrhotic with undiagnosed hyper vascular masses for the exclusion of HCC, which has led to a higher incidence of resected hamartomas, regenerative nodules, and small hemangiomas. There is a known higher incidence of hemangiomas present in patients with end stage liver failure from hepatitis C. Similar to the laparoscopic cholecystectomy, laparoscopic hepatic resection has provided an alternative to a traditional open resection with all of its inherent risk and pain. Dissemination of this procedure has increased referral of patients with symptomatic tumors that were previously not referred for open hepatic resection.

Often the introduction of new technology leads to the use of new technology. Since the inception of laparoscopic cholecystectomy, minimally invasive techniques have been applied to numerous other surgical procedures. This innovation has also seen a rise in the referral of patients for splenectomy, Nissen fundoplication, and even Heller myotomies. This increase is often not related to the rise in newly diagnosed patients but rather the perception of a surgical procedure by referring physicians, which is a slippery slope that must be avoided. Most current series of laparoscopic resection are highly selected and few mortalities have been reported. However, hepatic resection still carries significant morbidity, and yes, mortality despite the use of laparoscopy. To date, more than 3000 laparoscopic resections have been performed worldwide. The laparoscopic approach to benign tumors seems optimal because the efficacy of laparoscopic resection for cancer is still debated by some. Laparoscopic resection may increase the referral of patients for surgery, but surgeons must adhere to guidelines for the necessity of surgery.

SUMMARY

Advances in imaging techniques will dramatically decrease the number of undiagnosed tumors. New molecular techniques should allow the identification of pathologic factors that are predictive of complicated forms. Surgery should be limited to symptomatic benign tumors or those who have a risk for complication (hemorrhage, rupture, or degeneration). When surgery is indicated, patients with benign disease are the best candidates for laparoscopy.

REFERENCES

1. Foster JH. Survival after liver resection for cancer. Cancer 1970;26(3):493–502.
2. Shiu MH, Fortner JG. Current management of hepatic tumors. Surg Gynecol Obstet 1975;140(5):781–8.
3. Fortner JG, Shiu MH, Kinne DW, et al. Major hepatic resection using vascular isolation and hypothermic perfusion. Ann Surg 1974;180(4):644–52.
4. Almersjö O, Bengmark S, Hafström L. Liver resection for cancer. Acta Chir Scand 1976;142(2):139–44.
5. Schiff L. Hepatic neoplasia: selected clinical aspects. Semin Roentgenol 1983; 18(2):71–4.
6. Ishak KG, Rabin L. Benign tumors of the liver. Med Clin North Am 1975;59(4): 995–1013.
7. Takagi H. Diagnosis and management of cavernous hemangioma of the liver. Semin Surg Oncol 1985;1(1):12–22.
8. Lencioni R, Crocetti L, Della Pina MC, et al. Guidelines for imaging focal lesions in liver cirrhosis. Expert Rev Gastroenterol Hepatol 2008;2(5):697–703.
9. Yu JS, Chung JJ, Kim JH, et al. Large (>or=2 cm) non-hypervascular nodules depicted on MRI in the cirrhotic liver: fate and implications. Clin Radiol 2008; 63(10):1121–30.
10. Sun HY, Lee JM, Shin CI, et al. Gadoxetic acid-enhanced magnetic resonance imaging for differentiating small hepatocellular carcinomas (<or=2 cm in diameter) from arterial enhancing pseudolesions: special emphasis on hepatobiliary phase imaging. Invest Radiol 2010;45(2):96–103.
11. Macarini L, Milillo P, Cascavilla A, et al. MR characterisation of dysplastic nodules and hepatocarcinoma in the cirrhotic liver with hepatospecific superparamagnetic contrast agents: pathological correlation in explanted livers. Radiol Med 2009;114(8):1267–82.
12. Yu JS, Chung JJ, Kim JH, et al. Hypervascular focus in the nonhypervascular nodule ("nodule-in-nodule") on dynamic computed tomography: imaging evidence of aggressive progression in hepatocellular carcinoma. J Comput Assist Tomogr 2009;33(1):131–5.
13. Vandecaveye V, De Keyzer F, Verslype C, et al. Diffusion-weighted MRI provides additional value to conventional dynamic contrast-enhanced MRI for detection of hepatocellular carcinoma. Eur Radiol 2009;19(10):2456–66.
14. Mentha G, Rubbia-Brandt L, Howarth N, et al. Management of focal nodular hyperplasia and hepatocellular adenoma. Swiss Surg 1999;5(3):122–5.
15. De Carlis L, Pirotta V, Rondinara GF, et al. Hepatic adenoma and focal nodular hyperplasia: diagnosis and criteria for treatment. Liver Transpl Surg 1997;3(2):160–5.
16. Choi BY, Nguyen MH. The diagnosis and management of benign hepatic tumors. J Clin Gastroenterol 2005;39(5):401–12.

17. Ardito F, Tayar C, Laurent A, et al. Laparoscopic liver resection for benign disease. Arch Surg 2007;142(12):1188–93.
18. Dagher I, Di Giuro G, Lainas P, et al. Laparoscopic right hepatectomy with selective vascular exclusion. J Gastrointest Surg 2009;13(1):148–9.
19. Buell JF, Cherqui D, Geller DA, et al. World Consensus Conference on Laparoscopic Surgery. The international position on laparoscopic liver surgery: the Louisville Statement, 2008. Ann Surg 2009;250(5):825–30.
20. Vibert E, Kouider A, Gayet B. Laparoscopic anatomic liver resection. HPB (Oxford) 2004;6(4):222–9.
21. Gigot JF, Hubert C, Banice R, et al. Laparoscopic management of benign liver diseases: where are we? HPB (Oxford) 2004;6(4):197–212.
22. Assy N, Nasser G, Djibre A, et al. Characteristics of common solid liver lesions and recommendations for diagnostic workup. World J Gastroenterol 2009; 15(26):3217–27.
23. Bolondi L, Gaiani S, Celli N, et al. Characterization of small nodules in cirrhosis by assessment of vascularity: the problem of hypovascular hepatocellular carcinoma. Hepatology 2005;42(1):27–34.
24. Jang HJ, Yu H, Kim TK. Imaging of focal liver lesions. Semin Roentgenol 2009; 44(4):266–82.
25. Noda I, Kitamoto M, Nakahara H, et al. Regular surveillance by imaging for early detection and better prognosis of hepatocellular carcinoma in patients infected with hepatitis C virus. J Gastroenterol 2010;45(1):105–12.
26. Llovet JM, Bruix J. Novel advancements in the management of hepatocellular carcinoma in 2008. J Hepatol 2008;48(Suppl 1):S20–37.
27. Zuber-Jerger I, Schacherer D, Woenckhaus M, et al. Contrast-enhanced ultrasound in diagnosing liver malignancy. Clin Hemorheol Microcirc 2009;43(1): 109–18.
28. Seitz K, Strobel D, Bernatik T, et al. Contrast-Enhanced Ultrasound (CEUS) for the characterization of focal liver lesions - prospective comparison in clinical practice: CEUS vs. CT (DEGUM multicenter trial). Ultraschall Med 2009;30(4): 383–9.
29. Lencioni R, Piscaglia F, Bolondi L. Contrast-enhanced ultrasound in the diagnosis of hepatocellular carcinoma. J Hepatol 2008;48(5):848–57.
30. Jang HJ, Yu H, Kim TK. Contrast-enhanced ultrasound in the detection and characterization of liver tumors. Cancer Imaging 2009;6(9):96–103.
31. Goyal N, Jain N, Rachapalli V, et al. Non-invasive evaluation of liver cirrhosis using ultrasound. Clin Radiol 2009;64(11):1056–66.
32. Yoon SH, Lee JM, So YH, et al. Multiphasic MDCT enhancement pattern of hepatocellular carcinoma smaller than 3 cm in diameter: tumor size and cellular differentiation. AJR Am J Roentgenol 2009;193(6):W482–9.
33. Zacherl J, Pokieser P, Wrba F, et al. Accuracy of multiphasic helical computed tomography and intraoperative sonography in patients undergoing orthotopic liver transplantation for hepatoma: what is the truth? Ann Surg 2002;235(4):528–32.
34. Peterson MS, Baron RL, Marsh JW Jr, et al. Pretransplantation surveillance for possible hepatocellular carcinoma in patients with cirrhosis: epidemiology and CT-based tumor detection rate in 430 cases with surgical pathologic correlation. Radiology 2000;217(3):743–9.
35. Catalano O, Cusati B, Sandomenico F, et al. Multiple-phase spiral computerized tomography of small hepatocellular carcinoma: technique optimization and diagnostic yield. Radiol Med 1999;98(1–2):53–64.

36. Yoo HJ, Lee JM, Lee JY, et al. Additional value of SPIO-enhanced MR imaging for the noninvasive imaging diagnosis of hepatocellular carcinoma in cirrhotic liver. Invest Radiol 2009.

37. Burrel M, Llovet JM, Ayuso C, et al. Barcelona Clínic Liver Cancer Group. MRI angiography is superior to helical CT for detection of HCC prior to liver transplantation: an explant correlation. Hepatology 2003;38(4):1034–42.

38. Catalano OA, Choy G, Zhu A, et al. Differentiation of malignant thrombus from bland thrombus of the portal vein in patients with hepatocellular carcinoma: application of diffusion-weighted MR imaging. Radiology 2010; 254(1):154–62.

39. Goshima S, Kanematsu M, Matsuo M, et al. Malignant hepatic tumor detection with ferumoxide-enhanced magnetic resonance imaging: is chemical-shift-selective fat suppression necessary for fast spin-echo sequence? J Magn Reson Imaging 2004;20(1):75–82.

40. Kato H, Kanematsu M, Kondo H, et al. Ferumoxide-enhanced MR imaging of hepatocellular carcinoma: correlation with histologic tumor grade and tumor vascularity. J Magn Reson Imaging 2004;19(1):76–81.

41. Huynh LT, Kim SY, Murphy TF. The typical appearance of focal nodular hyperplasia in triple-phase CT scan, hepatobiliary scan, and Tc-99m sulfur colloid scan with SPECT. Clin Nucl Med 2005;30(11):736–9.

42. Weigand K, Weigand K. Percutaneous liver biopsy: retrospective study over 15 years comparing 287 inpatients with 428 outpatients. J Gastroenterol Hepatol 2009;24(5):792–9.

43. Padia SA, Baker ME, Schaeffer CJ, et al. Safety and efficacy of sonographic-guided random real-time core needle biopsy of the liver. J Clin Ultrasound 2009;37(3):138–43.

44. Cook JA, Harrison SA. Same day endoscopy and percutaneous liver biopsy: safety and cost-effectiveness. Dig Dis Sci 2009;54(8):1753–7.

45. Reddy KR, Kligerman S, Levi J, et al. Benign and solid tumors of the liver: relationship to sex, age, size of tumors, and outcome. Am Surg 2001;67(2):173–8.

46. Mergo PJ, Ros PR. Benign lesions of the liver. Radiol Clin North Am 1998;36(2): 319–31.

47. Trotter JF, Everson GT. Benign focal lesions of the liver. Clin Liver Dis 2001;5(1): 17–42.

48. Motohara T, Semelka RC, Nagase L. MR imaging of benign hepatic tumors. Magn Reson Imaging Clin N Am 2002;10(1):1–14.

49. Mortele KJ, Ros PR. Benign liver neoplasms. Clin Liver Dis 2002;6(1):119–45.

50. Semelka RC, Martin DR, Balci C, et al. Focal liver lesions: comparison of dual-phase CT and multisequence multiplanar MR imaging including dynamic gadolinium enhancement. J Magn Reson Imaging 2001;13(3):397–401.

51. Namimoto T, Yamashita Y, Sumi S, et al. Focal liver masses: characterization with diffusion-weighted echo-planar MR imaging. Radiology 1997;204(3):739–44.

52. Pain JA, Gimson AE, Williams R, et al. Focal nodular hyperplasia of the liver: results of treatment and options in management. Gut 1991;32(5):524–7.

53. Sadowski DC, Lee SS, Wanless IR, et al. Progressive type of focal nodular hyperplasia characterized by multiple tumors and recurrence. Hepatology 1995;21(4):970–5.

54. Wanless IR, Mawdsley C, Adams R. On the pathogenesis of focal nodular hyperplasia of the liver. Hepatology 1985;5(6):1194–200.

55. Gaffey MJ, Iezzoni JC, Weiss LM. Clonal analysis of focal nodular hyperplasia of the liver. Am J Pathol 1996;148(4):1089–96.

56. Nguyen BN, Flejou JF, Terris B, et al. Focal nodular hyperplasia of the liver: a comprehensive pathologic study of 305 lesions and recognition of new histologic forms. Am J Surg Pathol 1999;23(12):1441–54.

57. Terkivatan T, de Wilt JH, de Man RA, et al. Indications and long-term outcome of treatment for benign hepatic tumors: a critical appraisal. Arch Surg 2001;136(9):1033–8.

58. Kim TK, Jang HJ, Burns PN, et al. Focal nodular hyperplasia and hepatic adenoma: differentiation with low-mechanical-index contrast-enhanced sonography. AJR Am J Roentgenol 2008;190(1):58–66.

59. Terkivatan T, van den Bos IC, Hussain SM, et al. Focal nodular hyperplasia: lesion characteristics on state-of-the-art MRI including dynamic gadolinium-enhanced and superparamagnetic iron-oxide-uptake sequences in a prospective study. J Magn Reson Imaging 2006;24(4):864–72.

60. Grazioli L, Morana G, Kirchin MA, et al. Accurate differentiation of focal nodular hyperplasia from hepatic adenoma at gadobenate dimeglumine-enhanced MR imaging: prospective study. Radiology 2005;236(1):166–77.

61. Edmondson HA, Henderson B, Benton B. Liver-cell adenomas associated with use of oral contraceptives. N Engl J Med 1976;294(9):470–2.

62. Rooks JB, Ory HW, Ishak KG, et al. Epidemiology of hepatocellular adenoma. The role of oral contraceptive use. JAMA 1979;242(7):644–8.

63. Heinemann LA, Weimann A, Gerken G, et al. Modern oral contraceptive use and benign liver tumors: the German benign liver tumor case-control study. Eur J Contracept Reprod Health Care 1998;3(4):194–200.

64. Bagia S, Hewitt PM, Morris DL. Anabolic steroid-induced hepatic adenomas with spontaneous haemorrhage in a bodybuilder. Aust N Z J Surg 2000;70(9):686–7.

65. Dokmak S, Paradis V, Vilgrain V, et al. A single-center surgical experience of 122 patients with single and multiple hepatocellular adenomas. Gastroenterology 2009;137(5):1698–705.

66. Di Stasi M, Caturelli E, De Sio I, et al. Natural history of focal nodular hyperplasia of the liver: an ultrasound study. J Clin Ultrasound 1996;24(7):345–50.

67. Terkivatan T, de Wilt JH, de Man RA, et al. Treatment of ruptured hepatocellular adenoma. Br J Surg 2001;88(2):207–9.

68. Ruppert-Kohlmayr AJ, Uggowitzer MM, Kugler C, et al. Focal nodular hyperplasia and hepatocellular adenoma of the liver: differentiation with multiphasic helical CT. AJR Am J Roentgenol 2001;176(6):1493–8.

69. Krasinskas A. The significance of nodular regenerative hyperplasia in the transplanted liver. Liver Transpl 2007;13(11):1496–7.

70. Krasinskas AM, Eghtesad B, Kamath PS, et al. Liver transplantation for severe intrahepatic noncirrhotic portal hypertension. Liver Transpl 2005;11(6):627–34 [discussion: 610–1].

71. Mathieu D, Vasile N, Menu Y, et al. Budd-Chiari syndrome: dynamic CT. Radiology 1987;165(2):409–13.

72. Miller WJ, Federle MP, Straub WH, et al. Budd-Chiari syndrome: imaging with pathologic correlation. Abdom Imaging 1993;18(4):329–35.

73. Grazioli L, Alberti D, Olivetti L, et al. Congenital absence of portal vein with nodular regenerative hyperplasia of the liver. Eur Radiol 2000;10(5):820–5.

74. Menon KV, Shah V, Kamath PS. The Budd-Chiari syndrome. N Engl J Med 2004;350(6):578–85.

75. Vilgrain V, Lewin M, Vons C, et al. Hepatic nodules in Budd-Chiari syndrome: imaging features. Radiology 1999;210(2):443–50.

76. Nonomura A, Mizukami Y, Kadoya M. Angiomyolipoma of the liver: a collective review. J Gastroenterol 1994;29(1):95–105.
77. Ahmadi T, Itai Y, Takahashi M, et al. Angiomyolipoma of the liver: significance of CT and MR dynamic study. Abdom Imaging 1998;23(5):520–6.
78. Sawai H, Manabe T, Yamanaka Y, et al. Angiomyolipoma of the liver: case report and collective review of cases diagnosed from fine needle aspiration biopsy specimens. J Hepatobiliary Pancreat Surg 1998;5(3):333–8.
79. Rouquie D, Eggenspieler P, Algayres JP, et al. [Malignant-like angiomyolipoma of the liver: report of one case and review of the literature]. Ann Chir 2006; 131(5):338–41 [in French].
80. Parfitt JR, Bella AJ, Izawa JI, et al. Malignant neoplasm of perivascular epithelioid cells of the liver. Arch Pathol Lab Med 2006;130(8):1219–22.
81. Dalle I, Sciot R, de Vos R, et al. Malignant angiomyolipoma of the liver: a hitherto unreported variant. Histopathology 2000;36(5):443–50.
82. Cessna MH, Zhou H, Sanger WG, et al. Expression of ALK1 and p80 in inflammatory myofibroblastic tumor and its mesenchymal mimics: a study of 135 cases. Mod Pathol 2002;15(9):931–8.
83. Caramella T, Novellas S, Fournol M, et al. [Imaging of inflammatory pseudotumors of the liver]. J Radiol 2007;88(6):882–8 [in French].
84. Liu GJ, Lu MD, Xie XY, et al. Real-time contrast-enhanced ultrasound imaging of infected focal liver lesions. J Ultrasound Med 2008;27(4):657–66.
85. Wang WP, Ding H, Qi Q, et al. Characterization of focal hepatic lesions with contrast-enhanced C-cube gray scale ultrasonography. World J Gastroenterol 2003;9(8):1667–74.
86. Materne R, Van Beers BE, Gigot JF, et al. Inflammatory pseudotumor of the liver: MRI with mangafodipir trisodium. J Comput Assist Tomogr 1998;22(1):82–4.
87. Horiuchi R, Uchida T, Kojima T, et al. Inflammatory pseudotumor of the liver. Clinicopathologic study and review of the literature. Cancer 1990;65(7):1583–90.
88. Hagenstad CT, Kilpatrick SE, Pettenati MJ, et al. Inflammatory myofibroblastic tumor with bone marrow involvement. A case report and review of the literature. Arch Pathol Lab Med 2003;127(7):865–7.
89. Zavaglia C, Barberis M, Gelosa F, et al. Inflammatory pseudotumour of the liver with malignant transformation. Report of two cases. Ital J Gastroenterol 1996; 28(3):152–9.
90. Giannitrapani L, Soresi M, La Spada E, et al. Sex hormones and risk of liver tumor. Ann N Y Acad Sci 2006;1089:228–36.
91. Dourakis SP, Tolis G. Sex hormone preparations and the liver. Eur J Contracept Reprod Health Care 1998;3(1):7–16.
92. Lindberg MC. Hepatobiliary complication of oral contraceptives. J Gen Intern Med 1992;7(2):199–209.
93. Nagasue N, Kohno H. Hepatocellular carcinoma and sex hormones. HPB Surg 1992;6(1):1–6.
94. Scalori A, Tayani A, Gallus S, et al. Oral contraceptives and the risk of focal nodular hyperplasia of the liver: a case control study. Am J Obstet Gynecol 2002;186(2):195–7.
95. Mathieu D, Kobeiter H, Maison P, et al. Oral contraceptive use and focal nodular hyperplasia of the liver. Gastroenterology 2000;118(3):560–4.
96. Baum JK, Bookstein JJ, Holtz F, et al. Possible association between benign hepatomas and oral contraceptives. Lancet 1973;2(7835):926–9.
97. Lee NM, Brady CW. Liver disease in pregnancy. World J Gastroenterol 2009; 15(8):897–906.

98. Haram K, Svendsen E, Abildgaard U. The HEELP syndrome: clinical issues and management. BMC Pregnancy Childbirth 2009;9:8.

99. Kulungowski AM, Kashuk JL, Moore EE, et al. HEELP syndrome: when is surgical help needed? Am J Surg 2009;198(6):916–20.

100. Micchelli ST, Vivekanandan P, Boitnott JK, et al. Malignant transformation of hepatic adenomas. Mod Pathol 2008;21(4):491–7.

101. van der Windt DJ, Kok NF, Hussain SM, et al. Case oriented approach to the management of hepatocellular adenoma. Br J Surg 2006;93(12):1495–502.

Hepatic Resection Nomenclature and Techniques

Scott A. Celinski, MD[a], T. Clark Gamblin, MD, MS[b],*

KEYWORDS

- Liver resection • Nomenclature
- Parenchymal transection • Technique

Liver surgery has evolved significantly in the past 100 years, from the rare trauma operation to routine major hepatectomies. This rapid expansion has been greatly reliant on the understanding of the internal biliary and vascular anatomy of the liver. It was not until 1952 that the first true anatomic hemihepatectomy with vascular control signaled the start of modern hepatic surgery. Early on, only 4 anatomic resections existed: left lateral sectionectomy, right and left hemihepatectomies, and right trisectionectomy. An additional 30 years passed before Starzl[1] published a report on left hepatic trisectionectomy, completing the armamentarium of major liver resections. Methods have been developed to improve the safety and ease of liver resections including new anesthetic techniques, methods of vascular control, and methods of transection. Modern high-resolution imaging allows careful preoperative planning and spares many unresectable patients from the morbidity of a nontherapeutic operation. As we move forward, it is vital that a unified language is used regarding liver anatomy and resection.

NOMENCLATURE OF ANATOMY AND RESECTION

One of the major advances in hepatic surgery has been the understanding of the internal segmental anatomy of the liver. With a thorough comprehension of the internal architecture of the liver, complex resections may be performed with greater safety with less insult to the liver than was possible in the past (**Fig. 1**).

An understanding of the segmental anatomy of the liver is also important for a consistent description of liver resections. In 1998 the International Hepato-Pancreato-Biliary Association (IHPBA) established a Terminology Committee of 8

[a] Division of Surgical Oncology, Baylor University Hospital, Dallas, TX, USA
[b] Division of Surgical Oncology, Medical College of Wisconsin, 9200 West Wisconsin Avenue, Suite 3510, Milwaukee, WI 53226, USA
* Corresponding author.
E-mail address: tcgamblin@mcw.edu

Surg Clin N Am 90 (2010) 737–748
doi:10.1016/j.suc.2010.04.007   **surgical.theclinics.com**

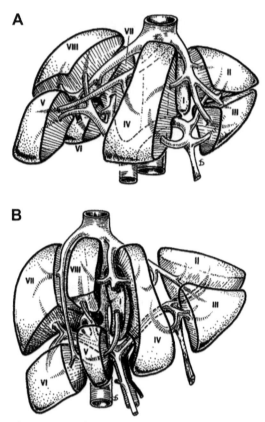

Fig. 1. The functional division of the liver and of the liver segments according to Couinaud's nomenclature. (*A*) As seen in the patient. (*B*) In the ex vivo position. (*From* Blumgart LH, editor. Surgery of the liver, biliary tract, and pancreas. 4th edition. Philadelphia: Saunders; 2006. p. 6; with permission.)

hepato-parcreato-biliary surgeons to standardize the terminology used for describing hepatic anatomy and liver resections. The resultant consensus was approved in 2000 at the IHPBA meeting in Brisbane, Australia, and is referred to as the Brisbane 2000 terminology. This terminology is useful for describing anatomy, as well as resections.[2,3]

Following the portal and biliary anatomy, the liver is divided into 9 segments. The definitions of these segments are the result of the cumulative anatomic work of Couinaud, Healey, and others.[4–10] There is some debate on whether the liver should be described as having 8 or 9 segments. The caudate lobe lies at the heart of the controversy. Traditionally referred to as segment 1, the caudate lobe has been divided into 2 segments: 1 and 9. Segment 1 refers to the Spiegel lobe, and segment 9 refers to the paracaval portion and caudate process.[11]

The liver anatomy is described in first-, second-, and third-order divisions. The third-order divisions, or segments (Sg), are referred to by Arabic numerals, not Roman numerals. Arabic numerals were chosen because many nonwestern countries do not use Roman numerals.

The first-order division divides the liver into the left and right hemiliver, or left and right liver. Th term lobe is not used because the division between the right and left hemiliver is not an externally apparent structure. The border, also referred to as a watershed, of the first-order division is referred to as the midplane of the liver and is defined by the plane between the inferior vena cava (IVC) and the gallbladder fossa. Cantlie line is a misnomer, because the division between the hemilivers is a three-dimensional space, and therefore technically a plane. The caudate lobe, also referred to as segment 1 is not included in the first-order division. The terminology for surgical resection at the first-order division is right or left hepatectomy or hemihepatectomy. To correctly classify the resection, whether or not segment 1 was included in the resection must be stipulated (**Fig. 2**).

The second-order division divides the liver into 4 sections based on the biliary and hepatic artery anatomy. The right liver is divided into the right anterior section (Sg 5,8) and the right posterior section (Sg 6,7). The left liver is divided into the left medial section (Sg 4) and the left lateral section (Sg 2,3). The terminology for resection is obtained by adding -ectomy to the anatomic term (ie, left lateral sectionectomy) (**Fig. 3**).

The Brisbane 2000 system also added an addendum for an alternate second-order division based on portal vein anatomy rather than biliary and arterial anatomy. The alternative second-order division uses the term sector rather than section. The right lobe is divided as in the addendum system, but given different names; segments 5 and 8 are referred to as the right anterior sector or the right paramedian sector, and segments 6 and 7 are referred to as the right posterior sector or right lateral sector. The left lobe has a different division in the addendum. Segments 3 and 4 are referred to as the left medial sector or the left paramedian sector and segment 2 is referred to as the left lateral sector or the left posterior sector.

The third-order division refers to the individual segments of the liver. The segments are referred to as segment 1 to segment 9. The traditional Couinaud classification contains only 8 segments and labels the entire caudate lobe as segment 1. However, the more recent description of the caudate divides the lobe into segment 1 (Spiegel lobe) and segment 9 (caudate process and paracaval portion).[4] The segments are divided by intersegmental planes that represent the borders or watersheds of the segments. Resection of a single segment is referred to as

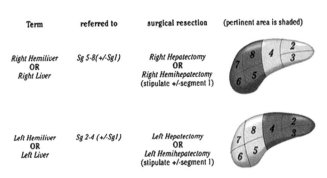

Term	referred to	surgical resection	(pertinent area is shaded)
Right Hemiliver OR Right Liver	Sg 5-8(+/-Sg1)	Right Hepatectomy OR Right Hemihepatectomy (stipulate +/-segment 1)	
Left Hemiliver OR Left Liver	Sg 2-4 (+/-Sg1)	Left Hepatectomy OR Left Hemihepatectomy (stipulate +/-segment 1)	

Border or watershed: The border or watershed of the first order division which separates the two hemilivers is a plane which intersects the gallbladder fossa and the fossa for the IVC and is called the midplane of the liver.

Fig. 2. First-order division. (*From* Strasberg SM. Nomenclature of hepatic anatomy and resections: a review of the Brisbane 2000 system. J Hepatobiliary Pancreat Surg 2005;12(5):354; with permission.)

Anatomical Term	Couinaud segments referred to	Term for surgical resection	Diagram (pertinent area is shaded)
Right Anterior Section	*Sg 5,8*	Add (-ectomy)to any of the anatomical terms as in *Right anterior sectionectomy*	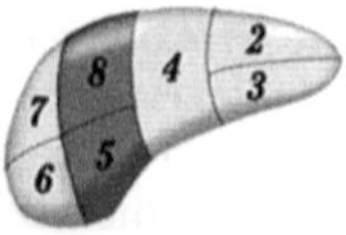
Right Posterior Section	*Sg 6,7*	*Right posterior sectionectomy*	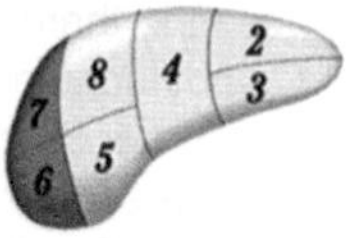
Left Medial Section	*Sg 4*	Left medial sectionectomy OR Resection segment 4 (also see Third order) OR Segmentectomy 4 (also see Third order)	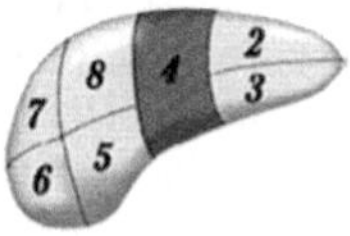
Left Lateral Section	*Sg 2,3*	Left lateral sectionectomy OR Bisegmentectomy 2,3 (also see Third order)	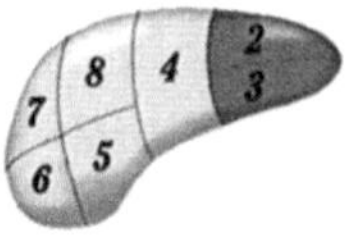

Fig. 3. Second-order divisions. (*From* Strasberg SM. Nomenclature of hepatic anatomy and resections: a review of the Brisbane 2000 system. J Hepatobiliary Pancreat Surg 2005;12(5):354; with permission.)

a segmentectomy and resection of any 2 contiguous segments is referred to as a bisegmentectomy (**Fig. 4**).

The term Reidel lobe refers to a "tongue-like projection of the anterior border of the right lobe of the liver to the right of the gallbladder" below the costal margin. It is not a true anatomic lobe, but is a normal variant of segments 5 and 6. Before cross-sectional imaging, the Reidel lobe was of greater clinical significance for inclusion in the differential diagnosis of a right-sided abdominal mass. It is important to include the most caudal aspect of the liver in imaging, because pathologic lesions may be present

Anatomical Term	Couinaud segments referred to	Term for surgical resection	Diagram (pertinent area is shaded)
Segments 1-9	*Any one of Sg 1 to 9*	*Segmentectomy* (e.g. segmentectomy 6)	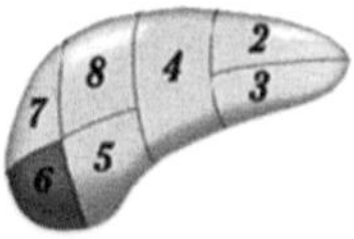
2 contiguous segments	*Any two of Sg 1 to Sg 9 in continuity*	*Bisegmentectomy* (e.g. bisegmentectomy 5,6)	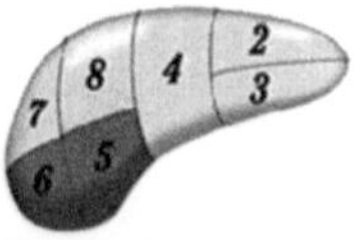

For clarity Sg. 1 and 9 are not shown. It is also acceptable to refer to ANY resection by its third-order segments, eg. right hemihepatectomy can also be called resection sg 5-8.

Border or watersheds: The borders or watersheds of the segments are planes referred to as intersegmental planes.

Fig. 4. Third-order divisions. (*From* Strasberg SM. Nomenclature of hepatic anatomy and resections: a review of the Brisbane 2000 system. J Hepatobiliary Pancreat Surg 2005;12(5):355; with permission.)

in the Reidel lobe. The incidence of Reidel lobe is between 3.3% and 65% depending on patient age and definition of Reidel lobe (below costal margin or below umbilicus).[12]

The Brisbane 2000 terminology also allows for other sectional liver resections. Resection of segments 4 to 8 ($\pm$ Sg 1) is referred to as a right trisectionectomy (preferred term) or extended right hepatectomy or extended right hemihepatectomy. Resection of segments 2 to 5 and 8 ($\pm$ Sg 1) is referred to as a left trisectionectomy (preferred term) or extended left hepatectomy or extended left hemihepatectomy (**Fig. 5**).

Although the Brisbane 2000 terminology brings liver surgery closer to a unifying language for discussion of hepatic anatomy and resection, it does not address the nomenclature of resections that do not encompass a complete segment, sometimes referred to as wedge resections or partial segmentectomies. In addition, it does not define gray zones between resections; that is, is a right hepatectomy that includes only a portion of segment 4 classified as a right hepatectomy or a right trisectionectomy?

RESECTION TECHNIQUE

In liver surgery, there are many aspects that contribute to enhancing the safety of the operation and optimizing the outcomes. The anesthetic contributions, vascular control options, and parenchymal transection options are discussed in this section. This discussion is meant to be a basic primer and is not an exhaustive review.

When performing liver resections, the concept of low central venous pressure (CVP) has become a cornerstone in the effort to reduce blood loss. Inflow to the liver may be controlled by ligation of the feeding portal vein and hepatic artery, but back-bleeding of the hepatic veins during parenchymal transection can be a source of significant blood loss. Early in the evolution of liver resection, the anesthesia strategy was to keep the patient euvolemic to hypervolemic in anticipation of high blood loss and subsequent hemodynamic lability, which was routine. This volume strategy distended the vena cava as well as the hepatic veins. Because there are no valves on the hepatic veins, the pressure of the venous bleeding is directly linked to the pressure in the vena cava (ie, CVP). The higher pressure and distended veins contribute to higher blood loss. By reducing the CVP during parenchymal transection, the venous back-bleeding may be significantly reduced.

With the technique of low CVP anesthesia, the operation is divided into 2 separate phases: the pre- and postparenchymal transection phase. For the pretransection

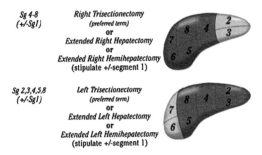

Sg 4-8 (+/-Sg1)
Right Trisectionectomy *(preferred term)* or *Extended Right Hepatectomy* or *Extended Right Hemihepatectomy* (stipulate +/-segment 1)

Sg 2,3,4,5,8 (+/-Sg1)
Left Trisectionectomy *(preferred term)* or *Extended Left Hepatectomy* or *Extended Left Hemihepatectomy* (stipulate +/-segment 1)

Border or watershed: The borders or watersheds of the sections are planes referred to as the *right and left intersectional planes.* The left intersectional plane passes through the umbilical fissure and the attachment of the falciform ligament. There is no surface marking of the right intersectional plane.

Fig. 5. Other sectional liver resections. (*From* Strasberg SM. Nomenclature of hepatic anatomy and resections: a review of the Brisbane 2000 system. J Hepatobiliary Pancreat Surg 2005;12(5):355; with permission.)

phase, the CVP is ideally maintained at less than 5 mm Hg, and this is accomplished by limiting the intraoperative fluids to occasional boluses for low urine output or hypotension. Occasionally low dose vasopressor drugs are used to maintain arterial blood pressure. Diuresis or vasodilators may be used to decrease CVP when necessary. The postparenchymal transaction phase begins after transaction and after all major bleeding from the transected surface is controlled. The patient is then returned to euvolemia with crystalloid, colloid, or blood products as deemed appropriate.[13,14]

Vascular Occlusion

Before the advent of low CVP anesthesia, vascular occlusion and exclusion were being used in hepatic resections in an attempt to reduce blood loss. More than 100 years ago, J.H. Pringle[15] published his seminal paper on liver trauma in which he described "the hepatic and portal vessels were grasped between fingers and thumb as soon as the abdomen was opened" achieving "perfect control of the bleeding areas of the liver." This technique of compression of the hepatoduodenal ligament to eliminate the inflow of blood to the liver has since been referred to as the Pringle maneuver.

Vascular occlusion techniques described in the literature use multiple combinations of total or partial occlusion of the hepatic inflow and outflow. Here inflow occlusion and total hepatic vascular exclusion are briefly discussed.

The hepatic inflow may be occluded for liver resection by encircling the hepatoduodenal ligament with a vessel loop or umbilical tape tourniquet, which is tightened down until the hepatic artery no longer has a pulse distal to the clamping. Occlusion may also be accomplished with a vascular clamp applied en mass to the portal triad; however, this is not our practice. Hemodynamic effects from this maneuver are minimal. In normothermic conditions, a healthy liver may tolerate continuous ischemia for as long as 60 minutes.[16] To facilitate longer periods of inflow occlusion, an intermittent clamping approach may be undertaken. This technique involves alternating 15- to 20-minute periods of inflow occlusion with 5-minute periods of reperfusion. Intermittent clamping can allow total ischemia times greater than 120 minutes.[17,18] Care must be taken when subjecting an abnormal liver to ischemia. Patients with cirrhosis have little hepatic reserve, and continuous clamping results in greater liver injury than intermittent clamping. There is evidence that a liver with steatosis or cirrhosis should be managed with intermittent portal occlusion because of lower rates of hepatic failure and mortality compared with a continuous occlusion technique.[19,20]

With inflow occlusion alone to the liver, there may still be significant bleeding from backflow through the hepatic veins. Hepatic vascular exclusion (HVE) removes the liver from the systemic circulation and may be helpful in situations of high CVP or large tumors encroaching on the hepatic veins or IVC. HVE requires the complete mobilization of the liver, including ligation of the right adrenal vein. Care must be taken to identify and control any accessory or replaced hepatic arteries. The infrahepatic IVC and suprahepatic IVC are surrounded just above the hepatic veins. The hepatoduodenal ligament, the infrahepatic IVC, and suprahepatic IVC are occluded to achieve complete exclusion. HVE may result in significant hemodynamic shifts, including decreased cardiac output and systolic blood pressure as well as increased systemic vascular resistance and heart rate. As a result of these changes, ~10% to 15% of patients are unable to tolerate HVE. To identify this population before beginning the liver transection, a trial clamping should occur. If the patient is able to tolerate clamping for 5 minutes without detrimental hemodynamic changes, the resection may commence, with HVE being safely applied for up to 60 minutes in a normal liver.[21]

Although there are many methods of hepatic vascular occlusion during liver resection, many complex resections may be safely completed without HVE, and HVE may not have an advantage over inflow occlusion alone.[22,23] Any surgeon performing hepatic surgery should be familiar with these techniques, and use them with discretion. It is our practice to surround the hepatoduodenal ligament and be prepared for inflow occlusion before beginning parenchymal transection, however, inflow occlusion is selectively performed as needed. Even extended resections may be accomplished with minimal blood loss and no vascular occlusion.

Parenchymal Transection Methods

The liver was long thought to be an inoperable organ because of its extreme propensity to bleed. A greater understanding of the internal vascular and biliary anatomy of the liver combined with the ability to control the inflow and outflow of blood from the liver has resulted in decreased blood loss with liver surgery. Despite these advances, bleeding remains the one of greatest challenges in liver surgery. Operative blood loss has been shown to be a risk factor for complications and tumor recurrence.[24,25]

There are many techniques that have been posited for parenchymal transection of the liver. In addition, many tools and devices have been used for liver transection. No single technique or tool is right for every resection. That being said, the results of the few randomized controlled trials do not show other methods to be advantageous over the clamp-crush technique.[26–31] Here, many of the widely used techniques and instruments for the parenchymal transection of the liver are discussed.

Clamp-crush

The clamp-crush technique is a modification of the finger fracture technique that was introduced by Lin in 1954. The finger fracture technique involved crushing the liver parenchyma with the surgeon's fingers to reveal the vascular and biliary structures. This technique evolved to use a clamp for the parenchymal crushing instead of fingers, resulting in finer control of the parenchymal transection. The skeletonized structures may then be cauterized, ligated, clipped, or sealed as appropriate before division. The clamp-crush technique has been the gold standard for comparisons, and to date, no randomized controlled trial has shown any other technique to be clearly and significantly superior to the clamp-crush method.

Many attempts have been made to improve the clamp-crush technique for blood loss, bile leaks, and speed using different instruments and technologies for ligation and division of the vessels and bile ducts encountered. Saline-cooled radiofrequency coagulation, bipolar vessel-sealing devices, ultrasonic shears, and other methods have been described. The bipolar vessel-sealing device was compared in 2 randomized trials with silk ligature. One study found no difference in operative time, blood loss, or complication rate, whereas the second study showed a decrease in operative time and blood loss without an increase in complications.[30,32,33]

Radiofrequency-assisted Liver Surgery

In 2002, a new technique for precoagulation of the liver parenchyma using radiofrequency energy was introduced. In this technique, a field of heat-induced necrosis is created using a radiofrequency probe. The treated parenchyma may then be divided using a scalpel or other device. It is important to clearly define the resection margins of the surface of the liver before beginning resection with this technique because the coagulated tissue has increased echogenicity, making ultrasound monitoring of the desired margin difficult. In addition, the ablated tissue becomes firm, making palpation of the tumor edges difficult. After the resection margins are defined, the radiofrequency probe is inserted in the liver along the planned resection plane and the tissue is ablated. This procedure is performed in an overlapping fashion to ensure coagulation of all targeted tissue. Once the coagulation is complete, the parenchyma may be divided using a scalpel, scissors, cautery, or other device with little to no bleeding.

In randomized trials and meta-analysis, radiofrequency-assisted liver surgery compared with the clamp-crush technique was found to have a longer operative time and a higher rate of complications, most notably abscess formation, which are likely a result of the extensive tissue necrosis induced by this technique.[31,34–36] Despite a higher rate of complications in unselected patients, this technique shows promise in resection of the cirrhotic liver.[37]

Tissue-sealing Devices

There are numerous tissue-sealing devices available on the market offering bipolar or ultrasonic energy sources to achieve sealing. These devices have been used in liver resections for many years.[38] No randomized trials have been performed using these tools alone for liver resection. The greatest use for such devices seems to be for segmental resections and laparoscopic resections.

Ultrasonic Dissection

Ultrasonic dissection coupled with aspiration has been used for liver parenchymal transection. The technique is used in a similar manner to that of the clamp-crush method. The ultrasonic dissector is used to free the hepatic parenchyma from vessels and bile ducts providing exposure for ligation. The vessels may then be addressed with cautery, ligation clips, or other methods.[39] This method is often used in the procurement of living donor livers. In meta-analysis, there was no difference in overall morbidity comparing ultrasonic dissection with clamp-crushing.[34]

Hydrojet

Another technique for removing the hepatic parenchyma for exposure of vessels is the hydrojet dissector. This instrument emits a high-pressure stream of water to remove the hepatic parenchyma from the vessels. The exposed vessels are then ligated. In a randomized trial comparing clamp-crushing with hydrojet, ultrasonic dissection, radiofrequency dissecting sealer, the clamp-crush technique was found to be faster with less blood loss and with a similar complication rate.[27]

Radiofrequency Dissecting Sealer

The radiofrequency dissecting sealer is an instrument that uses radiofrequency energy to divide and seal tissue. The radiofrequency energy is channeled to the tip, which is cooled with a continuous stream of saline to keep the temperature ~100°C to avoid eschar formation. This instrument is used to dissect the parenchyma and expose the vessels. The smaller vessels may be coagulated and divided by the instrument. Vessels larger than ~6 mm are controlled via ligation, clips, or vascular stapler. Excellent results using this instrument have been reported by our group in a series of 170 patients, however, in a randomized trial, the radiofrequency dissecting sealer was not found to be superior to clamp-crushing.[27,29,40,41] This device is also useful in achieving hemostasis of the cut surface of the liver when using other transection methods. The authors believe that its use is superior to that of the argon beam because there is no char formation, providing early effective hemostasis.

Vascular Staplers

The initial use of staplers in liver resection was for vascular control, but subsequently their use has expanded significantly.[42,43] The use of staplers offers an increase in speed as well as facilitating division of difficult pedicles. The use of staplers for liver parenchymal transection has been well established and multiple groups have published large series using the technique with minimal morbidity. Staple techniques in liver transection have been shown in nonrandomized studies to have a significant reduction in operative time and blood loss, however this has not been tested in a randomized controlled fashion against other techniques.[44–46]

Staplers may be used in many capacities for liver resection. Initially used in left lateral sectionectomies, a stapler may be used as the sole tool of division of the hepatic parenchyma, vessels and bile ducts. A popular technique for hemihepatectomy involves use of staplers to selectively ligate and divide the portal inflow and bile ducts, followed by the hepatic veins. The parenchyma is then divided with the stapler. At our institution, a Kelley clamp is used to probe the proposed tract of the stapler. Response to tactile feedback is important, because any resistance met is from vascular or biliary structures. The resistance-free path is then used for guiding the stapler. This method avoids unnecessary tearing of crossing vessels by using tactile feedback.[44]

Although much has been written on the subject of parenchymal transection of the liver, the literature is sparse in randomized controlled trials. Trials are difficult to compare with each other as the reporting and definitions of cirrhosis and steatosis are not standardized. In addition, reports tend to include major and minor as well as anatomic and nonanatomic resections together. It is likely that the method that is best for an anatomic hemihepatectomy will not be the best for complex nonanatomic resections. Although the literature does not show a significant advantage of the newer technologies over the clamp-crush technique, each of the available tools is useful in certain instances.

A surgeon who performs liver resections should be familiar with the available techniques and tools, because no single method is optimal in all situations. In addition, many surgeons now use the existing tools and techniques in combination. In nonrandomized case series, many groups are reporting either low complication rates or improved rates compared with nonrandomized clamp-crush controls.[24,33,47,48] Given the heterogeneity of liver resections, liver textures and tumor locations, and the difficulty of conducting a well-designed randomized trial of techniques, it is unlikely that a truly superior parenchymal transection method will emerge from those in existence at this time. As we move forward, patient selection, a strong understanding of the internal liver anatomy, and attention to detail are likely to be the most important factors in parenchymal transection.

SUMMARY

To facilitate accurate communication regarding liver anatomy and resections, the standardized Brisbane 2000 terminology should be used uniformly by investigators. When performing liver resection, blood loss should be minimized by using low CVP anesthesia and vascular occlusion as appropriate. There are many options for transection of the liver parenchyma, and although no technique has been shown to be superior to clamp-crushing, hepatic surgeons should be familiar with the available techniques.

REFERENCES

1. Starzl TE, Iwatsuki S. Liver resection for primary hepatic neoplasms. Acta Chirurgica Austriaca 1988;4:374–9.
2. The Terminology Committee of the IHPBA. The Brisbane 2000 terminology of hepatic anatomy and resections. HPB 2000;2:333–9.

3. Strasberg SM. Nomenclature of hepatic anatomy and resections: a review of the Brisbane 2000 system. J Hepatobiliary Pancreat Surg 2005;12(5):351–5.
4. Couinaud C. The paracaval segments of the liver. J Hepatobiliary Pancreat Surg 1994;1(2):145–51.
5. Couinaud C. Le foie: études anatomiques et chirurgicales. Paris: Masson; 1957.
6. Healey J Jr, Schroy P, Sorenson R. Distributions of the hepatic artery in man. J Int Coll Surg 1953;20:133–49.
7. Healey JE Jr. Clinical anatomic aspects of radical hepatic surgery. J Int Coll Surg 1954;22(5, Sect 1):542–50.
8. Healey JE Jr, Schroy PC. Anatomy of the biliary ducts within the human liver; analysis of the prevailing pattern of branchings and the major variations of the biliary ducts. AMA Arch Surg 1953;66(5):599–616.
9. Hjortsjo CH. The topography of the intrahepatic duct systems. Acta Anat (Basel) 1951;11(4):599–615.
10. Goldsmith NA, Woodburne RT. The surgical anatomy pertaining to liver resection. Surg Gynecol Obstet 1957;105(3):310–8.
11. Abdalla EK, Vauthey JN, Couinaud C. The caudate lobe of the liver: implications of embryology and anatomy for surgery. Surg Oncol Clin N Am 2002;11(4):835–48.
12. Gillard JH, Patel MC, Abrahams PH, et al. Riedel's lobe of the liver: fact or fiction? Clin Anat 1998;11(1):47–9.
13. Melendez JA, Arslan V, Fischer ME, et al. Perioperative outcomes of major hepatic resections under low central venous pressure anesthesia: blood loss, blood transfusion, and the risk of postoperative renal dysfunction. J Am Coll Surg 1998;187(6):620–5.
14. Rees M, Plant G, Wells J, et al. One hundred and fifty hepatic resections: evolution of technique towards bloodless surgery. Br J Surg 1996;83(11):1526–9.
15. Pringle JH. Notes on the arrest of hepatic hemorrhage due to trauma. Ann Surg 1908;48(4):541.
16. Huguet C, Gavelli A, Chieco PA, et al. Liver ischemia for hepatic resection: where is the limit? Surgery 1992;111(3):251–9.
17. Ishizaki Y, Yoshimoto J, Miwa K, et al. Safety of prolonged intermittent Pringle maneuver during hepatic resection. Arch Surg 2006;141(7):649–53 [discussion: 654].
18. Sakamoto Y, Makuuchi M, Takayama T, et al. Pringle's maneuver lasting 322 min. Hepatogastroenterology 1999;46(25):457–8.
19. Belghiti J, Noun R, Malafosse R, et al. Continuous versus intermittent portal triad clamping for liver resection: a controlled study. Ann Surg 1999;229(3):369–75.
20. Man K, Fan ST, Ng IO, et al. Prospective evaluation of Pringle maneuver in hepatectomy for liver tumors by a randomized study. Ann Surg 1997;226(6):704–11 [discussion: 711–3].
21. Abdalla EK, Noun R, Belghiti J. Hepatic vascular occlusion: which technique? Surg Clin North Am 2004;84(2):563–85.
22. Torzilli G, Makuuchi M, Midorikawa Y, et al. Liver resection without total vascular exclusion: hazardous or beneficial? An analysis of our experience. Ann Surg 2001;233(2):167–75.
23. Benoist S, Salabert AS, Penna C, et al. Portal triad clamping (TC) or hepatic vascular exclusion (VE) for major liver resection after prolonged neoadjuvant chemotherapy? A case-matched study in 60 patients. Surgery 2006;140(3):396–403.
24. Katz SC, Shia J, Liau KH, et al. Operative blood loss independently predicts recurrence and survival after resection of hepatocellular carcinoma. Ann Surg 2009;249(4):617–23.

25. Kooby DA, Stockman J, Ben-Porat L, et al. Influence of transfusions on perioperative and long-term outcome in patients following hepatic resection for colorectal metastases. Ann Surg 2003;237(6):860–9 [discussion: 869–70].
26. Takayama T, Makuuchi M, Kubota K, et al. Randomized comparison of ultrasonic vs clamp transection of the liver. Arch Surg 2001;136(8):922–8.
27. Lesurtel M, Selzner M, Petrowsky H, et al. How should transection of the liver be performed?: a prospective randomized study in 100 consecutive patients: comparing four different transection strategies. Ann Surg 2005;242(6):814–22 [discussion: 822–3].
28. Koo BN, Kil HK, Choi JS, et al. Hepatic resection by the Cavitron Ultrasonic Surgical Aspirator increases the incidence and severity of venous air embolism. Anesth Analg 2005;101(4):966–70 [table of contents].
29. Arita J, Hasegawa K, Kokudo N, et al. Randomized clinical trial of the effect of a saline-linked radiofrequency coagulator on blood loss during hepatic resection. Br J Surg 2005;92(8):954–9.
30. Saiura A, Yamamoto J, Koga R, et al. Usefulness of LigaSure for liver resection: analysis by randomized clinical trial. Am J Surg 2006;192(1):41–5.
31. Lupo L, Gallerani A, Panzera P, et al. Randomized clinical trial of radiofrequency-assisted versus clamp-crushing liver resection. Br J Surg 2007;94(3):287–91.
32. Ikeda M, Hasegawa K, Sano K, et al. The vessel sealing system (LigaSure) in hepatic resection: a randomized controlled trial. Ann Surg 2009;250(2): 199–203.
33. Patrlj L, Tuorto S, Fong Y. Combined blunt-clamp dissection and LigaSure ligation for hepatic parenchyma dissection: postcoagulation technique. J Am Coll Surg 2010;210(1):39–44.
34. Rahbari NN, Koch M, Schmidt T, et al. Meta-analysis of the clamp-crushing technique for transection of the parenchyma in elective hepatic resection: back to where we started? Ann Surg Oncol 2009;16(3):630–9.
35. Gurusamy KS, Pamecha V, Sharma D, et al. Techniques for liver parenchymal transection in liver resection. Cochrane Database Syst Rev 2009;1:CD006880.
36. Varshney S, Sharma S, Kapoor S, et al. Pitfalls of radiofrequency assisted liver resection. Hepatogastroenterology 2007;54(77):1539–41.
37. Curro G, Jiao L, Scisca C, et al. Radiofrequency-assisted liver resection in cirrhotic patients with hepatocellular carcinoma. J Surg Oncol 2008;98(6): 407–10.
38. Schmidbauer S, Hallfeldt KK, Sitzmann G, et al. Experience with ultrasound scissors and blades (UltraCision) in open and laparoscopic liver resection. Ann Surg 2002;235(1):27–30.
39. Aloia TA, Zorzi D, Abdalla EK, et al. Two-surgeon technique for hepatic parenchymal transection of the noncirrhotic liver using saline-linked cautery and ultrasonic dissection. Ann Surg 2005;242(2):172.
40. Hutchins R, Bertucci M. Experience with TissueLink–radiofrequency-assisted parenchymal division. Dig Surg 2007;24(4):318–21.
41. Geller DA, Tsung A, Maheshwari V, et al. Hepatic resection in 170 patients using saline-cooled radiofrequency coagulation. HPB (Oxford) 2005;7(3):208–13.
42. Fong Y, Blumgart LH. Useful stapling techniques in liver surgery. J Am Coll Surg 1997;185(1):93–100.
43. McEntee GP, Nagorney DM. Use of vascular staplers in major hepatic resections. Br J Surg 1991;78(1):40–1.
44. Balaa FK, Gamblin TC, Tsung A, et al. Right hepatic lobectomy using the staple technique in 101 patients. J Gastrointest Surg 2008;12(2):338–43.

45. Reddy SK, Barbas AS, Gan TJ, et al. Hepatic parenchymal transection with vascular staplers: a comparative analysis with the crush-clamp technique. Am J Surg 2008;196(5):760–7.

46. Schemmer P, Friess H, Hinz U, et al. Stapler hepatectomy is a safe dissection technique: analysis of 300 patients. World J Surg 2006;30(3):419–30.

47. Aldrighetti L, Pulitano C, Arru M, et al. "Technological" approach versus clamp crushing technique for hepatic parenchymal transection: a comparative study. J Gastrointest Surg 2006;10(7):974–9.

48. El Moghazy WM, Hedaya MS, Kaido T, et al. Two different methods for donor hepatic transection: cavitron ultrasonic surgical aspirator with bipolar cautery versus cavitron ultrasonic surgical aspirator with radiofrequency coagulator-A randomized controlled trial. Liver Transpl 2009;15(1):102–5.

Laparoscopic Liver Resection—Current Update

Kevin Tri Nguyen, MD, PhD, David A. Geller, MD*

KEYWORDS

- Laparoscopic liver resection • Laparoscopic hepatic resection
- Liver cancer • HCC • Colorectal cancer metastases

Laparoscopic hepatic resection is an emerging option in the field of hepatic surgery. With almost 3000 laparoscopic hepatic resections reported in the literature for benign and malignant tumors, with a combined mortality of 0.3% and morbidity of 10.5%, there will be an increasing demand for minimally invasive liver surgery.[1] Multiple series have been published on laparoscopic liver resections; however, no randomized controlled trial has been reported that compares laparoscopic with open liver resection. Large series, meta-analyses, and reviews have thus far attested to the feasibility and safety of minimally invasive hepatic surgery for benign and malignant lesions.[2–17] The largest single-center experience was published by Koffron and colleagues[3] and describes various minimally invasive approaches to liver resection, including pure laparoscopic, hand-assisted laparoscopic, and laparoscopic-assisted open (hybrid) techniques. The choice of the minimally invasive approach should depend on surgeon experience, tumor size, location, and the extent of liver resection.

This article reviews the literature on reports comparing laparoscopic with hepatic resections. Special emphasis is on the cumulative world literature on laparoscopic liver surgery, the consensus meeting on laparoscopic liver resection, the learning curve on laparoscopic liver resection, laparoscopic major hepatectomies, short-term benefits after laparoscopic liver resection, and survival outcomes for laparoscopic liver resection of hepatocellular carcinoma (HCC) and colorectal liver metastasis. Finally, financial cost comparisons are evaluated to determine the cost advantages or disadvantages of the laparoscopic approach.

WORLD REVIEW

Since the first laparoscopic liver resection was reported in 1992, there has been an exponential increase in the number of reported laparoscopic liver resection, with more than 127 published articles, totaling almost 3000 reported cases of laparoscopic liver resection.[1] Half of the reported cases were performed for malignant lesions and 45% for

---

Department of Surgery, Starzl Transplant Institute, UPMC Liver Cancer Center, University of Pittsburgh, 3459 Fifth Avenue, UPMC Montefiore, 7 South, Pittsburgh, PA 15213-2582, USA
* Corresponding author.
E-mail address: gellerda@upmc.edu

doi:10.1016/j.suc.2010.04.008
surgical.theclinics.com

benign lesions. In addition, laparoscopic live donor hepatectomy was performed in 1.7% of cases. Several variations of the minimally invasive approach have been described, with the most commonly performed variation the pure laparoscopic approach (75%), followed distantly by the hand-assisted approach (17%) and the hybrid approach (2%). A hybrid approach is when the operation is started laparoscopically to mobilize the liver and perform the initial hilar dissection. Then, the parenchymal transection is completed through a small open incision or slight extension of the hand port incision.[18] The conversion rate from a laparoscopic approach to an open procedure was 4.1%. The most common type of laparoscopic liver resection performed is a wedge resection or segmentectomy (45%), followed by left lateral sectionectomy (20%). Major anatomic hepatectomies are still less frequently performed: right hepatectomy (9%) and left hepatectomy (7%). Cumulative morbidity and mortality was 10.5% and 0.3%.

INTERNATIONAL CONFERENCE ON LAPAROSCOPIC LIVER SURGERY

The first consensus meeting on laparoscopic liver surgery was held at the University of Louisville in Louisville, Kentucky, in November 2008, incorporating the opinions of the world's experts in laparoscopic and open liver surgery. The conference consisted of more than 125 liver surgeons from more than a dozen countries with 25 invited faculty members. From this meeting, consensus statements on laparoscopic liver surgery were formulated[19]:

1. Three terms should be used to describe laparoscopic liver resection: pure laparoscopy, hand-assisted laparoscopy, and the hybrid technique.
2. As in open hepatic resection, several different technical approaches for performing major laparoscopic liver resection have evolved. Similar to open liver surgery, no single method of parenchymal transection has been shown superior.
3. Major laparoscopic liver resections have been performed with safety and efficacy equal to that of open surgery in highly specialized centers.
4. The best indications for laparoscopic liver resection are in patients with solitary lesions, 5 cm or less, located in peripheral liver segments (segments 2–6). Major liver resections should be reserved for experienced surgeons already facile with more limited laparoscopic resections.
5. Conversion to an open liver resection should be performed for lack of case progression or patient safety.
6. Indications for surgery for benign hepatic lesions should not be expanded.
7. Resection (laparoscopic or open) remains the gold standard for the treatment of colorectal liver metastases.
8. When local resection for HCC is undertaken, it should be an anatomic segmental resection because this is associated with reduced local recurrence.
9. Laparoscopic live-donor hepatectomy remains the most controversial application of laparoscopic liver surgery and should only proceed in the confines of a worldwide registry.
10. A prospective randomized trial may be impractical due to difficulties defining the relevant study questions, the size of the study population, and the length of time to perform the trial. A cooperative patient registry may be more practical to help understand the role and safety of laparoscopic liver surgery.

THE LEARNING CURVE OF LAPAROSCOPIC LIVER RESECTION

Successful laparoscopic liver surgery requires expertise in advance laparoscopy and hepatobiliary surgery. An unknown number of cases, however, need to be performed to surpass the initial learning curve. The learning curve effect has been described for laparoscopic colorectal surgery and hernia repairs,[20-25] but until recently, no such study had been described for laparoscopic liver resection. Vigano and colleagues[26] evaluated the learning curve of laparoscopic liver resection. After adjusting for case-mix and potential confounders using the cumulative sum analysis, they showed that the learning curve for laparoscopic minor hepatectomies could be overcome with 60 cases. They showed that over 3 time periods in a 12-year span (1996–1999, 2000–2003, and 2004–2008), they performed a higher proportion of laparoscopic cases (17.5%, 22.4%, and 24.2%), laparoscopic resection for HCC (17.6%, 25.6, and 39.4%), laparoscopic resection of colorectal liver metastasis (0%, 6.4%, and 13%), and major hepatectomies (1.1%, 9.1%, and 8.5%). In addition, intraoperative outcomes were improved over time with less operative time (210, 180, and 150 minutes), less blood loss (300, 200, and 200 mL), and less conversion to open rate (15.5%, 10.3%, and 3.4%). Likewise, the Northwestern University group reported an increase in the percentage of total liver cases performed laparoscopically from 10% in 2002 to 80% in 2007.[3]

LAPAROSCOPIC MAJOR HEPATECTOMY

In the reported world literature, approximately 75% of cases performed were wedge resections, segmentectomies, or bisegmentectomies; however, 16% were anatomic hemihepatectomies.[1] The first reported major hepatectomies were reported by Hüscher and colleagues.[27] Widespread dissemination of laparoscopic major hepatectomies has been hindered by fears of major hemorrhage and the technical challenges of portal, caval, and hepatic vein dissection. Recently, Dagher and colleagues[28] reported an international, prospective study on 210 laparoscopic major liver resections (136 right and 74 left hepatectomies) in 5 medical centers (3 European, 2 United States, and 1 Australian) from 1997 to 2008. They showed an increasing number of laparoscopic major liver resections were performed each year. A pure laparoscopic approach was used in 43.3% of cases whereas a hand-assisted approach was used in 56.7% of cases. Conversion to laparotomy was required in 12.4% of cases. Mortality occurred in 1% of patients, and specific morbidity (hemorrhage, ascites, or biloma) occurred in 8.1% of patients. For patients with malignant disease, negative margins (R0 resections) were achieved in 97.4% of patients. Comparing the early experience (n = 90) with the late experience (n = 120), operative time, blood loss, portal clamping time, conversion rate, and hospital length of stay were improved over time. The investigators concluded from this multicenter, international study that laparoscopic major hepatectomy was feasible in selected patients, performed by surgeons already advanced in laparoscopic minor hepatectomies.

HEPATOCELLULAR CARCINOMA

HCC is the most common primary liver cancer worldwide with risk factors that include long-term excessive alcohol consumption, hepatitis B virus infection, hepatitis C virus infection, and metabolic liver diseases. For eligible patients, liver transplantation offers the highest recurrence-free survival rate; however, liver transplantation is limited due to a worldwide shortage of organs. For patents who do not meet transplantation criteria, liver resection offers the next best survival rate.

In the world literature, HCCs accounted for 52% of laparoscopic liver resections for malignant lesions.[1] Several studies have provided outcomes of laparoscopic resection for HCC (**Table 1**). Belli and colleagues[29] provide the largest matched comparison of laparoscopic (n = 54) with open liver resection (n = 125) of HCC in

Table 1
Overall survival after laparoscopic liver resection for HCC studies

Authors	Year	No. of Patients	OS 1 Year (%)	OS 2 Years (%)	OS 3 Years (%)	OS 4 Years (%)	OS 5 Years (%)
Belli et al[29]	2009	54	—	—	67	—	—
Lai et al[30]	2009	30	—	—	—	—	50
Santambrogio et al[31]	2009	22	—	—	—	50	—
Sasaki et al[32]	2009	37	90	—	73	—	53
Cai et al[33]	2008	24	95.5	–	67.5	—	56.2
Chen et al[14]	2008	116	94.7	—	74.2	—	61.7
Dagher et al[34]	2008	32	—	—	71.9	—	—
Belli et al[35]	2007	23	—	86.9	—	—	—
Cherqui et al[36]	2006	27	—	—	93	—	—
Tang et al[37]	2006	17	86	59	—	—	—
Vibert et al[11]	2006	16	85	–	66	—	—
Kaneko et al[38]	2005	30	—	—	—	—	61
Teramoto et al[39]	2005	15	100	—	80	—	—
Laurent et al[40]	2003	13	—	—	89	—	—
Teramoto et al[41]	2003	11	—	—	—	—	75
Gigot et al[42]	2002	10	83.5	62.5	—	—	—
Shimada et al[43]	2001	17	85	—	70	—	50

Abbreviation: OS, overall survival.

patients with cirrhosis. Mortalities at 30 days were similar between the two groups; however, morbidity was significantly lower in the laparoscopic group (19% vs 36%, $P = .02$). From an oncologic standpoint, the 3-year overall survival (67% vs 62%, $P = .347$) and disease-free survival (52% vs 59%, $P = .864$) between the laparoscopic and open groups were not significantly different. This important study supports the short-term benefits without the oncologic disadvantages of laparoscopic liver resection over open liver resection for HCC. These results are comparable with results of other studies showing an overall 3-year survival of 60% to 93% and 3-year disease-free survival of 52% to 64% after laparoscopic liver resection for HCC.[34,36,44]

Sarpel and colleagues[45] from the Mt Sinai group matched 20 laparoscopic liver resections for HCC to 56 open resections for HCC. Patients were well matched for age, gender, degree of cirrhosis, and tumor size. There were no significant differences in operative time or rates of blood transfusion whereas the laparoscopic patients had a shorter length of stay. There was no significant difference in positive margins or disease-free or overall survival between the groups. Five-year overall survival rates were also comparable in recent matched comparison studies of laparoscopic (50%–95%) with open (47%–75%) hepatic resection for HCC.[33,46,47]

Laparoscopic liver resection also facilitated subsequent liver transplantation after liver resection for HCC. Laurent and colleagues[48] performed 24 orthotopic liver transplants after prior liver resection for HCC (12 laparoscopic and 12 open liver resections). Indications for liver transplantation were recurrent HCC ($n = 19$) or planned bridge to transplant ($n = 5$). The same experienced liver transplant team performed the minimally invasive or open hepatic resection as well as subsequent liver transplantation. The laparoscopic group of patients had significantly fewer adhesions and facilitated the subsequent liver transplantation. Specifically, those patients who underwent prior laparoscopic liver resection had significantly less hepatectomy time (2.5 hours vs 4.5 hrs, $P<.05$), less total operating room time (6.2 hours vs 8.5 hours, $P<.05$), less blood loss (1.2 L vs 2.3 L, $P<.05$), and less blood transfusion (3 units vs 6 units packed red blood cells, $P<.05$) compared with the open group.

COLORECTAL CANCER LIVER METASTASIS

The new paradigm for surgical therapy of colorectal liver metastasis is resection, if possible, of all liver metastases with a negative margin while maintaining sufficient functional liver parenchyma with adequate inflow and outflow.[49] The standard approach to liver resection remains the open approach. The use of laparoscopy has, in the past, been limited to diagnostic laparoscopy to rule out extrahepatic disease that would preclude proceeding with open hepatic resection of the liver metastasis. Recent reports indicate that laparoscopic liver resection for colorectal liver metastasis is used in select patients with increasing frequency although not as often as laparoscopic hepatic resection for HCC (35% vs 52% of all reported laparoscopic liver resection for malignancy).[1] Major concerns about laparoscopic resection for colorectal cancer metastases include possible adhesions from prior intra-abdominal operation and the oncologic integrity of the resection. Data are emerging, however, to support minimally invasive hepatic resection for colorectal liver metastases. Nguyen and colleagues[2] reported a multi-institutional, international study on laparoscopic liver resection for metastatic colorectal cancer in 109 patients, 95% of whom had prior intra-abdominal operations. Oncologically, negative margins were achieved in 94.4% of patients and overall survivals at 1, 3, and 5 years were 88%, 69%, and 50% whereas disease-free survivals at 1, 3, and 5 years were 65%, 43%, and 43%. Other recent studies also report similar 5-year survival rates of 46% to

64% after laparoscopic liver resection of colorectal cancer metastases.[32,50] These 5-year survival results after laparoscopic liver resection of colorectal cancer metastases are comparable with overall 5-year survival results of 37% to 50% reported in modern open hepatic resection series from large liver cancer centers (**Table 2**). This study supports the safety and oncologic integrity of laparoscopic liver resection for colorectal cancer metastases in experienced centers.

The only head-to-head comparison of laparoscopic with open hepatectomy for colorectal liver metastases was performed by Castaing and colleagues.[51] They compared two groups (60 patients each) from two highly specialized liver surgery centers in France. From an oncologic standpoint, the laparoscopic approach was comparable with, if not better than, the open approach on several parameters. First, the laparoscopic group had a greater margin-free resection rate than the open group (87% vs 72%, $P = .04$). Second, the two groups had comparable overall survival, with 1-, 3-, and 5-year rates of 97%, 82%, and 64% in the laparoscopic group, and 97%, 70%, and 56% in the open group (log rank $P = .13$). Third, disease-free survival was comparable between the two groups with 1-, 3-, 5-year rates of 70%, 47%, and 35% in the laparoscopic group and 70%, 40%, and 27% in the open group (log rank $P = .32$). A limitation of this study is that the open hepatic resections were performed in a large volume hepatobiliary center, whereas the laparoscopic approach was performed by a single master minimally invasive surgery surgeon (BG). It is unclear whether or not these same results can be achieved on a broader scale. Nonetheless, the data support equivalent 5-year survival results of laparoscopic versus open hepatic resection for colorectal liver metastasis in selected patients.

BENEFITS OF LAPAROSCOPIC LIVER RESECTION

No prospective, randomized controlled trials have been established to compare laparoscopic with open liver resections. Several studies, however, have retrospectively compared laparoscopic with open liver resection. Many groups have shown decreased blood loss with laparoscopic versus open liver resection.[3,17,29,47,52,58–67] Postoperative pain control was better in laparoscopic cases with fewer days of required narcotic pain medication[52,68] and decreased total amount of pain medication required.[33,46,60,67,69,70]

More importantly, almost all the studies comparing laparoscopic with open liver resection consistently showed a significant earlier discharge to home after laparoscopic liver resection. Lengths of stay were variable based on the country of origin of the studies but were consistently shorter for laparoscopic liver resection. Three studies published in the United States[3,59,67] presented a length of stay of 1.9 to 4.0 days after laparoscopic liver resection. Studies from Europe[17,29,35,40,47,51,62–64,68,69,71–73] showed an average length of stay of 3.5 to 10 days whereas those from Asia[30,33,38,46,60,61,70] reported an average of length of stay of 4 to 20 days after laparoscopic liver resection.

COST ANALYSIS

There are concerns that the minimally invasive approach to liver resection may be associated with increased cost due to laparoscopic equipment/instrumentation. Koffron and colleagues[3] showed that the operating room costs for minimally invasive liver resections cases were significantly higher than those of open liver resection cases; however, these added expenses was more than offset by lower nonoperating room costs for the laparoscopic group, with the biggest factor a shorter length of stay. In their analysis, the operating room cost for right hemihepatectomy was 36% of total hospital costs for open cases compared with 47% of total hospital costs for minimally

Table 2
Laparoscopic versus open hepatic resection for colorectal cancer metastases

Authors (Laparoscopic)	Year	Journal	No. of Patients	OS 3 Years (%)	OS 5 Years (%)
Kazaryan et al[50]	2010	Arch Surg	96	79	46
Nguyen et al[2]	2009	Ann Surg	109	69	50
Castaing et al[51]	2009	Ann Surg	60	82	64
Sasaki et al[32]	2009	Br J Surg	39	64	64
Ito et al[52]	2009	J Gastrointest Surg	13	72	—
Robles et al[53]	2008	Surg Endosc	21	80	—
Vibert et al[11]	2006	Br J Surg	41	87	—
O'Rourke and Fielding[8]	2004	J Gastrointest Surg	22	75 (2 y)	—
Gigot et al[42]	2002	Ann Surg	27	100 (2 y)	—
Authors (Open)	**Year**	**Journal**	**No. of Patients**	**OS 3 Years (%)**	**OS 5 Years (%)**
Ito et al[54]	2008	Ann Surg	1067	65	45
Blazer et al[55]	2008	J Clin Oncol	305	65	42
Adam et al[56]	2008	J Clin Oncol	738	61	45
Zakaria et al[57]	2007	Ann Surg	662	55	37

Abbreviation: OS, overall survival.

invasive cases; however, the nonoperating room costs were less with the minimally invasive group. Specifically, the nonoperating room costs for right hemihepatectomy were 64% of total hospital costs for open cases compared with 35% of total hospital costs for minimally invasive cases. This cost differential was significantly dependent on length of hospital stay (P<.0001).[3] Rowe and colleagues[66] showed that the costs of stapler/trocar devices were similar between the laparoscopic and the open groups whereas Polignano and colleagues[64] showed that disposable instruments and other devices were significantly higher for laparoscopic hepatic resection versus open hepatic resection (P<.0001). Two studies confirmed, however, that overall hospital costs were less for the laparoscopic group due to shorter lengths of stay (P≤.04).[64,67] Vanounou and colleagues[74] used deviation-based cost modeling to compare the costs of laparoscopic with open left lateral sectionectomy at the University of Pittsburgh Medical Center. They compared 29 laparoscopic with 40 open cases and showed that patients who underwent the laparoscopic approach faired more favorably with a shorter length of stay (3 vs 5 days, P<.0001), significantly less postoperative morbidity (P = .001), and a weighted-average median cost savings of $1527 to $2939 per patient compared with patients who underwent open left lateral sectionectomy.

CANCER OUTCOMES
Surgical Margins

Initial concerns about the adequacy of surgical margins and possible tumor seeding prevented the widespread adoption of laparoscopic resection approaches for liver cancers. In comparison studies, there were no differences in margin-free resections between laparoscopic and open liver resection.[17,29,33,35,40,45–47,51,52,60,64–67,72] In addition, no incidence of port-site recurrence or tumor seeding has been reported. With more than 3000 cases of minimally invasive hepatic resection reported in the literature (and no documentation of any significant port-site or peritoneal seeding), the authors conclude that this concern should not prevent surgeons from accepting a laparoscopic approach.

Survival Outcomes

There were no significant differences in overall survival in the 13 studies that compared laparoscopic liver resection with open liver resection for cancer.[29,30,33,35,38,40,43,45–47,51,52,60] For example, Cai and colleagues[33] showed that the 1-, 3-, and 5-year survival rates after laparoscopic resection of HCC were 95.4%, 67.5%, and 56.2% versus 100%, 73.8%, and 53.8% for open resection. For resection of colorectal cancer liver metastasis, Ito and colleagues[52] showed a 3-year survival of 72% after laparoscopic liver resection and 56% after open liver resection whereas Castaing and colleagues[51] showed a 5-year survival of 64% after laparoscopic liver resection versus 56% after open liver resection.

DISCUSSION

Compared with open liver resections, laparoscopic liver resections are associated with less blood loss, less pain medication requirement, and shorter length of hospital stay. A randomized controlled clinical trial is the best method to compare laparoscopic with open liver resection; however, such a trial may be difficult to conduct because patients are unlikely to subject themselves to an open procedure when a minimally invasive approach has been shown feasible and safe in experienced hands. In addition, many patients would have to be accrued to detect a difference in complications that occur infrequently. Short of a large randomized clinical trial, meta-analysis and matched comparisons provide the next best option to compare laparoscopic with open liver resection.

For laparoscopic resection of HCC or colorectal cancer metastases, there has been no difference in 5-year overall survival compared with open hepatic resection. In addition, from a financial standpoint, the minimally invasive approach to liver resection may be associated with higher operating room costs; however, the total hospital costs were offset or improved due to the associated shorter length of hospital stay with the minimally invasive approach.

SUMMARY

Minimally invasive hepatic resection for benign and malignant liver lesions is safe and feasible with short-term benefits, no economic disadvantage, and no compromise to oncologic principles. These results indicate that laparoscopic hepatic resection is an important part of the armamentarium in hepatic resection surgery in selected patients.

REFERENCES

1. Nguyen KT, Gamblin TC, Geller DA. World review of laparoscopic liver resection—2,804 patients. Ann Surg 2009;250(5):831–41.
2. Nguyen KT, Laurent A, Dagher I, et al. Minimally invasive liver resection for metastatic colorectal cancer: a multi-institutional, international report of safety, feasibility, and early outcomes. Ann Surg 2009;250(5):842–8.
3. Koffron AJ, Auffenberg G, Kung R, et al. Evaluation of 300 minimally invasive liver resections at a single institution: less is more. Ann Surg 2007;246(3):385–92.
4. Koffron AJ, Geller DA, Gamblin TC, et al. Laparoscopic liver surgery: Shifting the management of liver tumors. Hepatology 2006;44(6):1694–700.
5. Gamblin TC, Holloway SE, Heckman JT, et al. Laparoscopic resection of benign hepatic cysts: a new standard. J Am Coll Surg 2008;207(5):731–6.
6. Buell JF, Thomas MT, Rudich S, et al. Experience with more than 500 minimally invasive hepatic procedures. Ann Surg 2008;248(3):475–86.
7. Descottes B, Glineur D, Lachachi F, et al. Laparoscopic liver resection of benign liver tumors. Surg Endosc 2003;17(1):23–30.
8. O'Rourke N, Fielding G. Laparoscopic right hepatectomy: surgical technique. J Gastrointest Surg 2004;8(2):213–6.
9. Are C, Fong Y, Geller DA. Laparoscopic liver resections. Adv Surg 2005;39:57–75.
10. Cai XJ, Yu H, Liang X, et al. Laparoscopic hepatectomy by curettage and aspiration. Experiences of 62 cases. Surg Endosc 2006;20(10):1531–5.
11. Vibert E, Perniceni T, Levard H, et al. Laparoscopic liver resection. Br J Surg 2006;93(1):67–72.
12. Dagher I, Proske JM, Carloni A, et al. Laparoscopic liver resection: results for 70 patients. Surg Endosc 2007;21(4):619–24.
13. Simillis C, Constantinides VA, Tekkis PP, et al. Laparoscopic versus open hepatic resections for benign and malignant neoplasms—a meta-analysis. Surgery 2007; 141(2):203–11.
14. Chen HY, Juan CC, Ker CG. Laparoscopic liver surgery for patients with hepatocellular carcinoma. Ann Surg Oncol 2008;15(3):800–6.
15. Cho J, Han H, Yoon Y, et al. Experiences of laparoscopic liver resection including lesions in the posterosuperior segments of the liver. Surg Endosc 2008;22(11):2344–9.

16. Pulitanò C, Aldrighetti L. The current role of laparoscopic liver resection for the treatment of liver tumors. Nat Clin Pract Gastroenterol Hepatol 2008;5(11): 648–54.

17. Topal B, Fieuws S, Aerts R, et al. Laparoscopic versus open liver resection of hepatic neoplasms: comparative analysis of short-term results. Surg Endosc 2008;22(10):2208–13.

18. Koffron AJ, Kung RD, Auffenberg GB, et al. Laparoscopic liver surgery for everyone: the hybrid method. Surgery 2007;142(4):463–8.

19. Buell JF, Cherqui D, Geller DA, et al. The international position on laparoscopic liver surgery: the Louisville Statement, 2008. Ann Surg 2009;250(5):825–30.

20. Lal P, Kajla RK, Chander J, et al. Laparoscopic total extraperitoneal (TEP) inguinal hernia repair: overcoming the learning curve. Surg Endosc 2004;18(4):642–5.

21. Bencini L, Sánchez LJ. Learning curve for laparoscopic ventral hernia repair. Am J Surg 2004;187(3):378–82.

22. Haidenberg J, Kendrick ML, Meile T, et al. Totally extraperitoneal (TEP) approach for inguinal hernia: the favorable learning curve for trainees. Curr Surg 2003; 60(1):65–8.

23. Edwards CC 2nd, Bailey RW. Laparoscopic hernia repair: the learning curve. Surg Laparosc Endosc Percutan Tech 2000;10(3):149–53.

24. Tekkis PP, Senagore AJ, Delaney CP, et al. Evaluation of the learning curve in laparoscopic colorectal surgery: comparison of right-sided and left-sided resections. Ann Surg 2005;242(1):83–91.

25. Schlachta CM, Mamazza J, Seshadri PA, et al. Defining a learning curve for laparoscopic colorectal resections. Dis Colon Rectum 2001;44(2):217–22.

26. Vigano L, Laurent A, Tayar C, et al. The learning curve in laparoscopic liver resection: improved feasibility and reproducibility. Ann Surg 2009;250(5):772–82.

27. Hüscher CG, Lirici MM, Chiodini S, et al. Current position of advanced laparoscopic surgery of the liver. J R Coll Surg Edinb 1997;42(4):219–25.

28. Dagher I, O'Rourke N, Geller DA, et al. Laparoscopic major hepatectomy: an evolution in standard of care. Ann Surg 2009;250(5):856–60.

29. Belli G, Limongelli P, Fantini C, et al. Laparoscopic and open treatment of hepatocellular carcinoma in patients with cirrhosis. Br J Surg 2009;96(9):1041–8.

30. Lai EC, Tang CN, Yang GP, et al. Minimally invasive surgical treatment of hepatocellular carcinoma: long-term outcome. World J Surg 2009;33(10):2150–4.

31. Santambrogio R, Aldrighetti L, Barabino M, et al. Laparoscopic liver resections for hepatocellular carcinoma. Is it a feasible option for patients with liver cirrhosis? Langenbecks Arch Surg 2009;394(2):255–64.

32. Sasaki A, Nitta H, Otsuka K, et al. Ten-year experience of totally laparoscopic liver resection in a single institution. Br J Surg 2009;96(3):274–9.

33. Cai XJ, Yang J, Yu H, et al. Clinical study of laparoscopic versus open hepatectomy for malignant liver tumors. Surg Endosc 2008;22(11):2350–6.

34. Dagher I, Lainas P, Carloni A, et al. Laparoscopic liver resection for hepatocellular carcinoma. Surg Endosc 2008;22(2):372–8.

35. Belli G, Fantini C, D'Agostino A, et al. Laparoscopic versus open liver resection for hepatocellular carcinoma in patients with histologically proven cirrhosis: short- and middle-term results. Surg Endosc 2007;21(11):2004–11.

36. Cherqui D, Laurent A, Tayar C, et al. Laparoscopic liver resection for peripheral hepatocellular carcinoma in patients with chronic liver disease: midterm results and perspectives. Ann Surg 2006;243(4):499–506.

37. Tang CN, Tsui KK, Ha JP, et al. A single-centre experience of 40 laparoscopic liver resections. Hong Kong Med J 2006;12(6):419–25.

38. Kaneko H, Takagi S, Otsuka Y, et al. Laparoscopic liver resection of hepatocellular carcinoma. Am J Surg 2005;189(2):190–4.

39. Teramoto K, Kawamura T, Takamatsu S, et al. Laparoscopic and thoracoscopic approaches for the treatment of hepatocellular carcinoma. Am J Surg 2005; 189(4):474–8.

40. Laurent A, Cherqui D, Lesurtel M, et al. Laparoscopic liver resection for subcapsular hepatocellular carcinoma complicating chronic liver disease. Arch Surg 2003;138(7):763–9.

41. Teramoto K, Kawamura T, Takamatsu S, et al. Laparoscopic and thoracoscopic partial hepatectomy for hepatocellular carcinoma. World J Surg 2003;27(10):1131–6.

42. Gigot JF, Glineur D, Santiago Azagra J, et al. Laparoscopic liver resection for malignant liver tumors: preliminary results of a multicenter European study. Ann Surg 2002;236(1):90–7.

43. Shimada M, Hashizume M, Maehara S, et al. Laparoscopic hepatectomy for hepatocellular carcinoma. Surg Endosc 2001;15(6):541–4.

44. Lai EC, Tang CN, Ha JP, et al. Laparoscopic liver resection for hepatocellular carcinoma: ten-year experience in a single center. Arch Surg 2009;144(2):143–7.

45. Sarpel U, Hefti MM, Wisnievsky JP, et al. Outcome for patients treated with laparoscopic versus open resection of hepatocellular carcinoma: case-matched analysis. Ann Surg Oncol 2009;16(6):1572–7.

46. Endo Y, Ohta M, Sasaki A, et al. A comparative study of the long-term outcomes after laparoscopy-assisted and open left lateral hepatectomy for hepatocellular carcinoma. Surg Laparosc Endosc Percutan Tech 2009;19(5):e171–4.

47. Tranchart H, Di Giuro G, Lainas P, et al. Laparoscopic resection for hepatocellular carcinoma: a matched-pair comparative study. Surg Endosc 2010;24(5):1170–6.

48. Laurent A, Tayar C, Andréoletti M, et al. Laparoscopic liver resection facilitates salvage liver transplantation for hepatocellular carcinoma. J Hepatobiliary Pancreat Surg 2009;16(3):310–4.

49. Mayo SC, Pawlik TM. Current management of colorectal hepatic metastasis. Expert Rev Gastroenterol Hepatol 2009;3(2):131–44.

50. Kazaryan AM, Pavlik Marangos I, Rosseland AR, et al. Laparoscopic liver resection for malignant and benign lesions: ten-year Norwegian single-center experience. Arch Surg 2010;145(1):34–40.

51. Castaing D, Vibert E, Ricca L, et al. Oncologic results of laparoscopic versus open hepatectomy for colorectal liver metastases in two specialized centers. Ann Surg 2009;250(5):849–55.

52. Ito K, Ito H, Are C, et al. Laparoscopic versus open liver resection: a matched-pair case control study. J Gastrointest Surg 2009;13(12):2276–83.

53. Robles R, Marín C, Abellán B, et al. A new approach to hand-assisted laparoscopic liver surgery. Surg Endosc 2008;22(11):2357–64.

54. Ito H, Are C, Gonen M, et al. Effect of postoperative morbidity on long-term survival after hepatic resection for metastatic colorectal cancer. Ann Surg 2008;247(6):994–1002.

55. Blazer DG 3rd, Kishi Y, Maru DM, et al. Pathologic response to preoperative chemotherapy: a new outcome end point after resection of hepatic colorectal metastases. J Clin Oncol 2008;26(33):5344–51.

56. Adam R, Wicherts DA, de Haas RJ, et al. Complete pathologic response after preoperative chemotherapy for colorectal liver metastases: myth or reality? J Clin Oncol 2008;26(10):1635–41.

57. Zakaria S, Donohue JH, Que FG, et al. Hepatic resection for colorectal metastases: value for risk scoring systems? Ann Surg 2007;246(2):183–91.

58. Lesurtel M, Cherqui D, Laurent A, et al. Laparoscopic versus open left lateral hepatic lobectomy: a case-control study. J Am Coll Surg 2003;196(2):236–42.
59. Buell JF, Thomas MJ, Doty TC, et al. An initial experience and evolution of laparoscopic hepatic resectional surgery. Surgery 2004;136(4):804–11.
60. Lee KF, Cheung YS, Chong CN, et al. Laparoscopic versus open hepatectomy for liver tumours: a case control study. Hong Kong Med J 2007;13(6):442–8.
61. Mamada Y, Yoshida H, Taniai N, et al. Usefulness of laparoscopic hepatectomy. J Nippon Med Sch 2007;74(2):158–62.
62. Abu Hilal M, McPhail MJ, Zeidan B, et al. Laparoscopic versus open left lateral hepatic sectionectomy: a comparative study. Eur J Surg Oncol 2008;34(12):1285–8.
63. Aldrighetti L, Pulitanò C, Catena M, et al. A prospective evaluation of laparoscopic versus open left lateral hepatic sectionectomy. J Gastrointest Surg 2008;12(3):457–62.
64. Polignano FM, Quyn AJ, de Figueiredo RS, et al. Laparoscopic versus open liver segmentectomy: prospective, case-matched, intention-to-treat analysis of clinical outcomes and cost effectiveness. Surg Endosc 2008;22(12):2564–70.
65. Dagher I, Di Giuro G, Dubrez J, et al. Laparoscopic versus open right hepatectomy: a comparative study. Am J Surg 2009;198(2):173–7.
66. Rowe AJ, Meneghetti AT, Schumacher PA, et al. Perioperative analysis of laparoscopic versus open liver resection. Surg Endosc 2009;23(6):1198–203.
67. Tsinberg M, Tellioglu G, Simpfendorfer CH, et al. Comparison of laparoscopic versus open liver tumor resection: a case-controlled study. Surg Endosc 2009; 23(4):847–53.
68. Mala T, Edwin B, Gladhaug I, et al. A comparative study of the short-term outcome following open and laparoscopic liver resection of colorectal metastases. Surg Endosc 2002;16(7):1059–63.
69. Farges O, Jagot P, Kirstetter P, et al. Prospective assessment of the safety and benefit of laparoscopic liver resections. J Hepatobiliary Pancreat Surg 2002; 9(2):242–8.
70. Tang CN, Tai CK, Ha JP, et al. Laparoscopy versus open left lateral segmentectomy for recurrent pyogenic cholangitis. Surg Endosc 2005;19(9):1232–6.
71. Rau HG, Buttler E, Meyer G, et al. Laparoscopic liver resection compared with conventional partial hepatectomy–a prospective analysis. Hepatogastroenterology 1998;45(24):2333–8.
72. Morino M, Morra I, Rosso E, et al. Laparoscopic vs open hepatic resection: a comparative study. Surg Endosc 2003;17(12):1914–8.
73. Troisi R, Montalti R, Smeets P, et al. The value of laparoscopic liver surgery for solid benign hepatic tumors. Surg Endosc 2008;22(1):38–44.
74. Vanounou T, Steel J, Nguyen KT, et al. Comparing the clinical and economic impact of laparoscopic versus open liver resection. Ann Surg Oncol 2010; 17(4):998–1009.

Robotic Liver Surgery

Kamran Idrees, MD, David L. Bartlett, MD*

KEYWORDS

• Robotic • Liver • Resection • Hepaticojejunostomy • Surgery

The introduction of minimally invasive techniques has dramatically transformed surgery in the past 2 decades. This approach is shown to be beneficial in reducing the length of hospital stay, improving cosmetic results, and decreasing postoperative pain in all the surgical specialties compared with conventional open operations.[1–3] These advanced minimally invasive procedures require surgeons to have highly developed laparoscopic skills, including suturing, knot tying, and complex bimanual manipulation. However, conventional laparoscopic surgery has its own limitations, including reduced freedom of movement within the abdominal cavity and 2-dimensional view of a 3-dimensional operative field. In addition, the laparoscopic instruments provide surgeons with reduced precision and poor ergonomics.[4–6] These limitations translate into a significant learning curve, requiring a lot of time and effort to develop and maintain such advanced laparoscopic skills.[6,7] These shortcomings of laparoscopic surgery were the impetus behind the development of robotic surgery.

Robotic surgery allows surgeons to perform advanced laparoscopic procedures with greater ease. Similar to a human hand, the robotic articulating laparoscopic instruments translate the natural movements of the surgeon's hand into precise movements inside the abdominal cavity. The 3-dimensional view of the operative field along with 7° of freedom and tremor filtration allows the surgeon with wristlike dexterity to perform delicate dissection and precise intracorporeal suturing. These significant advantages of robotic surgery have expanded the scope of surgical procedures that can be performed through minimally invasive techniques.

Liver surgery was nonexistent in the beginning of the twentieth century because of the high propensity for bleeding and inherent friability of the liver. The improved understanding of liver anatomy and knowledge of its regenerative capability set the stage for the development of liver surgery in the middle of the twentieth century. Subsequent advancements in anesthesia, critical care, transfusion medicine, postoperative care, and enhanced diagnostic imaging by computed tomography and magnetic resonance imaging scans have transformed liver surgery to be performed routinely with reduced morbidity and mortality by the end of the last century. The technological advancements in the liver parenchymal transection techniques with the help of precoagulating

Division of Surgical Oncology, Department of Surgery, University of Pittsburgh Medical Center Cancer Pavilion, 5150 Centre Avenue, Suite 414, Pittsburgh, PA, USA
* Corresponding author.
E-mail address: bartdl@upmc.edu

Surg Clin N Am 90 (2010) 761–774
doi:10.1016/j.suc.2010.04.020   surgical.theclinics.com
0039-6109/10/$ – see front matter © 2010 Elsevier Inc. All rights reserved.

devices, ultrasonic aspiration dissector, improved surface coagulators along with improved patient selection, and radiographic staging have paved the way for laparoscopic liver surgery. Laparoscopic liver surgery is increasingly being performed over the past several years, although it was more slowly embraced than the minimally invasive surgery revolution in gastrointestinal surgery.[8–13] Laparoscopic liver surgery offers the same universal benefits of minimally invasive surgery, such as better cosmesis, reduced duration of hospitalization, and less postoperative pain.[14–16] The technique has been shown to be as safe and feasible in experienced hands. However, the restrictive movement of laparoscopic instruments, limited by fixed pivot point with only 4° of freedom and 2-dimensional view, limits its utility in hepatobiliary surgery with a complex repertoire of operations. Robotic surgery was developed to address some of these inherent limitations of laparoscopic surgery and in this article the authors' preview the potential scope of robotics in hepatobiliary surgery.

ADVANTAGES AND DISADVANTAGES OF ROBOTIC SURGERY

The da Vinci Surgical System (Intuitive Surgical, Inc, Sunnyvale, CA, USA) is the only commercially available therapeutic robotic system in the market, which was approved by the US Food and Drug Administration for use in surgery. The system is being used in various surgical subspecialties, including urology, gynecology, and colorectal and cardiothoracic surgery. The robotic surgical platform has several pros and cons (**Table 1**). The system provides more fluid movement because of tremor filtration, scaling of the movements, and articulating instruments with 7° of freedom, which results in increased dexterity to perform delicate dissection and precise intracorporeal suturing. This additional dexterity provided by wristed instruments is also of paramount importance in complex surgical procedures in difficult anatomic locations (**Fig. 1**). The 3-dimensional stereoscopic view with adjustable magnification provides superior visualization compared with standard laparoscopy and open surgery. The camera is on a stable camera platform and directly controlled by the surgeon, eliminating the need for an assistant to hold the video camera. The comfortable seated operating posture reduces fatigue and physical stress on the surgeon as compared with conventional laparoscopy, which often requires the surgeon to assume unnatural postures (**Fig. 2**). The coaxial alignment of eyes, hands, and tool tip images along with intuitive translation of the instrument handle to the tip movement not only eliminates mirror-image effect but also improves hand-eye coordination. The surgical robots are, however, not without their own disadvantages. These systems are costly; are bulky, requiring a lot of operating room space and an inefficient switch of instruments; have limited trocar placement options, making it difficult to switch operative fields during a procedure; and most importantly lack tactile feedback.[17–19] Acquisition

Table 1	
Pros and cons of robotic surgery	
Pros	**Cons**
• Advanced technology	• Expense
• Complex movements	• Learning curve
• Improved visibility	• Increased duration of case
• Better camera control	• Lack of tactile feedback
• Enhanced suturing capability	• Need for skilled assistant
• Future improvements in technology	• Difficult conversion to open

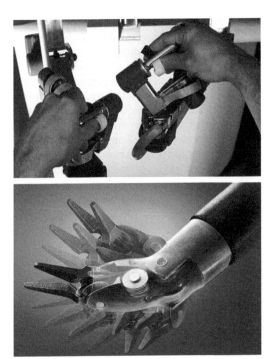

Fig. 1. The hand controls for the da Vinci system and the degrees of movement of the robotic instruments are demonstrated here. (*Courtesy of* Intuitive Surgical, Inc, Sunnyvale, CA, USA; with permission.)

and annual maintenance of these surgical robots is an expensive proposition. Operating times are greatly increased if the operative field is switched during the procedure, requiring patient repositioning, moving, and redocking of the robot. The absence of tactile feedback can result in tissue injury as well as breaking of suture.

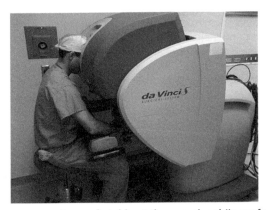

Fig. 2. The primary surgeon sits comfortably at the console while performing the robotic surgery.

Many surgeons attempt to assess or question the advantages of robotic surgery over straight laparoscopic surgery. Although patient outcome is improved with a minimally invasive approach, the use of a robot does not provide incremental improvement over straight laparoscopy for most procedures. Many skilled laparoscopists can perform complex suturing and complex procedures without the aid of the robot. However, the lesson learned from the prostate experience is that the use of a robot leads to an easier and faster sutured urethral anastomosis and more surgeons can perform this anastomosis safer and faster robotically than with straight laparoscopy.[20,21] The robot should be looked at as a new advanced tool to improve the minimally invasive approach for complex procedures such as liver resections.

ROBOTIC LIVER RESECTION

Technological advancement and improvement in laparoscopy have resulted in exponential increase in the number of laparoscopic liver resections across the world in the past few years.[8–13] Improved cosmetic results, shorter hospitalization, and less postoperative pain are compelling reasons to perform minimally invasive liver resection, especially for benign hepatic lesions. An international consensus conference was convened to evaluate the status of laparoscopic liver surgery.[22] According to this consensus report, the best indications for laparoscopic liver resection were solitary lesions, 5 cm or less, located in the peripheral liver segments (segments 2–6), whereas lesions adjacent to major vessels or near the liver hilum were not considered suitable for laparoscopic liver resection because of the potential risk of massive bleeding and the potential need for biliary reconstruction. Malignant tumors (colorectal liver metastases and hepatocellular carcinoma [HCC]) are not a contraindication to minimally invasive resection as demonstrated in various comparative studies, as long as there is no compromise in the oncologic integrity of the procedure. Although robotic liver surgery was not discussed in the consensus conference manuscript, the same rules can be applied to the technique as long as patient safety and oncologic results are not compromised.

Robotic liver surgery will broaden the scope of minimally invasive liver surgery by overcoming some of the limitations of conventional laparoscopy, including the difficulty to suture bleeding hepatic parenchyma laparoscopically, to perform complex hilar dissections, and to perform liver resections requiring biliary-enteric reconstructions, and by minimizing the learning curve for these complex procedures. One of the major concerns of laparoscopic liver resection is major bleeding from vascular structures within the parenchyma. This fear of uncontrolled bleeding has deterred liver surgeons from performing major liver resections using a minimally invasive technique. Several features of the da Vinci robot are extremely useful in controlling and definitely managing bleeding without conversion to an open surgery. These features include the use of 3 robotic arms by the same operating surgeon with use of articulating instruments to be locked in place as vascular clamps with the ability to perform intracorporeal suturing and tying in difficult locations. The capability of locking the articulating instruments in place as a substitute for vascular clamp is invaluable because it gives the anesthesia team time to resuscitate the patient and the surgical team to formulate a plan to manage the situation. The da Vinci surgical robot was used to repair a large vena caval tear after a staple misfire during a robot-assisted liver resection.[23]

With an increase in the incidence of HCC as a result of hepatitis C and the nonalcoholic steatohepatitis epidemic, more patients will benefit from minimally invasive surgical resection because of limited availability of liver allografts.[22] Minimally invasive liver surgery, which results in less postoperative adhesions making subsequent dissection relatively easy, is especially useful in patients with HCC who may require repetitive surgery or future transplantation. Two case series have shown the feasibility of robot-assisted left lateral hepatic segmentectomies.[24,25] As surgeons' experience with robotics improves, major hepatectomies will be more commonplace at busy liver centers. The delicate dissection that can be performed with the robotic platform to achieve inflow and outflow control and safe parenchymal transection will be recognized as a distinct advantage over laparoscopic instruments for major liver resections. Although robotic liver surgery is in its infancy, the advantages offered by surgical robots will undoubtedly expand its use for this purpose in the future.

ROBOTIC BILIARY-ENTERIC RECONSTRUCTION

The precision, steadiness, and manual dexterity conferred by robotic surgery make it ideal for biliary dissection and biliary-enteric anastomosis. Hence, the technique can be used for a multitude of benign conditions including choledochal cyst excision, benign common bile duct strictures, and biliary atresia.[26–28] One can not only perform fine dissection within the portal triad but also carry out intricate suturing required for the Roux-en-Y bilioenteric anastomosis. The anastomosis has to be performed meticulously so as to not compromise the anastomotic integrity and to avoid any technical errors that result in anastomotic stricture formation from improper suturing or vascular compromise. Several case reports and series have been published reporting the safety and feasibility of robotic biliary surgery in adults as well as in pediatric population for choledochal cyst disease and biliary atresia. Successful accomplishment of cyst excision along with biliary-enteric anastomosis and Kasai portoenterostomy has been reported in these studies.[26–28] Despite the fact that the first laparoscopic choledochal cyst excision with Roux-en-Y hepaticojejunostomy was performed in 1995, these procedures are still not routinely performed, which is an attestation to the fact that although these complex biliary procedures can be performed with conventional laparoscopic technique they are extremely difficult and challenging.[29] This disadvantage is secondary to the restrictive movement of laparoscopic instruments, combined with the fulcrum effect of laparoscopy, poor ergonomics, and compromised dexterity.

Robotic surgery overcomes all these shortcomings of conventional laparoscopy. Another advantage of performing these procedures through a minimally invasive technique as opposed to an open surgery is less postoperative adhesions, making subsequent surgery such as liver transplantation after failed Kasai procedure possibly easier. Robotic surgery does have its own set of disadvantages as discussed earlier, including the lack of tactile sensation, which makes it difficult for the surgeon to gauge the tension while manipulating and maneuvering tissue or suture.

COMBINED ROBOT-ASSISTED LIVER AND COLORECTAL RESECTION

Liver metastases are diagnosed simultaneously in 15% to 20% of newly diagnosed colorectal cancers.[30–32] Simultaneous colorectal and liver resection is performed at specialized institutes with low morbidity and mortality in carefully selected patients. This approach has shown to be advantageous in terms of oncologic outcomes, quality of life, as well as cost-effectiveness.[33,34] Laparoscopic colorectal surgery is being increasingly performed ever since adequacy of oncologic resections has been found to be similar in several large prospective randomized trials.[35,36] Based on comparable oncologic results and added advantages of improved visualization, enhanced dexterity, and great ergonomics, robotic surgery is being used more often in colorectal cancer, especially in rectal surgery. Wristed articulating instruments with a 3-dimensional view along with 7° of freedom provides increased maneuverability in anatomically challenging locations such as a narrow male pelvis and infradiaphragmatic hepatic vein isolation. Another benefit of robotic surgery is the ability to accurately suture intracorporeally to ligate bleeding vessels or to reinforce staple line in the pelvis. This minimally invasive approach has the potential advantage of improved early outcome after a major operation and thus allows for early administration of adjuvant chemotherapy. A pilot study has been performed demonstrating the safety and feasibility of robot-assisted simultaneous liver and colorectal resection.[37]

ROBOTIC HEPATIC ARTERY INFUSION PUMP PLACEMENT

Liver is the most common site of metastasis for colorectal cancer, and 60% of patients with colorectal cancer eventually develop hepatic metastases.[30,31] Together, HCC and intrahepatic cholangiocarcinoma account for most primary liver cancers.[38,39] Surgical resection is the most effective therapy for colorectal liver metastases as well as primary liver cancers; however, only a subset of patients are candidates for curative resection. Unlike systemic chemotherapy for colorectal metastases, the results of systemic therapy for primary liver cancers are disappointing.[40–42] Liver-directed therapy with the help of a surgically implanted hepatic arterial infusion pump provides an attractive option because it is not limited by tumor size, location, multifocality, or proximity to vascular structures, and higher doses can be given with little systemic side effects.[43] Hepatic artery infusion (HAI) therapy has been shown to be effective and safe for unresectable, isolated colorectal liver metastases and primary liver cancers.[44–46] However, the need for an open operation through a midline or subcostal incision and the associated surgical morbidity are the major disadvantages with HAI pump placement. This weakness can be circumvented with robotic placement of the infusion pump.

HAI pump has been placed successfully with laparoscopic techniques but requires a high level of laparoscopic skills.[47,48] The use of long instruments with amplification of hand tremor, only 4° of motion, and a 2-dimensional operative field view makes the required meticulous dissection of the hepatic artery demanding and difficult. Advancement of the catheter in the gastroduodenal artery is especially challenging because of the fulcrum effect. The robotic platform imparts improved depth perception secondary to magnified 3-dimensional view, negated hand tremor, and enhanced manual dexterity, giving the surgeon an unparalleled level of precision and control to perform dissection with finesse. Accurate arteriotomy and intracorporeal suturing are key components of this procedure as well as for advancement of the cannula through the arteriotomy and have been successfully performed and reported.[49]

UNIVERSITY-OF-PITTSBURGH EXPERIENCE WITH ROBOTIC LIVER SURGERY

Since 2007, we have been performing complex surgical oncology procedures with the robot. Our experience now includes more than 150 procedures, including liver resections, bile duct resections, pancreaticoduodenectomies, distal pancreatectomies, total and partial gastrectomies, adrenalectomies, colectomies, low anterior resections, abdominoperineal resections, oophorectomies, hysterectomies, and retroperitoneal tumor resections. Although these procedures are also performed with straight laparoscopy, we prefer the robotic instruments, especially when complex suturing is required or when visibility is difficult, such as with the deep pelvis. The lack of tactile feedback is not a significant drawback because the visual cues are extremely strong, but the most significant disadvantages are the setup time and the need for a skilled assistant at the table.

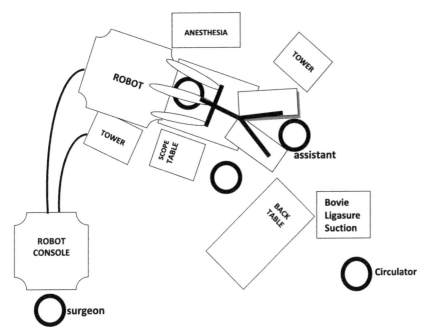

Fig. 3. The operating room schematic for liver surgery.

We have performed 15 liver resections (including 1 right hepatic lobectomy, 1 caudate lobectomy, left lateral sectionectomies, complex segmentectomies, and wedge excisions), more than 30 hepaticojejunostomies, and 3 hepatic arterial infusion pump implants. The patient is positioned supine on a split-leg table, with the table in

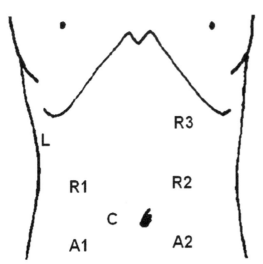

Fig. 4. The recommended port site location for hepatic resections. These ports can be rotated to the patient's right for right-sided wedge resections. A, assistant ports; C, camera ports; L, optional liver retractor; R, robotic ports.

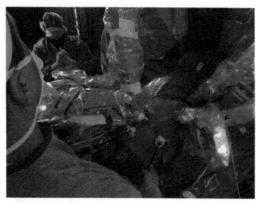

Fig. 5. Assistant surgeon standing between the patient's legs and using the assistant ports during the operation.

reverse Trendelenburg position. It is helpful to have the table, robotic arms, anesthesia, and nursing carefully arranged from the beginning to avoid delays while docking. A typical operating room setup is demonstrated in **Fig. 3**.

The patient is first explored laparoscopically, and ultrasonography of the liver is performed to ensure the feasibility of resection. Three robotic arm ports and a camera port are inserted as demonstrated in **Fig. 4**. The assistant ports are placed inferiorly, and the assistant stands between the split legs (**Fig. 5**). An additional liver retractor port can be placed if needed. The ports can be rotated depending on the location of the resection. We generally perform the liver mobilization and division of the triangular ligament and peritoneal attachments laparoscopically, which sometimes requires movement of the camera port higher in the abdomen and this flexibility is better performed laparoscopically. The need for a hand assist is not necessary, but the tumor margins must be carefully outlined and constantly reexamined with the intraoperative ultrasound.

The robot is then brought to the field and docked. The portal dissection can be performed using the hook cautery, a Maryland dissector, and standard grasping

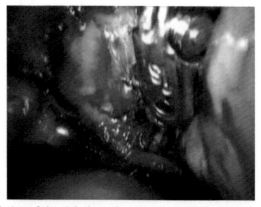

Fig. 6. Robotic isolation of the right hepatic artery in the porta hepatis using the Maryland dissector.

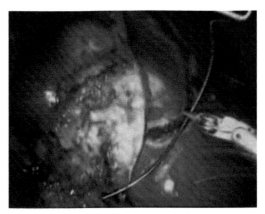

Fig. 7. Robotic placement of large chromic retracting sutures.

instruments (**Fig. 6**). We use a combination of robotic monopolar cautery, bipolar cautery, and a cauterizing dissecting device handled by the assistant surgeon. The main portal vein branches are divided with the endovascular stapler, and robotic locking clips are used for the artery and bile ducts. These can easily be reinforced with silk ties or sutures. The hepatic veins can be dissected extrahepatically or intrahepatically. We have performed both procedures and found that, as with open liver resection, each case has different issues that need to be considered. We use large chromic sutures through the liver for retraction (**Fig. 7**). These sutures can be held by the robot's third arm and greatly aid in the parenchymal dissection by opening the dissection plane. The capsule of the liver is divided with the hook cautery, and parenchymal dissection is accomplished using a crush technique with robotic dissectors (**Figs. 8** and **9**). Small vessels are controlled with bipolar cautery, whereas larger vessels are isolated and clipped, tied, or sutured. Large pedicles or hepatic veins are carefully isolated using robotic dissection, then stapled with an endovascular stapler through the assistant port. It is helpful to have silk and Prolene sutures loaded and ready to pass, in case of bleeding during the parenchymal dissection. The enhanced range of motion achieved with the robotic instruments allow for easy suturing and tying within the parenchyma.

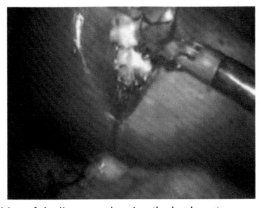

Fig. 8. Robotic incision of the liver capsule using the hook cautery.

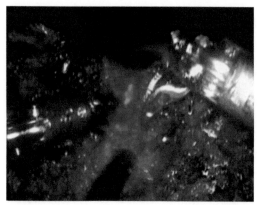

Fig. 9. Robotic parenchymal dissection using a crush technique with the Maryland dissector and bipolar cautery. The assistant uses the suction to keep the field dry.

For hepaticojejunostomies, we generally perform the Roux-en-Y anastomosis laparoscopically and place the end of the jejunum through the transverse colon mesentery before docking the robot. This operation can be performed quickly and easily laparoscopically using stapling devices without the need for suturing. The robot is then

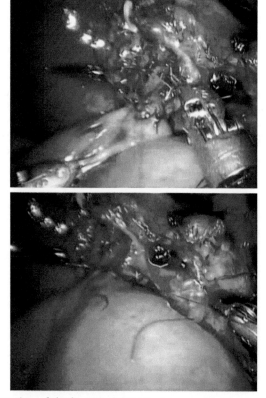

Fig. 10. Robotic suturing of the hepaticojejunostomy.

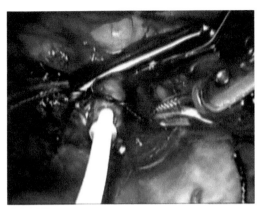

Fig. 11. Robotic placement of the hepatic arterial catheter connected to an infusion pump.

docked and the resection performed. The anastomosis is performed as we do open procedures, with a running posterior layer and an interrupted anterior layer (**Fig. 10**). Corner stitches are placed first and can be held by the third robotic arm for improved visualization. The time efficiency of this anastomosis greatly depends on the skill of the assistant and operating room technician in passing and cutting suture. The hepatic arterial pump insertions are performed exactly as for open procedures. We use small vascular clamps that can be placed with laparoscopic instruments and adjusted with the robotic instruments. Advancing the pump catheter using the robotic arms is much easier than in the straight laparoscopic approach, as is tying the holding sutures around the catheter and vessel (**Fig. 11**).

SUMMARY

Surgery of the liver has progressed tremendously because of a clearer understanding of its functional anatomy, improved knowledge of its regenerative capability, and its functional reserve. Better patient staging and selection, as a result of significant advances in imaging technology, have had a profound effect on the safety of major hepatic resection. Improved techniques to achieve vascular control and technological advancements have facilitated parenchymal transection, resulting in decreased mortality and morbidity from liver surgery. All of this knowledge and technology has been used to extend the scope of liver surgery to incorporate minimally invasive techniques (laparoscopic and robotic) to practically all types of hepatic resections. In addition to the advantages of laparoscopic liver surgery, robotic surgery offers improved visualization and enhanced functionality and maneuverability, thus extending the horizon of minimally invasive liver surgery. The development of new sophisticated surgical robots that are smaller, cheaper, more streamlined, and with tactile feedback, will make robotic surgery more common and popular for these kinds of complex procedures.

In the beginning of the twentieth century, fear of uncontrollable bleeding and friability of the liver parenchyma made the surgeons shy away from open liver surgery; the very same reasons are the grounds for surgeons' hesitance to perform minimally invasive surgery on the liver today. Liver surgery has advanced remarkably and will continue to do so. As in the words of Fortner and Blumgart[50] "It is well to remember that, in the 19th century, surgery was thought to have reached its apogee – but the best is yet to come."

REFERENCES

1. Jones DB, Provost DA, DeMaria EJ, et al. Optimal management of the morbidly obese patient. SAGES appropriateness conference statement. Surg Endosc 2004;18(7):1029–37.
2. Katkhouda N, Mason RJ, Towfigh S, et al. Laparoscopic versus open appendectomy: a prospective randomized double-blinded study. Ann Surg 2005;242(3): 439–48.
3. Hewett PJ, Allardyce RA, Bagshaw PF, et al. Short-term outcomes of the Australian randomized clinical study comparing laparoscopic and conventional open surgical treatments for colon cancer: the ALCCaS trial. Ann Surg 2008;248(5): 728–38.
4. Cadiere GB, Himpens J, Germay O, et al. Feasibility of robotic laparoscopic surgery: 146 cases. World J Surg 2001;25(11):1467–77.
5. Berguer R, Rab GT, Abu-Ghaida H, et al. A comparison of surgeon's posture during laparoscopic and open surgical procedures. Surg Endosc 1997;11(2): 139–42.
6. Ballantyne GH. The pitfalls of laparoscopic surgery: challenges for robotics and telerobotic surgery. Surg Laparosc Endosc Percutan Tech 2002;12(1):1–5.
7. Cusick RA, Waldhausen JH. The learning curve associated with pediatric laparoscopic splenectomy. Am J Surg 2001;181(5):393–7.
8. Koffron AJ, Auffenberg G, Kung R, et al. Evaluation of 300 minimally invasive liver resections at a single institution: less is more. Ann Surg 2007;246(3):385–92.
9. Gamblin TC, Holloway SE, Heckman JT, et al. Laparoscopic resection of benign hepatic cysts: a new standard. J Am Coll Surg 2008;207(5):731–6.
10. Gayet B, Cavaliere D, Vibert E, et al. Totally laparoscopic right hepatectomy. Am J Surg 2007;194(5):685–9.
11. O'Rourke N, Fielding G. Laparoscopic right hepatectomy: surgical technique. J Gastrointest Surg 2004;8(2):213–6.
12. Nguyen KT, Gamblin TC, Geller DA. World review of laparoscopic liver resection-2,804 patients. Ann Surg 2009;250(5):831–41.
13. Dagher I, O'Rourke N, Geller DA, et al. Laparoscopic major hepatectomy: an evolution in standard of care. Ann Surg 2009;250(5):856–60.
14. Farges O, Jagot P, Kirstetter P, et al. Prospective assessment of the safety and benefit of laparoscopic liver resections. J Hepatobiliary Pancreat Surg 2002; 9(2):242–8.
15. Huscher CG, Lirici MM, Chiodini S. Laparoscopic liver resections. Semin Laparosc Surg 1998;5(3):204–10.
16. Lesurtel M, Cherqui D, Laurent A, et al. Laparoscopic versus open left lateral hepatic lobectomy: a case-control study. J Am Coll Surg 2003; 196(2):236–42.
17. Hanley EJ, Talamini MA. Robotic abdominal surgery. Am J Surg 2004;188: 19S–26.
18. Delaney CP, Lynch AC, Senagore AJ, et al. Comparison of robotically performed and traditional laparoscopic colorectal surgery. Dis Colon Rectum 2003;46(12): 1633–9.
19. Anvari M, Birch DW, Bamehriz F, et al. Robotic-assisted laparoscopic colorectal surgery. Surg Laparosc Endosc Percutan Tech 2004;14(6):311–5.
20. Ahlering TE, Skarecky D, Lee D, et al. Successful transfer of open surgical skills to a laparoscopic environment using a robotic interface: initial experience with laparoscopic radical prostatectomy. J Urol 2003;170(5):1738–41.

21. Berryhill R Jr, Jhaveri J, Yadav R, et al. Robotic prostatectomy: a review of outcomes compared with laparoscopic and open approaches. Urology 2008; 72(1):15–23.
22. Buell JF, Cherqui D, Geller DA, et al. The international position on laparoscopic liver surgery: the Louisville statement, 2008. Ann Surg 2009;250(5):825–30.
23. Boggi U, Moretto C, Vistoli F, et al. Robotic suture of a large caval injury caused by endo-GIA stapler malfunction during laparoscopic wedge resection of liver segments VII and VIII en-bloc with the right hepatic vein. Minim Invasive Ther Allied Technol 2009;1:1–5.
24. Choi SB, Park JS, Kim JK, et al. Early experiences of robotic-assisted laparoscopic liver resection. Yonsei Med J 2008;49(4):632–8.
25. Vasile S, Sgarbură O, Tomulescu V, et al. The robotic-assisted left lateral hepatic segmentectomy: the next step. Chirurgia 2008;103(4):401–5.
26. Kang CM, Chi HS, Kim JY, et al. A case of robot-assisted excision of choledochal cyst, hepaticojejunostomy, and extracorporeal Roux-en-y anastomosis using the da Vinci surgical system. Surg Laparosc Endosc Percutan Tech 2007;17(6): 538–41.
27. Meehan JJ, Elliott S, Sandler A. The robotic approach to complex hepatobiliary anomalies in children: preliminary report. J Pediatr Surg 2007;42(12):2110–4.
28. Woo R, Le D, Albanese CT, et al. Robot-assisted laparoscopic resection of a type I choledochal cyst in a child. J Laparoendosc Adv Surg Tech A 2006;16(2): 179–83.
29. Farello GA, Cerofolini A, Rebonato M, et al. Congenital choledochal cyst: video-guided laparoscopic treatment. Surg Laparosc Endosc 1995;5(5):354–8.
30. Weiss L, Grandmann E, Torhost J, et al. Hematogenous metastatic patterns in colonic carcinoma: an analysis of 1541 necropsies. J Pathol 1986;150(3): 195–203.
31. Fong YC, Fortner AM, Enker JG, et al. Liver resection for colorectal metastases. J Clin Oncol 1997;15(3):938–46.
32. Nordlinger B, Guiguet M, Vaillant JC, et al. Surgical resection of colorectal carcinoma metastases to the liver. A prognostic scoring system to improve case selection, based on 1568 patients. Association Francaise de Chirurgie. Cancer 1996; 77(7):1254–62.
33. Adam R. Colorectal cancer with synchronous liver metastases. Br J Surg 2007; 94(2):129–31.
34. Capussotti L, Ferrero A, Vigano L, et al. Major liver resections synchronous with colorectal surgery. Ann Surg Oncol 2007;14(1):195–201.
35. The Clinical Outcomes of Surgical Therapy Study Group. A comparison of laparoscopically assisted and open colectomy for colon cancer. N Engl J Med 2004; 350(20):2050–9.
36. Jayne DG, Guillou PJ, Thorpe H, et al. Randomized trial of laparoscopic-assisted resection of colorectal carcinoma: 3-year results of the UK MRC CLASICC Trial Group. J Clin Oncol 2007;25(21):3061–8.
37. Patriti A, Ceccarelli G, Bartoli A, et al. Laparoscopic and robot-assisted one-stage resection of colorectal cancer with synchronous liver metastases: a pilot study. J Hepatobiliary Pancreat Surg 2009;16(4):450–7.
38. Endo I, Gonen M, Yopp AC, et al. Intrahepatic cholangiocarcinoma: rising frequency, improved survival, and determinants of outcome after resection. Ann Surg 2008;248(1):1–13.
39. Fong Y, Sun RL, Jarnagin W, et al. An analysis of 412 cases of hepatocellular carcinoma at a Western center. Ann Surg 1999;229(6):790–9.

40. Knox JJ, Hedley D, Oza A, et al. Combining gemcitabine and capecitabine in patients with advanced biliary cancer: a phase II trial. J Clin Oncol 2005; 23(10):2332–8.
41. Andre T, Tournigand C, Rosmorduc O, et al. Gemcitabine combined with oxaliplatin (GEMOX) in advanced biliary tract adenocarcinoma: a GERCOR study. Ann Oncol 2004;15(9):1339–43.
42. Abou-Alfa GK, Schwartz L, Ricci S, et al. Phase II study of sorafenib in patients with advanced hepatocellular carcinoma. J Clin Oncol 2006;24(26):4293–300.
43. Ong ES, Poirier M, Espat NJ. Hepatic intra-arterial chemotherapy. Ann Surg Oncol 2006;13(2):142–9.
44. Kemeny N, Huang Y, Cohen AM, et al. Hepatic arterial infusion of chemotherapy after resection of hepatic metastases from colorectal cancer. N Engl J Med 1999; 341(27):2039–48.
45. Kemeny MM, Adak S, Gray B, et al. Combined-modality treatment for resectable metastatic colorectal carcinoma to the liver: surgical resection of hepatic metastases in combination with continuous infusion of chemotherapy, an intergroup study. J Clin Oncol 2002;20(6):1499–505.
46. Jarnagin WR, Schwartz LH, Gultekin DH, et al. Regional chemotherapy for unresectable primary liver cancer: results of a phase II clinical trial and assessment of DCE-MRI as a biomarker of survival. Ann Oncol 2009;20(9):1589–95.
47. Urbach DR, Herron DM, Khajanchee YS, et al. Laparoscopic hepatic artery infusion pump placement. Arch Surg 2001;136(6):700–4.
48. Franklin ME Jr, Gonzalez JJ Jr. Laparoscopic placement of hepatic artery catheter for regional chemotherapy infusion: technique, benefits, and complications. Surg Laparosc Endosc Percutan Tech 2002;12(6):398–407.
49. Hellan M, Pigazzi A. Robotic-assisted placement of a hepatic artery infusion catheter for regional chemotherapy. Surg Endosc 2008;22(2):548–51.
50. Fortner JG, Blumgart LH. A historic perspective of liver surgery for tumors at the end of the millennium. J Am Coll Surg 2001;193(2):210–22.

Current Management of Hepatic Trauma

Greta L. Piper, MD[a], Andrew B. Peitzman, MD[b],*

KEYWORDS

- Hepatic trauma • Liver resection • Trauma • Liver injury
- Operative techniques

The liver is the most commonly injured abdominal organ. With the sweeping shift toward nonoperative management, most hepatic injuries are successfully observed.[1–9] In addition, the mortality from hepatic injury has declined over the past several decades. Richardson and colleagues[8] proposed that the major reasons for the decrease in mortality for hepatic trauma over the past 25 years are: improved results with packing and reoperation, use of arteriography and embolization, advances in operative techniques for major hepatic injuries, and decrease in the number of hepatic venous injuries undergoing surgery. Patients with blunt hepatic injury tend to present either hemodynamically stable and can be observed, or hemodynamically unstable, requiring urgent laparotomy to control hemorrhage from a major hepatic injury. Because most injuries to the liver are minor (grade I or II), most blunt hepatic injuries can be safely observed (**Table 1**).[10] On the other hand, as many as two-thirds of higher-grade hepatic injuries (grades III, IV, V) may require laparotomy for control of hemorrhage.[2–4,7,11,12] Even at busy trauma centers, high-grade hepatic injuries, particularly juxtahepatic venous injuries, are uncommon. Thus, operations required for liver injury can be challenging in decision making and operative technique.

MECHANISM OF INJURY AND ANATOMIC CONSIDERATIONS

The liver is suspended by superior attachments to the diaphragm, and anterior attachments of the coronary ligaments, triangular ligaments, and the falciform ligament. It is also attached to the lesser curve of the stomach.[13] Deceleration injuries result in tears at these sites of fixation. A common deceleration injury creates a fracture between the posterior segments and the anterior segments of the right lobe. A crushing mechanism or a focused blunt injury to the right upper quadrant compresses the ribs into the liver causing a stellate-type laceration across the dome and anterior surface of the right lobe, often termed a "bear-claw injury." Anterior-posterior forces can produce

[a] Department of Surgery, University of Pittsburgh, F-1265, UPMC-Presbyterian, Pittsburgh, PA 15213, USA
[b] Department of Surgery, University of Pittsburgh, F-1281, UPMC-Presbyterian, Pittsburgh, PA 15213, USA
* Corresponding author.
E-mail address: peitzmanab@upmc.edu

Surg Clin N Am 90 (2010) 775–785
doi:10.1016/j.suc.2010.04.009
0039-6109/10/$ – see front matter © 2010 Elsevier Inc. All rights reserved.

surgical.theclinics.com

Table 1
Liver organ injury scale

Grade		Description
I	Hematoma	Subcapsular, <10% surface area
	Laceration	Capsular tear, <1 cm parenchymal depth
II	Hematoma	Subcapsular, 10%–50% surface area; intraparenchymal, <10 cm in diameter
	Laceration	1–3 cm parenchymal depth, <10 cm in length
III	Hematoma	Subcapsular, >50% surface area or expanding; ruptured subcapsular or parenchymal hematoma
	Laceration	>3 cm parenchymal depth
IV	Hematoma	Parenchymal disruption involving 25%–75% of hepatic lobe or 1–3 Couinaud segments within a single lobe
V	Laceration	Parenchymal disruption involving >75% of hepatic lobe or >3 Couinaud segments within a single lobe
	Vascular	Juxtahepatic venous injuries; ie, retrohepatic vena cava/central major hepatic vein
VI		Hepatic avulsion

Data from Moore EE, Shackford SR, Pachter HL. Organ injury scaling: spleen, liver and kidney. J Trauma 1995;38:323–4.

a split-liver, often through the line of Cantlie. In general, blunt trauma more commonly affects the right hepatic lobe.

INITIAL PRESENTATION AND ASSESSMENT

Patients with abdominal trauma who are unstable at presentation or become unstable in the trauma bay despite resuscitative efforts should be taken immediately to the operating room for laparotomy. In contrast, the stable patient should undergo a rapid physical examination and portable chest radiography. Although outward signs of injury are nonspecific and the absence of such findings do not exclude injury, seatbelt signs or other marks, regions of tenderness, and obvious penetrating wounds must be noted. Patients with a seatbelt sign have a 3.1-fold higher incidence of liver injury than those patients presenting without a seatbelt sign.[14] Right-sided rib fractures or pulmonary contusion should also raise suspicion for hepatic injury.

The focused assessment by ultrasound for trauma (FAST) has become a routine diagnostic tool in the trauma bay. The hemodynamically unstable patient with a positive FAST is transported immediately to the operating room for laparotomy.

Diagnostic peritoneal lavage (DPL) is a sensitive but nonspecific study that can be performed rapidly in the trauma bay or in the operating room. An unstable patient who has sustained blunt abdominal trauma belongs in the operating room. However, in the patient with blunt injury with another reason for hypotension, pelvic fracture, or a significant extremity fracture, DPL can accurately identify significant intraabdominal injuries.[15] DPL has 98.5% accuracy for detection of hemoperitoneum.[16]

Computerized tomography (CT) is the standard diagnostic modality for stable trauma patients with a suspected abdominal injury. CT has a sensitivity of 92% to 97% and a specificity of 98.7% for detection of liver injury.[1] The type and grade of liver injury, the volume of hemoperitoneum, and differentiation between clotted blood and active bleeding can be identified. CT scan also allows diagnosis of associated intraperitoneal and retroperitoneal injuries, including splenic, renal, bowel, and chest trauma, and pelvic fractures.

NONOPERATIVE MANAGEMENT

The current approach to hepatic trauma has evolved to nonoperative management in more than 80% of cases.[2] Several contributing factors have been recognized: (1) realization that more than 50% of liver injuries stop bleeding spontaneously, (2) the precedent of successful nonoperative management in pediatric patients, (3) knowledge that the liver has tremendous capacity to heal after injury, and (4) improvements in liver imaging with CT.[3]

Criteria for nonoperative management include foremost, hemodynamic stability, absence of other abdominal injuries that require laparotomy, immediate availability of resources including a fully staffed operating room, and a vigilant surgeon. In general, any patient who is stable enough to have a CT scan performed is likely to be successfully managed nonoperatively.[1,2] Grade I and II hepatic injuries should be observed in a monitored setting with serial hematocrit evaluations and bed rest. Higher-grade injuries in stable patients should be observed in an intensive care unit setting with optimization of all coagulation factors.

The current reported success rate of nonoperative management of hepatic trauma ranges from 82% to 100%. Twenty-five percent of patients with blunt hepatic injury managed nonoperatively, 92% of whom have grade IV or V injury, will require an intervention for complications.[6,7] Interventional radiology may be needed to perform an angiogram and embolization for bleeding or to percutaneously drain an abscess or biloma. An endoscopic retrograde cholangiopancreatogram (ERCP) and stent placement may be required for biliary leak. Even when such complications of the liver injury develop, only 15% require operative intervention. Hepatic artery angiography with embolization is an important tool for the stable patient with contrast extravasation who is being managed nonoperatively. It can also be invaluable for the postoperative patient who has been stabilized by perihepatic packing or who has rebled after an initial period of stability. Angioembolization has a greater than 90% success rate in the control of bleeding with a low risk of rebleeding and a reduction in required volume of transfusion.[6,17–20]

Bile leaks are a frequent complication in the nonoperative management of liver injuries, occurring in 6% to 20% of cases. Biliary complications are variable in their time of presentation and may require multiple treatment strategies (**Fig. 1**). Ultrasound and CT scan are used to diagnose a biloma, whereas a hepatobiliary iminodiacetic acid scan is used to show an active bile leak. Most collections can be managed by simple ultrasound- or CT-guided percutaneous drainage. Carillo and colleagues[6] determined that one-third of patients diagnosed with a biloma required ERCP and stent placement in addition to radiologic drainage to manage the bile leak.

A less common complication is hemobilia, caused by an abnormal communication between an intrahepatic blood vessel, usually an artery, and the biliary tree. The incidence after trauma is less than 3% and is more often associated with blunt trauma than with penetrating injuries. Hemobilia presents as gastrointestinal bleeding with or without abdominal pain and jaundice caused by bile ducts occluded by blood clots. It has been reported immediately after the initial trauma or up to 4 months later,[21] and Croce and colleagues[22] noted that 80% of patients with hemobilia also had bile leaks detected on hepatobiliary scans. Angiography permits precise identification and selective embolization of the appropriate branch vessel as opposed to the surgical alternative of ligation of a main hepatic artery or hepatic resection, thereby preserving more functional hepatic parenchyma.[21]

Reported predictors of failure of nonoperative management include hypotension on admission, high CT grades of injury, and the need for blood transfusion. Fang and

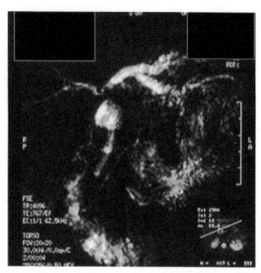

Fig. 1. MRI of a 23-year-old woman sent to us 4 years after injury to her liver from a motor vehicle crash. At the outside facility, she had multiple stents placed across the injury to her left hepatic duct and repeated bouts of cholangitis. The study shows a stricture in the left hepatic duct with associated dilatation. A left lobectomy was performed for her atrophic left lobe.

colleagues[23] regard hemodynamically stable patients with intraperitoneal contrast extravasation and hemoperitoneum in 6 compartments on CT at high risk for the need of operation after blunt hepatic trauma. The risk for failure of nonoperative management approaches 96% in the presence of (1) a splenic or renal injury with a positive FAST result, (2) an estimated amount of free fluid on CT of greater than 300 mL, and (3) the requirement for blood transfusion. If all of these factors are absent, the risk for nonoperative management failure is only 2%.[5]

OPERATIVE MANAGEMENT

Operations for liver injury are necessary in the setting of complex hepatic injury and generally indicated for hypotension and significant bleeding; these operations are often challenging. In part, because of this difficulty, paradigm shifts have occurred in our operative approach to hepatic trauma. Madding and Kennedy[24] wrote that before World War II, "house surgeons advocated expectant or conservative treatment, or no treatment at all for the majority of wounds of the liver." During World War II, drainage of liver injuries and abandonment of the use of gauze packs decreased mortality from 30% to 17%. Temporary packing and damage control with the goals to control bleeding and gastrointestinal contamination with an abbreviated laparotomy have made a resurgence and are invaluable when appropriately used.[25–28] It is critical that surgical bleeding is controlled before truncating any operation on the liver. Damage control with packing is appropriate only for medical bleeding (coagulopathy, acidosis, hypothermia).

Anesthesia must ensure that blood products are already in the room. The massive transfusion protocol should be activated so that the blood bank is always ahead of the patient's needs for packed red blood cells, fresh frozen plasma, platelets, and cryoprecipitate. Adequate vascular access and arterial blood pressure monitoring are essential. It is important to preferentially have venous access above the diaphragm. Resuscitation fluids infused under pressure through femoral access will exacerbate hepatic venous bleeding, at times dramatically so. Massive transfusion protocols should be activated early to prevent any delay in resuscitation with blood products.

As with every trauma laparotomy, the patient should be widely prepped, chin to knees and table to table laterally. A generous midline incision is made. For injuries to the right lobe or right hepatic vein, a transverse incision branched to the right off the midline incisions is essential.[29] Although others have reported use of sternotomy or thoracotomy for exposure of hepatic injury, we have found these are rarely needed. Self-retaining retractors are essential. The most easily and quickly used retractor in the patient exsanguinating from a liver injury is the Rochard retractor. In a less critically ill patient, many self-retaining retractors will work. Exposure is needed in a cephalad direction, but equally importantly, lifting the ribcage anteriorly.

The 4 quadrants are quickly packed with lap pads. This allows anesthesia to achieve effective intraoperative resuscitation. The lower quadrants are unpacked first, the bowel is quickly examined, and contamination is quickly temporized. The left upper quadrant is evaluated next. If an injury to the spleen is noted, it is removed. The right upper quadrant packs can then be removed to allow evaluation of the liver injury.

If significant liver bleeding is seen, initial methods to temporize the hemorrhage can also be diagnostic. The liver should first be manually closed and compressed. How this is conceptualized and performed is important. Packs placed in an anterior-posterior axis will often distract the injured liver further and worsen the bleeding. The lobes of the liver must be compressed back to normal position, essentially back toward midline. Simultaneously, the liver is pushed toward the diaphragm. Maintenance of this anatomic compression by the first or second assistant is critical to reduce bleeding as the surgeon assesses the liver injury or mobilizes the liver. Perihepatic packing can help to maintain this tamponade. Most minor venous bleeding and small lacerations to the parenchyma can be temporized by this maneuver. Hemostatic agents such as surgicell, thrombin-soaked gel foam, or fibrin glue are useful adjuncts. The argon beam coagulator is also an effective means of hemostasis in this case. Omentum can be placed over the liver defect as a more permanent packing method. If these simple maneuvers are effective, the operation should be truncated and the patient taken to the intensive care unit for further resuscitation (**Box 1**).

In an unstable patient, delay to control of hemorrhage will negatively affect outcome. As an independent predictor of outcome, the mortality doubles (25%–50%) as the patient's transfusion requirement increases from 10 to 20 units of packed red blood cells acutely. Ideally, the bleeding should be staunched as early as possible within this time frame. Avoidance of hypothermia, acidosis, and coagulopathy is best accomplished by early control of hemorrhage. Once the decision has been made to operate on an unstable patient with a known or suspected liver injury, the procedure of choice is often damage-control laparotomy.[30] The goals of a damage-control

---

Box 1
Goals in the operating room

Control hemorrhage

Control bile leak

Debride/resect devitalized liver

Drainage

laparotomy are twofold: to control hemorrhage and to control contamination. Perihepatic packing will control bleeding in up to 80% of patients undergoing laparotomy and allow for transfer to the intensive care unit for resuscitation and warming. Folded laparotomy packs are inserted over the diaphragmatic surfaces of the liver, never within a laceration, to promote a tamponade effect. Underpacking or inappropriate packing lead to worsened patient outcomes.[28] Excessive packing can also be detrimental, leading to renal vein and vena caval compression and subsequent abdominal compartment syndrome.

If hemorrhage continues in the operating room, the Pringle maneuver should be applied with placement of an atraumatic vascular clamp across the porta hepatis. If this controls the bleeding, an injury to a branch of the portal vein or hepatic artery is the likely source. A major injury to the hepatic veins or vena cava is less likely. However, when the Pringle maneuver fails to control bleeding from within a liver injury or dark venous bleeding persists from behind a hepatic lobe, a juxtahepatic venous injury is likely. If simple sutures and compression are performed and bleeding is still profuse, experienced judgment is crucial to decide whether to proceed with further exploration and attempted repair or perihepatic packing (**Box 2**).

Once the decision is made to perform a major operation, adequate exposure of the liver is essential. Injury high in the dome of the liver will likely require mobilization of the right lobe. The falciform and triangular ligaments are taken down with simultaneous compression of the liver. If the midline incision has not been extended to a subcostal incision, it can be extended at this time.

Hepatotomy and selective vascular ligation is one technique for management of major hepatic venous, portal venous, and arterial injuries. With Pringle control, the injured portion of the liver is further fractured with the surgeon's finger or with a Kelly clamp or the stapling devices to allow direct ligation of the bleeding vessels. This must be done, and should be done early and expediently in the operation. The finger fracture technique has been well described by Pachter and colleagues.[4] We commonly use the stapling devices to perform this hepatotomy. Intermittent release of the Pringle clamp with effective suction may allow identification of deep bleeding sites and control by direct suture.[4,11,25]

Nonanatomical resection refers to removal of injured parenchyma along the line of the injury rather than along a standard anatomic plane. In many cases, this involves the completion of an already extensive avulsion injury. Vascular stapling devices are the most rapid means of dividing tissue and controlling major veins. As with elective hepatic surgery, the stapling devices have been a major advance in the treatment of hepatic trauma. A case is presented to make this important point (**Fig. 2**A, B). A 20-year-old woman is involved in a motor vehicle crash. She is hypotensive and

---

Box 2
Major hepatic injury: critical decisions for the surgeon

- Do not be in the operating room unless clearly indicated.
- In hemodynamically unstable patients, do only what is essential to stop bleeding at the first operation. If simple maneuvers work, pack and truncate the operation (damage control).
- If major resection is required, the decision must be made early in the operation.
- Once you are committed to a major resection, technical/clinical expertise and speed are critical.
- Plan delayed resection in selected patients.

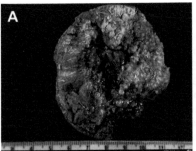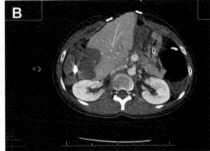

Fig. 2. (*A*) A nonanatomic right lobectomy was performed rapidly using the stapling device. The right lobe has essentially imploded with all vascular structures bleeding through the 3-cm laceration high on the dome of the liver. Once the right lobe was resected, bleeding sites were controlled with sutures or the GIA. (*B*) CT scan on postoperative day 1 showing the nonanatomic right lobectomy and the packed abdomen following the damage-control laparotomy.

collapses at the scene. She is intubated, lines are placed, intravenous fluids including blood are started during her helicopter flight. Despite this, she arrives in the trauma resuscitation area with a systolic blood pressure of 68 mm Hg and heart rate of 100 beats/min. Her chest radiograph is normal and her FAST is positive for hemoperitoneum. She leaves the Emergency Department for the operating room within 7 minutes. At laparotomy, she has 1 L of hemoperitoneum. Her abdomen is quickly packed with temporary control of bleeding. She has no visible abdominal injury on first look. However, on palpation, she has a 3-cm cruciate hole high on the dome of the right lobe of her liver, which we can feel but cannot visualize. She bleeds twice through packing. What do we do at this point? We quickly mobilized the right lobe of the liver and used the GIA stapling device to perform a nonanatomic right lobectomy within minutes. We could then clearly see that her right lobe had imploded and she was exsanguinating from all structures within the right lobe (see **Fig. 2**A). With the liver bisected and exposure provided, we then sutured or stapled all vascular and biliary structures. We packed her abdomen, closed it definitively in 2 days, and she was discharged home 14 days after injury (see **Fig. 2**B).

Anatomic resection involves removal of injured liver segments along standard anatomic places.[13,31,32] Hepatic resection for an injured segment of the liver definitively controls bleeding, potential bile leak, and removes devitalized tissue. However, the role of hepatic resection in the management of liver injury remains controversial. Trunkey stated in 2004, "there is a disturbing trend in the literature for too many liver injuries to be managed nonoperatively or without debridement or resection. This has led to increased morbidity."[7] This is corroborated by a report from Menegaux and colleagues,[9] evaluating the impact of a protocol that emphasized a conservative approach, with less frequent use of resection, whether anatomic or nonanatomic. The perioperative mortality increased from 24% to 34% with the less aggressive operative approach. The frequency of liver resection is 2% to 5% in most series, including our own from 2008.[2,4,8]

The mortality for liver resection was 80% in 1900.[7] With advances in operative technique, McClelland and Shires[33] reported in 1965 that 10% of 259 patients were treated by liver resection, with 20% mortality. Twenty years ago, Cogbill and colleagues[34] and Beal[11] reported greater than 50% mortality for liver resection for trauma, with an operative mortality of 46% for grade IV injury and 80% for grade V injury. As recently as

2004, Duane and colleagues[35] reported an operative mortality of 66% for trauma patients undergoing laparotomy for grade IV and V liver injury; 59% of these were from uncontrolled bleeding. As outlined in the articles in this issue, our understanding of liver anatomy, technologic advances (diagnostic and operative), have made hepatic resection routine and safe in many centers. Strong and colleagues[36] reported a liver-related mortality of 8% and hepatic complication rate of 19% following liver resection for trauma. Tsugawa and colleagues[37] reported on 100 patients undergoing liver resection for trauma, 20% of the liver injuries in their series, which is unusually high. After resection, liver-related mortality was 24% and morbidity was 25%.

We recently reported a 15-year series of 1049 adults with liver injury from the University of Pittsburgh.[2] Two hundred and sixteen of these patients had complex hepatic injury (grades III, IV, V). Two-thirds of these high-grade liver injuries underwent surgery; 33% were managed nonoperatively. Fifty-six of this series underwent liver resection; 25% of the patients required surgery for these complex liver injuries. In this group undergoing liver resection, the mechanism of injury was blunt in 62.5% and penetrating in 37.5%. The average injury severity score was 34 ± 11, indicating the severity of their injuries. The mean systolic blood pressure on presentation was 95 ± 38 mm Hg. Most of these patients had multiple abdominal injuries requiring operative repair. Sixteen of the 56 (29%) had concomitant hepatic venous injury. The median transfusion requirement in the first 24 hours for the patients undergoing liver resection was 14 units of packed red blood cells (range 7–211 units). The resections included 21 segmentectomies, 8 right lobectomies, 3 left lobectomies, 23 nonanatomic resections, and 1 total hepatectomy with liver transplantation. It is not essential to perform liver resection at the first laparotomy, if bleeding has been effectively controlled. Planned delayed reoperation for resection was applied in 16% of our patients. Seven patients underwent reoperation for planned removal of liver packing, 3 for bleeding and 2 patients for major bile leak. Morbidity related to liver resection was 30%. The mortality related to liver resection was 9%; overall mortality was 17.8%.

The mortality for grade IV and V hepatic injuries, which generally comprise only 15% of liver injuries, is greater than 50% in most series.[2,4,12,34,35,38] As a rule, these patients are hypotensive on presentation and require urgent laparotomy. The corollary is that most blunt hepatic injuries requiring surgery are hemodynamically unstable patients, with grade IV or V injury, a third of whom have an associated hepatic vascular injury.[2] Exsanguination is the cause of death, usually on the operating room table. Grade V hepatic injury has 2 subtypes, which are very different in anatomy and outcome. A grade V laceration is parenchymal disruption involving more than 75% of the hepatic lobe or more than 3 Couinaud segments within a single lobe. The patients may be hemodynamically stable and some will do well with nonoperative management. A grade V vascular injury is a juxtahepatic venous injury (retrohepatic inferior vena cava [IVC]/central major hepatic veins). These patients are exsanguinating and require urgent operation in 92% of cases. These hepatic venous and retrohepatic injuries are technically difficult to manage in the operating room and carry 50% to 80% mortality in most series, particularly when from blunt injury.[4,38,39] Presumably, high-grade liver injury from a blunt mechanism produces more severe parenchymal disruption than penetrating injury from low-velocity civilian weapons.[2,12,38–40]

In an interesting paper in 2000, Buckman discussed 2 types of juxtahepatic injury. Most juxtahepatic venous injuries involve an intraparenchymal laceration of a hepatic vein with associated parenchymal injury (type A juxtahepatic venous injury).[38] Type A venous injuries bleed through the injury in the liver. Reinforcement and restoration of torn containment around a type A juxtahepatic venous injury, either by packing or suturing, is generally effective. This approach is also safer and easier than direct exposure and vascular control. Several authors have reported intrahepatic vascular clamping with these type A injuries, leaving the clamps in situ, and packing the abdomen.[41] We have not found this approach to be necessary. Type B juxtahepatic venous injury is avulsion of the extrahepatic portion of the hepatic vein with uncontained hemorrhage around the liver. Type B injuries require direct exposure and control. Applying these principles for the 2 types of hepatic venous injury, mortality for these grade V injuries was 25% in a recent series from our institution.[2]

Approach to these injuries may require total vascular isolation of the liver by clamping the suprahepatic IVC, the suprarenal IVC, and the porta hepatis.[32] The liver can then be fully mobilized allowing exposure of the venous injuries followed by primary repair or ligation. Rapid control of the suprahepatic IVC can be obtained by incising the peritoneum between the esophagus and IVC at the diaphragm, follow the plane between the crura and the esophagus to the patient's left, and caudate lobe/IVC on the patient's right. The plane can be followed with your index finger around and then encircling the suprahepatic IVC. Another technique for rapid control of the suprahepatic IVC is incision in the central diaphragm/pericardium and a vascular clamp placed on the intrapericardial IVC. We do not advocate venovenous bypass or the atriocaval shunt in the management of these injuries. Adequate exposure through sufficient incisions (broad subcostal or midline with right subcostal extension), self-retaining retractors, and help experienced in hepatic surgery are necessary and sufficient. Assistance from an experienced liver or liver transplant surgeon is invaluable in these cases.

If the decision is made to truncate the operation after initial damage control, the abdomen is temporarily closed with a rapid skin-only closure or a negative-pressure vacuum-assisted closure dressing, and the patient is transferred to the intensive care unit. Aggressive resuscitation and warming is required to correct coagulopathy. On the other hand, maintenance of a low central venous pressure may minimize hepatic bleeding and swelling. Once the patient has been stabilized, reexploration and possible definitive repair in the operating room must be planned. Suggested end points of resuscitation include a systemic lactate concentration less than 2.5 mmol/L, base deficit less than 4 mmol/L, core temperature greater than 35°C and an internationalized normalized ratio of less than 1.25.[22] Optimal timing for pack removal is controversial. Caruso and colleagues[26] showed that rebleeding from the liver was significantly increased when packs were removed within 36 hours rather than waiting until after 36 hours. In addition to rebleeding, packing for liver trauma has also been associated with increased rates of abdominal sepsis and bile leaks. Nicol and colleagues.[27] demonstrated that the duration of packing is not associated with these complications and that a second-look laparotomy should only be performed after 48 hours. We generally return these patients to the operating room for pack removal 48 hours after damage-control laparotomy.

SUMMARY

A multidisciplinary approach to the management of hepatic injuries has evolved over the last few decades, but the basic principles of trauma continue to be observed. Diagnostic and therapeutic endeavors are chosen based mainly on the stability of the patient. Stable patients with reliable examinations and available resources can be managed nonoperatively. Unstable patients belong in the operating room and should never be taken to the CT scanner. Once in the operating room, simple maneuvers are attempted first followed by an early decision to proceed with resection if necessary. More experienced liver surgeons are invaluable resources when they are available. Interventional radiological techniques can prevent and treat complications of nonoperative and operative management of liver injuries. Successful management of patients with complex liver trauma depends on aggressive correction of hypothermia, coagulopathy, and acidosis, and rapid critical decision making and experienced judgment. Liver resection, either anatomic or nonanatomic, should be used in appropriate patients with complex liver injury (25% in our series), and can be accomplished with low morbidity and mortality. The stapling devices and clear understanding of hepatic anatomy facilitate operative management.

REFERENCES

1. Hoff WS, Holevar M, Nagy KK, et al. Practice management guidelines for the evaluation of blunt abdominal trauma: the EAST practice management guidelines work group. J Trauma 2002;53:602–15.
2. Polanco P, Leon S, Pineda J, et al. Hepatic resection in the management of complex injury to the liver. J Trauma 2008;65(6):1264–9 [discussion: 1269–70].
3. Badger SA, Barclay R, Diamond T, et al. Management of liver trauma. World J Surg 2009;33:2522–37.
4. Pachter HL, Spencer FC, Hofstetter SR, et al. Significant trends in the treatment of hepatic injuries. Experience with 411 injuries. Ann Surg 1992;215:492–500.
5. Velmahos GC, Toutouzas KG, Radin R, et al. Nonoperative treatment of blunt injury to solid abdominal organs: a prospective study. Arch Surg 2003;138(8):844–51.
6. Carillo EH, Spain DA, Wohltmann CD, et al. Interventional techniques are useful adjuncts in nonoperative management of hepatic injuries. J Trauma 1999;46:619–22.
7. Trunkey DD. Hepatic trauma: contemporary management. Surg Clin North Am 2004;84:437–50.
8. Richardson JD, Franklin GA, Lukan JK, et al. Evolution in the management of hepatic trauma: a 25-year perspective. Ann Surg 2000;232:324–30.
9. Menegaux F, Langlois P, Chigot JP. Severe blunt trauma of the liver: study of mortality factors. J Trauma 1993;35:865–9.
10. Moore EE, Shackford SR, Pachter HL. Organ injury scaling: spleen, liver and kidney. J Trauma 1995;38:323–4.
11. Beal SL. Fatal hepatic hemorrhage: an unresolved problem in the management of complex liver injuries. J Trauma 1990;30(2):163–9.
12. Asensio JA, Demetriades D, Chahwan S, et al. Approach to the management of complex hepatic injuries. J Trauma 2000;48:66–9.
13. Skandalakis JE, Skandalakis LJ, Skandalakis PN, et al. Hepatic surgical anatomy. Surg Clin North Am 2004;84:413–35.
14. Sharma OP, Oswanski MF, Kaminski BP, et al. Clinical implications of the seat belt sign in blunt trauma. Am Surg 2009;75(9):822–7.
15. Gomez GA, Alvarez R, Plasencia G, et al. Diagnostic peritoneal lavage in the management of blunt abdominal trauma: a reassessment. J Trauma 1987;27(1):1–5.
16. Fischer RP, Beverlin BC, Engrav LH, et al. Diagnostic peritoneal lavage: fourteen years and 2586 patients later. Am J Surg 1978;136:701–4.
17. Sclafani SJ, Shaftan GW, McAuley J, et al. Interventional radiology in the management of hepatic trauma. J Trauma 1984;24:256.
18. Wahl WL, Ahrns KS, Brandt MM, et al. The need for early angiographic embolisation in blunt liver injuries. J Trauma 2002;52:1097–101.

19. Mohr AM, Lavery RF, Barone A, et al. Angiographic embolisation for liver injuries: low mortality, high morbidity. J Trauma 2003;55:1077–81.
20. Misselbeck TS, Teicher EJ, Cipolle MD, et al. Hepatic angioembolization in trauma patients: indications and complications. J Trauma 2009;67(4):769–73.
21. Forlee MV, Krige JE, Welman CJ, et al. Haemobilia after penetrating and blunt liver injury: treatment with selective hepatic artery embolisation. Injury 2004; 35(1):23–8.
22. Croce MA, Fabian TC, Spiers AP, et al. Traumatic hepatic artery pseudoaneurysm with hemobilia. Am J Surg 1994;138:235–8.
23. Fang JF, Wong YC, Lin BC, et al. The CT risk factors for the need of operative treatment in initially hemodynamically stable patients after blunt hepatic trauma. J Trauma 2006;61(3):547–53 [discussion: 553–4].
24. Madding GF, Kennedy PA. Trauma to the liver. Philadelphia: WB Saunders; 1971.
25. Krige JEJ, Bornman PC, Terblanche J. Liver trauma in 446 patients. S Afr J Surg 1997;1:10–5.
26. Caruso DM, Battistella FD, Owings JT, et al. Perihepatic packing of major liver injuries. Arch Surg 1999;134:958–63.
27. Nicol AJ, Hommes M, Primrose R, et al. Packing for control of hemorrhage in major liver trauma. World J Surg 2007;31(3):569–74.
28. Aydin U, Yazici P, Zeytunlu M, et al. Is it more dangerous to perform inadequate packing? World J Emerg Surg 2008;14(3):1.
29. Berney T, Morel P, Huber O, et al. Combined midline-transverse surgical approach for severe blunt injuries to the liver. J Trauma 2000;48:349–53.
30. Loverland JA, Boffard KD. Damage control in the abdomen and beyond. Br J Surg 2004;91:1095–101.
31. Liau KH, Blumgart LH, DeMatteo RP. Segment-oriented approach to liver resection. Surg Clin North Am 2004;84:543–61.
32. Abdalla EK, Noun R, Belghiti J. Hepatic vascular occlusion: which technique? Surg Clin North Am 2004;84:563–85.
33. McClelland RN, Shires GT. Management of liver trauma in 259 consecutive cases. Ann Surg 1965;161:248–56.
34. Cogbill TH, Moore EE, Jurkovich GJ, et al. Severe hepatic trauma: a multicenter experience with 1335 liver injuries. J Trauma 1988;28:1433–8.
35. Duane TM, Como JJ, Bochicchio GV, et al. Reevaluating the management and outcomes of severe blunt liver injury. J Trauma 2004;57:494–500.
36. Strong RW, Lynch SV, Wall DR, et al. Anatomic resection for severe liver trauma. Surgery 1998;123:251–7.
37. Tsugawa K, Koyanagi N, Hashizume M, et al. Anatomic resection for severe blunt liver injury in 100 patients: significant differences between young and elderly. World J Surg 2002;26:544–9.
38. Buckman RF Jr, Miraliakbari R, Badellino MM. Juxtahepatic venous injuries: a critical review of reported management strategies. J Trauma 2000;48:978–84.
39. Chen R-J, Fang J-F, Lin B-C, et al. Factors determining operative mortality of Grade V blunt hepatic trauma. J Trauma 2000;49:886–91.
40. Chen R-J, Fang J-F, Lin B-C, et al. Surgical management of juxtahepatic venous injuries in blunt hepatic trauma. J Trauma 1995;38:886–90.
41. Carillo EH, Spain DA, Miller FB, et al. Intrahepatic vascular clamping in complex hepatic vein injuries. J Trauma 1997;43:131–3.

Bile Duct Injuries in the Era of Laparoscopic Cholecystectomies

Yuhsin V. Wu, MD[a], David C. Linehan, MD[b],*

KEYWORDS

- Bile duct injury • Laparoscopic cholecystectomy
- Prevention • Management • Biliary-enteric anastomosis

Compared with open cholecystectomy, laparoscopic cholecystectomy has the benefit of decreased postoperative pain, decreased lengths of stay, and a faster recovery period. However, since its introduction and routine use in the 1990s, the incidence of biliary injuries has doubled from 0.2% to 0.4% and remained constant despite advances in knowledge, technique, and technology.[1–3] These preventable injuries can be devastating, increasing the morbidity, mortality, and medical cost, while decreasing the patient's quality of life.[1,4] Biliary injuries will always exist, and we need to be aware of the best methods to avoid, evaluate, and treat them.

AVOIDING BILE DUCT INJURY: "CHANGING THE CULTURE OF CHOLECYSTECTOMY"

Although bile duct injuries can be repaired with a high level of success and most patients return to preinjury quality of life, it is obvious that prevention is preferable to remediation. In the early days of laparoscopic cholecystectomy, Hunter[5] described several techniques to minimize the risk of injury, including the use of a 30° scope, avoidance of electrocautery near the common duct, dissection near the cystic duct-gallbladder junction, and avoidance of dissection of the cystic duct-common duct junction. Bile duct injuries are associated with significant perioperative morbidity and even mortality, not to mention high rates of subsequent litigation. Many factors

[a] Division of General Surgery, Department of Surgery, Washington University School of Medicine, Surgery House Staff Office, 1701 West Building, Campus Box 8109, 660 South Euclid Avenue, St Louis, MO 63110, USA
[b] Section of Hepatobiliary Pancreatic and Gastrointestinal Surgery, Department of Surgery, Washington University School of Medicine, Suite 1160 NW Tower, 660 South Euclid Avenue, Box 8109, St Louis, MO 63110, USA
* Corresponding author.
E-mail address: linehand@wudosis.wustl.edu

Surg Clin N Am 90 (2010) 787–802
doi:10.1016/j.suc.2010.04.019
0039-6109/10/$ – see front matter © 2010 Published by Elsevier Inc.

surgical.theclinics.com

are associated with the occurrence of bile duct injury, and efforts to understand causation are likely to result in decreased incidence.

Risk Factors

There are several risk factors associated with bile duct injury, and these can be characterized as patient factors, local factors, and extrinsic factors. Patient factors include but are not limited to obesity, advanced age, male sex, and adhesion. Local factors include severe inflammation and/or infection, aberrant anatomy, and hemorrhage. Extrinsic factors include surgeon's experience and properly functioning equipment. The presence of any of these risk factors should alert the surgeon to the increased possibility of encountering a potentially dangerous situation during laparoscopic cholecystectomy. Even tired residents have been implicated as a risk factor by the suggestion that resident work hour restrictions are a protective factor for bile duct injuries.[6] The association of decreased incidence of bile duct injury with the institution of work hour restrictions is likely a correlation without causality.

Causes of Bile Duct Injuries

Error analyses in large series of patients who have had bile duct injury have shown that misidentification of the common bile duct, the common hepatic duct, or an aberrant duct (usually on the right side) is the most common cause of bile duct injury.[7] Because misidentification is the cause of most injuries, the goal of dissection should be the conclusive identification of the cystic structures within the Calot triangle. If the cystic duct and cystic artery are conclusively and correctly identified before dividing, more than 70% of bile duct injuries would be avoided.

Misidentification, however, is not the only cause. Technical failure such as slippage of clips placed on the cystic duct, inadvertent thermal injury to the common bile duct, tenting of the common duct during clip placement with subsequent stricture, and disruption of a bile duct entering directly into the gallbladder fossa are other less common causes of injury.

Technique

Four methods for identification of the cystic structures during cholecystectomy have been described:[8,9] the routine cholangiography, critical view technique, infundibular technique, and dissection of the main bile duct with visualization of the cystic duct or common duct insertion. The authors advocate the critical view technique and often selectively use cholangiography as an adjunct to duct identification. The infundibular technique, although widely used, is prone to failure in situations where the cystic duct is hidden because of difficulty retracting the gallbladder as a result of severe inflammation or one or more large stones effacing or fusing the cystic duct-common duct junction. In such a situation, the area where the infundibulum narrows can be interpreted to be the cystic duct when it is actually the cystic duct and the common duct together (Fig. 1).[10] Similarly, the authors do not advocate the fourth approach, that is, the dissection of the common duct, because of the increased likelihood of either thermal or retraction injury to the common bile duct. Aberrant insertion of the cystic duct (eg, on the medial aspect of the common duct) can also complicate this approach.

In the critical view technique, the cystic duct and cystic artery are identified through dissection of the upper border of the Calot triangle along the underside of the gallbladder. With cephalad traction of the fundus and lateral traction on the infundibulum, dissection is performed on the medial and lateral aspects of the gallbladder until the cystic artery and cystic duct are seen as the only 2 structures entering the gallbladder

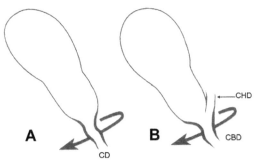

Fig. 1. (*A*) The usual anatomy when the infundibular technique is applied. The cyst duct-gall-bladder junction is characterized by a flaring tunnel shape (*bold lines*). Arrow represents circumferential dissection of the the CD-gallbladder junction during the infundibular technique. (*B*) Inflammation can pull the CBD onto the gallbladder creating a similar flaring tunnel shape. As a result, the CBD is mistaken for the cystic duct, resulting in classic injuries. CD, cystic duct; CHD, common hepatic duct. (*Reprinted from* Strasberg S. Error traps and vasculo-biliary injury in laparoscopic and open cholecystectomy. J Hepatobiliary Pancreat Surg 2008;15(3):285; with permission.)

(**Fig. 2**). This critical view of safety is obtained before any structures are clipped and divided.[8,9]

Since Strasberg and colleagues[8] originally described the critical view technique in 1995, many groups have adopted this strategy. However, in an evaluation of protocol uniformity for laparoscopic cholecystectomy in The Netherlands, Wauben and colleagues[11] reported that most surgeons had not adopted this technique, despite published guidelines from several international societies (The Society of American Gastrointestinal and Endoscopic Surgeons, European Association for Endoscopic Surgery) advocating its routine use to optimize safety. Yegiyants and Collins[12] conducted a large retrospective study to determine whether the routine use of the critical view technique reduced the observed-to-expected ratio of major bile duct injuries over a 5-year period. These investigators found that since the adoption of the critical view

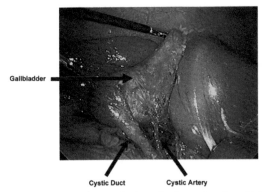

Fig. 2. The critical view of safety is obtained when the lateral and medial aspects of the gall-bladder (*horizontal arrow*) have been dissected free, and only 2 structures are seen entering the gallbladder; the cystic artery and the cystic duct (*slanted arrows*).

technique, the safety of laparoscopic cholecystectomy had improved by an order of magnitude.

Intraoperative Cholangiography

The use of routine cholangiography remains somewhat controversial because there are no prospective randomized trials showing a decreased incidence of bile duct injury when intraoperative cholangiography (IOC) is routinely used. However, there are several large, retrospective population-based studies showing that the incidence is higher in patients who did not have IOC performed.[1,3] Although IOC itself cannot prevent a bile duct injury, as a general rule the additional information gained (especially in a difficult cholecystectomy associated with anatomic ambiguity) may lower the risk.[13] Many investigators advocate the routine use of IOC, although the cost-effectiveness and efficacy of this approach have been questioned by others.[14]

Although IOC is an excellent and widely used method for avoiding misidentification of the cystic duct, it has its limitations. IOC images can be interpreted as normal if an aberrant right posterior sectoral duct inserts into the cystic duct. In such a situation the aberrant duct is cannulated, and the cholangiogram of the intrahepatic ducts can look normal even to the experienced eye (**Fig. 3**).

Intraoperative Ultrasound

Machi and colleagues[15] published a multicenter study advocating the routine use of intraoperative laparoscopic ultrasound (IOUS) to decrease the incidence of bile duct injury. The use of IOUS was studied in more than 1300 patients at 5 institutions. The investigators concluded that the routine use of laparoscopic ultrasound is effective because no major bile duct injuries were observed. It is unclear from this study whether a standardized technique was used for laparoscopic cholecystectomy. The conclusions are further confounded by the fact that more than one-third of the patients

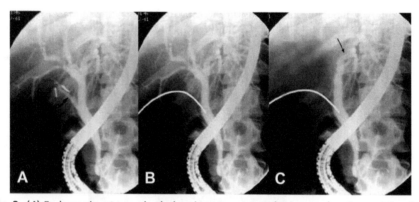

Fig. 3. (A) Endoscopic retrograde cholangiopancreatography image showing a right aberrant duct from segment 5. The cystic duct enters the aberrant duct near the clips (arrow). (B) Reconstruction of the image of what a cholangiogram would look like if the aberrant duct was cannulated. Few surgeons would realize that one segmental duct is missing and that an injury to the right aberrant duct has occurred. (C) Reconstruction of the image of what a cholangiogram would look like if the right main hepatic bile duct was cannulated. Note the much more obvious absence of the right hepatic ducts. The arrow points to the left hepatic duct. (Reprinted from Strasberg SM. Biliary injury in laparoscopic surgery: part 2. Changing the culture of cholecystectomy. J Am Coll Surg 2005;201(4):608; with permission.)

also had IOC performed. Little information is given on the technique of bile duct and cystic duct identification, and it is likely that the effectiveness of this technique is highly operator-dependent. The authors sometimes use IOUS for evaluation of choledocholithiasis, but do not advocate its use as an alternative to the critical view technique or for the avoidance of bile duct injury.

Changing the Culture of Cholecystectomy: Stopping Rules

Safety and avoiding bile duct injury should be of paramount concern to the surgeon performing laparoscopic cholecystectomy. It is important to remember that gallbladder disease is typically a benign condition that is rarely life threatening, and laparoscopic cholecystectomy can be converted to an open procedure or even aborted if local conditions present unacceptable risks of danger. As Strasberg[9] points out, the negative effects of conversion or even aborting the procedure and placing a cholecystostomy tube are minor compared with the negative effect of a bile duct injury. When difficulty is encountered during a laparoscopic cholecystectomy, persistence of the laparoscopic approach should be questioned by the surgeon. Failure of progression of the dissection, inability to grasp and retract the gallbladder, anatomic ambiguity, poor visualization of the field due to hemorrhage, and other factors should trigger the surgeon to consider an alternate approach.

Conversion to an open procedure, proceeding with partial cholecystectomy, or even aborting the procedure and placing a cholecystostomy tube are all viable options that decrease the likelihood of injury. Severe inflammation can preclude safe removal of the gallbladder, and partial cholecystectomy, leaving a portion of the infundibulum (ie, staying away from the inflamed cystic duct or common duct), is often a reasonable alternative. This partial procedure is a viable option especially in the setting of gangrenous necrosis of the gallbladder wall.

Sharp and colleagues[16] reported excellent long-term results using this technique in 26 cases (of 828 cholecystectomies performed). At a median follow-up of 1 year, no ongoing complaints attributable to biliary disease were reported. On rare occasions, the authors have had to perform completion cholecystectomy for a symptomatic remnant gallbladder, but this can be accomplished safely and with minimal morbidity when the local environment is more hospitable. When performing partial cholecystectomy, the authors advocate opening the gallbladder and visualizing the mucosa of the infundibulum where the cystic duct aperture can often be seen. This procedure will guide the extent of resection, and a mucosal purse-string suture can be placed in viable mucosa inside the infundibulum as close as possible to the cystic duct. Sharp and colleagues[16] reported a bile leak rate of 12% after partial cholecystectomy; therefore, leaving an intra-abdominal drain in the gallbladder fossa is advised.

Similarly, aborting a cholecystectomy in the setting of unfavorable local conditions is encouraged when the risk of bile duct injury is high, especially in the absence of gangrenous necrosis. In such a situation, the authors recommend the placement of a cholecystostomy drainage tube through the fundus of the gallbladder, which is secured with a double-layer purse-string suture. This procedure almost always temporizes the situation and improves the patient's symptoms. Endoscopic retrograde cholangiopancreatography (ERCP) may also be required if there is clinical evidence of choledocholithiasis. The authors then wait for at least 8 to 10 weeks to perform an interval cholecystectomy, which can often still be performed laparoscopically once the acute inflammation has resolved.

During a difficult cholecystectomy, the authors also strongly advocate early intraoperative consultation with an experienced surgical colleague, because it is logical that the chances of injury would be lower in the presence of 2 trained surgeons.

Intraoperative consultation is routinely done, especially in any operation that is characterized by failure to progress, anatomic ambiguity, inability to obtain optimal exposure, or excessive bleeding.

DIAGNOSIS

Recognition and proper diagnosis of bile duct injuries is advantageous in preventing serious complications and obtaining high repair success rates.[17] In 10% to 30% of the time, bile duct injuries are recognized at the time of surgery.[18,19] Injuries are suspected or diagnosed when a bile leak is visualized, seen during IOC, or realized after further dissection to clarify the anatomy. Once recognized, the surgeon can assess its severity and determine if there are any associated vascular injuries. Most surgeons have the skill set to repair simple injuries such as cystic duct leak, gallbladder bed leak, and partial duct lacerations. These injuries can be repaired immediately if the surgeon has the expertise required.[9] For more complex injuries, multiple studies have shown that an early referral to a hepatobiliary surgeon with extensive experience in such injuries improves prognosis.[20–22] A delay in referral leads to an increased complication rate after the definitive repair, and a 1.5% mortality rate.[21–23] The success rate of first-time repairs of a hepatobiliary surgeon was also found to be higher than that of the primary surgeon (79% vs 27%).[1,18] Despite these data, as much as 87% of repairs are still currently performed by the primary surgeon. If the complex injury is incurred in an institution without the capacity to treat these injuries, laparoscopic placement of a drain in the surgical bed is preferred. Conversion to a laparotomy for diagnosis or drainage and/or other endoscopic interventions is discouraged. Fischer and colleagues[21] found that 49% of interventions performed at the initial institution were inappropriate. Quick transfer to a facility capable of and experienced in managing these injuries prevents delays in care and decreases the need for reoperations.

Unfortunately, most bile duct injuries are not recognized intraoperatively, and most patients are sent home immediately after or within 24 hours. Patients who fail to recover within the first few days or develop progressive vague abdominal symptoms should be evaluated for a bile duct injury. There are 2 general types of injuries—biliary obstructions and bile leaks—and sometimes both can occur simultaneously. In addition to bile duct injury, concomitant vascular injuries are often present, and resultant ischemia can complicate matters, especially if immediate repair is performed and the vascular injury goes unrecognized.

Obstructed patients present with vague abdominal pain, anorexia, jaundice, and liver enzyme elevation. Through an unknown mechanism, pneumoperitoneum itself can cause a transient liver enzyme elevation and hyperbilirubinemia. Therefore, elevated laboratory values do not predict complication after laparoscopic cholecystectomy.[24–26] This transient increase resolves after 1 week, but it may contribute to an average delay of 1 to 2 weeks in the diagnosis.[18] Obstructions secondary to biliary strictures appear weeks to months later and may present as recurrent cholangitis, obstructive jaundice, or secondary biliary cirrhosis.[23]

Because hepatic bile is isotonic in nature and contains lower concentrations of bile salts than gallbladder bile, bile leaks do not cause extreme peritoneal irritation. Patients often complain of vague symptoms, such as nonspecific abdominal fullness, distension, nausea, vomiting, abdominal pain, fever, and chills. These symptoms may re-present and lead to bilomas, biliary fistulas, cholangitis, sepsis, or multiorgan system failure.[23] To make the diagnosis more difficult, results of laboratory tests can be normal or show only slight elevation in bile leaks.

To improve prognosis and outcomes for bile duct reconstruction, expedient evaluation of suspected bile duct injury is necessary. There should be a low threshold for requesting necessary imaging studies.

WORKUP
Bile Duct Injury

Radiological imaging is extremely useful and is the preferred way to evaluate for the presence of bile duct injury. The initial radiological imaging technique is commonly abdominal ultrasound or computed tomography (CT). Ultrasound and CT are capable of detecting intra-abdominal fluid collections and ductal dilations. Small fluid collections in the gallbladder fossa are found in 10% to 14% of patients after cholecystectomy, and are usually irrelevant.[27–29] However, large fluid collections outside of the gallbladder fossa are of concern for bile duct injuries. One disadvantage of ultrasound and CT is their inability to distinguish among postoperative seroma, lymphocele, hematoma, and bile leak.

In determining whether the intra-abdominal fluid collection is in continuity with the biliary tree (bile leak), hepatobiliary scintigraphy (HIDA) or aspiration and drainage of the fluid collection is necessary.[30] The authors typically perform image-guided drainage rather than HIDA, because it is diagnostic and therapeutic, and lack of filling on an HIDA scan does not preclude a biloma. Once found, bile collections should be adequately drained because undrained collections can progress to bile peritonitis, sepsis, abscess formation, and cardiopulmonary complications. The earlier the collection is drained, the less chance it has to get infected.[19] Despite demonstrating the presence of a leak, HIDA is not capable of identifying the exact location of the leak or the extent of the injury. Cholangiography will be necessary for a more detailed evaluation.

Cholangiography is the gold standard for evaluating bile duct injuries. Percutaneous transhepatic cholangiography (PTC), ERCP, or magnetic resonance cholangiopancreatography (MRCP) can be used. Each has its own advantages and disadvantages.

The advantage of ERCP is its ability to detect the exact location of the bile leak and simultaneously treat it. Endoscopically placed stents serve 2 purposes. First, stents decrease the pressure gradient between the biliary system and duodenum, creating a path of least resistance that allows the bile to flow away from the site of the leak. Second, stents can bridge and occlude a defect, allowing it time to heal and prevent strictures.[31] The disadvantage of ERCP is its inability to evaluate proximal bile duct injuries when there is a complete common bile duct or common hepatic duct occlusion. In addition, it provides no information about accompanying vascular injuries.

When ERCP is incapable of evaluating the proximal duct, PTC is used to map out the proximal biliary system.[32] This map provides useful information for future biliary-enteric reconstruction. Besides providing diagnostic information, it can also be used for therapeutic purposes such as drainage procedures, dilations, and stent placements. The major disadvantage of this procedure is its invasiveness. Complication rates can be as high as 6.9%, and complications include bleeding, bile duct injury, and cholangitis. However, in experienced hands, even nondilated intrahepatic ducts can be cannulated safely.[33]

MRCP offers a noninvasive way to evaluate the biliary system, proximal and distal to the injury. Some investigators suggest that it is superior to PTC or ERCP in providing information for operative repair.[34,35] Besides imaging the biliary system, it can also detect other associated intra-abdominal injuries, intra-abdominal fluid collections, associated vascular injuries, and hepatic ischemia or necrosis.[36,37]

Vascular Injury

A complete evaluation of the vascular system is as important as that of biliary injury. Although the true incidence of concomitant bile duct injury and vascular injury is unknown, it is estimated to be around 7% to 32%.[38,39] The right hepatic artery is most commonly injured because it can be mistaken for a posterior cystic artery.[40] Frequently, injury to the hepatic artery does not affect the liver because of its dual blood supply. However, hilar vascular injury with disruption of the hilar collateral system can lead to liver atrophy, necrosis, and formation of abscesses, requiring hemihepatectomy or liver transplant or even resulting in death.[41–43] Even though the liver may not be affected, studies have shown that vascular injuries result in proximal propagation of the bile duct injury secondary to bile duct ischemia and are associated with poorer overall outcomes. These patients have higher rates of hemobilia, abscess formation, postoperative bile leaks, and anastomotic stricture rates.[40,44] It is therefore extremely important to evaluate for concomitant vascular injuries. Duplex ultrasound can be effective but is operator-dependent, and the authors prefer MRCP with angiography when vasculobiliary injury is suspected.

CLASSIFICATION

Many classification systems have been proposed to help standardize the description, guide the treatment, and compare the outcomes of biliary injuries. However, no single classification system is universally accepted as the standard. The earliest was proposed by Bismuth and colleagues in 1982. It was designed to categorize strictures according to its anatomic location. Type 1 lesions are low common hepatic duct lesions with a hepatic duct stump greater than 2 cm. Type 2 lesions are proximal common hepatic duct lesions with a hepatic duct stump less than 2 cm. Type 3 and 4 lesions are strictures at or above the level of the left and right hepatic duct confluence. In type 3 lesions, both sides of the duct are still patent and communicating, whereas in type 4 lesions, the ducts are not communicating. Type 5 injuries describe involvement of an aberrant right sectoral duct injury concomitant with a common hepatic duct stricture.[45] The anatomic location of these injuries guides the surgeon regarding which type of open repair is feasible and appropriate to drain all sections of the liver.[46]

As laparoscopic cholecystectomies became more popular, bile duct injuries became more complicated and more proximal. Strasberg and colleagues[8] proposed a classification system that encompassed injuries commonly incurred during laparoscopic cholecystectomies. Instead of simply describing strictures it included leaks, partial transections, and complete occlusions (**Fig. 4**). This classification system maintained its usefulness in guiding the type of repair necessary.

Since then, many other classification systems have tried to improve on that of Strasberg by adding subcategories to describe more types of injuries. The system proposed by Neuhaus and colleagues[47] separated out leaks from the cystic duct (A1) from leaks from the liver bed (A2), separated strictures (E) versus complete obstruction (B), and subcategorized partial (B1), complete (B2), and transactions (D) of common bile duct.[45] These subcategories give clearer descriptions of the injury but do not change much in terms of picking treatment modalities.

An advantage of newer classification systems such as the Stewart-Way and the Hanover system is the classification of concomitant vascular injuries. Vascular injuries can disrupt the blood supply to the bile duct and compromise the success of biliary reconstruction.[48] Stewart and Way[40] proposed a system that groups injuries according to anatomic pattern and causation. The system describes the close proximity of

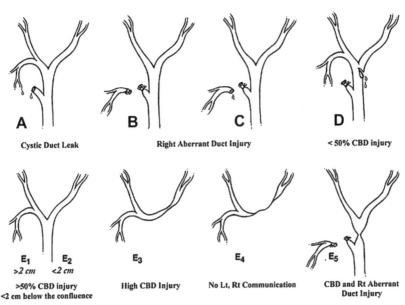

Fig. 4. Strasberg's classification of bile duct injuries. Type A injuries, which are cystic duct or gallbladder fossa leaks, are treated endoscopically. Right aberrant duct injuries (types B and C) require drainage procedures of the right liver. Type D injuries are amendable by primary repair. A near complete or complete injury to the low common bile duct are type E1 and E2 injuries. E3-5 are high common bile duct injuries. CBD, cystic duct-common bile duct; Lt, left; Rt, right. (*From* Strasberg S, Hertl M, Soper N. An analysis of the problem of biliary injury during laparoscopic cholecystectomy. J Am Coll Surg 1995;180(1):101–25; with permission.)

the cystic artery and duct to the right hepatic artery and duct, which can result in misidentification and injury. There are a few disadvantages of the Stewart-Way classification: it does not describe lesions that occur late, such as strictures; it does not classify transections at or above the bifurcation; and it does not classify injury to right sectoral ducts. These disadvantages limit its use in planning right aberrant duct or high bile duct repairs.[49] The Hanover classification incorporates the detailed classification of Neuhaus with its associated vascular injury; however, it can be overwhelming and complex.[49] Considering that most vascular injuries do not require repair, the authors use the Strasberg classification system because it gives just enough description of the injury relevant to their treatment modalities.[38,40]

MANAGEMENT

The management of bile duct injuries can be categorized into nonoperative versus operative repairs and early versus delayed repairs. The method and timing of the repair depends on several factors. The extent of the injury, the expertise of the operating surgeon and team, the amount of acute inflammation in the area, and the hemodynamic stability of the patient are the most important factors in achieving a successful repair.[20,23] The timing of the operation, the patient's presenting symptoms, or the history of prior attempts at repair does not affect the incidence of perioperative complications.[23,50,51] In all cases a complete, detailed diagnosis of the injury and associated vascular injuries should be achieved before attempted repair.

Intraoperative and Early Repair

Immediate or early repair (<1 week) is favored when a complete diagnosis is achieved for a stable patient without any intra-abdominal bile collection and without associated vascular injury. Asymptomatic obstruction of secondary branches does not require any intervention. When a simple bile duct injury is detected intraoperatively, immediate repair is advised.[9] Cystic stump leaks can be laparoscopically ligated, and Luschka duct leaks can be oversewn.[52] When a partial transection of the common bile duct (type D) is encountered, the authors favor primary repair with absorbable monofilament sutures over a T tube or endoscopic sphincterotomy and stenting. More complex injuries such as type E injuries can be repaired with a hepaticojejunostomy if a hepatobiliary surgeon is available and conditions are suitable. In the absence of a hepatobiliary surgeon, the operative bed should be adequately drained and the patient referred to a tertiary center. Repair of complex bile duct injuries by the primary surgeon is only 20% successful and should be avoided.[20]

Delayed repair is advised in situations involving complex bile duct injuries, concomitant arterial injury, severe local inflammation, or in the presence of bile collection. Surgery should only be contemplated when the infection is controlled and the patient is stable, because reconstruction during peritonitis is associated with worse outcomes.[44,53]

Preoperative Optimization

During the delay, patients need to be adequately optimized for their surgery. The initial management is focused on adequate resuscitation of the patient and drainage of any intra-abdominal collections to avoid and control sepsis. Fluid collections can be easily drained percutaneously, whereas proximal or intrahepatic bile duct dilations secondary to obstruction will require PTC drains. It is also advantageous to place PTC drains in all bile ducts that need reconstruction immediately before surgery. The drains will help in locating the bile ducts intraoperatively.

Bile contains electrolytes, bile acids, and bile salts. Its main purpose is to help in the digestion and absorption of food, mainly lipids. When bile is diverted from the gastrointestinal tract as a result of drains, patients can become nutritionally depleted and have electrolyte abnormalities. It is important to correct any electrolyte abnormalities, maintain a good nutritional status, and supplement fat-soluble vitamins, because these measures will improve outcomes.

Delayed Operative Repair

Once sepsis and leaks are controlled, the bile duct injury is adequately classified, and the patient is stable and nutritionally optimized, repair of the bile duct injury can be considered. A delay of 2 to 3 months is preferable in most cases. This delay allows time for inflammation in the area to decrease and devascularized bile ducts to "die back." All bile duct injuries in discontinuity with the bowel require surgical repair. Certain general principles are necessary for a successful biliary injury repair. The repair needs to be tension-free and widely patent, with a mucosa-to-mucosa anastomosis using well-vascularized bile ducts and monofilament absorbable sutures. The repair should also drain all aspects of the liver.[54] In the authors' institution, a side-to-side hepaticojejunostomy is preferred, because direct duct-to-duct anastomosis is associated with a 50% failure rate and late stenosis secondary to loss of substance and devascularization of the duct during dissection.[4,55]

The Hepp-Couinaud side-to-side biliary-enteric anastomosis takes advantage of the long extrahepatic location of the left hepatic duct to make a hepaticojejunostomy.[56] It has the advantage of requiring less extensive and potentially devascularizing dissection of the duct and allowing a wider anastomosis compared with an end-to-side anastomosis. This technique is preferred when concomitant vascular injuries are involved, so as to avoid devascularization of the bile ducts.[57] However, the continuity between the left and right hepatic ducts is required for this repair to drain all aspects of the liver.

Strasberg[50,54] was able to extend the Hepp-Couinaud principle into repairing injuries where the right and left sides are not in communication (eg, type E_4 or right aberrant duct injuries—E_5). With this technique, the anterior surface of the right hepatic duct is visualized, and a side-to-side biliary-enteric anastomosis can be easily created. The authors start by using the dissected-out left hepatic duct coronal plane and extending the dissection toward the right. Once the union of the cystic plate to the right portal pedicle sheath is encountered, the cystic plate is divided and that portion of the liver is lifted off the pedicle, exposing the right hepatic duct.[50,54] For better exposure, partial resection of segments 4b or 5 is sometimes needed. A side-to-side approach was accomplished in 92% of the patients, with 95% achieving excellent long-term anastomotic function of more than 4 years. Of the patients characterized as having a poor outcome, stents were placed for 7 to 11 months secondary to strictures, and none required a reoperation. Forty percent of these postoperative strictures were in small aberrant right ducts that were found incidentally on the cholangiogram. These results are superior to other published end-to-side results where restricture rates are as high as 12.8%, 5.5% of which required reoperation.[50,54]

In instances where a side-to-side repair cannot be achieved, that is, for ducts less than 3 mm in diameter or a short right duct, an anterior slit on the duct can be made. The duct is then sewn in an end-to-side manner to the jejunum.[50] If the duct cannot be repaired by either method, the final option is to perform a hemihepatectomy, which is rarely required.

Stenting in Bilioenteric Anastomosis

Controversy exists in stenting across a biliary-enteric anastomosis. Stents can prevent postoperative bile leaks and anastomotic stenosis. Many surgeons argue that if a safe anastomosis is done, there is no reason for the use of stents. Other surgeons selectively use stents when the duct is scarred, inflamed, or less than 4 mm in diameter. In these situations the anastomosis has a high probability of dysfunction, leakage, and even occlusion from postoperative edema. However, stents are associated with higher complication rates. They can cause pressure necrosis on the duct, promote scar formation, or cause arteriobiliary fistula formation.[58,59] The authors routinely use a Silastic (Dow Corning Corporation, Midland, MI, USA) infant feeding tube to stent across a biliary-enteric anastomosis. As an alternative, the previously placed PTC catheter can be advanced and left in place across the newly constructed anastomosis.

Associated Vascular Injuries

Many investigators have suggested that associated vascular injuries should not be repaired, because right hepatic artery ligation in an otherwise healthy liver rarely causes a problem.[38,40] In experienced hands, biliary repair can be successfully accomplished without the need to reconstruct the vasculature.[40,57] However, other investigators suggest that reconstruction of arterial injuries when found early may avoid rare but devastating consequences such as liver ischemia, atrophy, necrosis, and failure.[36,41,60] In delayed operations, vascular repair is rarely indicated or possible. Because the authors typically delay repair when vascular injury is suspected, hepatic arterial reconstruction is rarely performed.

Endoscopic or PTC Stenting

Endoscopic or PTC stenting is an alternative treatment modality in dealing with bile duct injuries. It is the preferred way to treat simple injuries such as cystic stump leaks, Luschka duct leaks, small partial common bile duct transections, and strictures less than 1 cm in diameter.[50] Success is more likely if the injury is peripheral, extrahepatic, and not associated with an abscess or biloma.[31,61] However, for longer strictures, wider transections, and central leaks, the success rate is much lower than that of operative repair (61% vs 94%).[31,62,63] Even with lower success rates and undetermined long-term results, some investigators recommend ERCP as the first-line treatment for patients in an effort to avoid the increased morbidity associated with open surgery.[30] Endoscopic or PTC stenting may be the only option for patients who are not candidates for operative repair or who have undergone multiple attempts at operative repair without success.

OUTCOME

Although endoscopic and surgical results are favorable for bile duct repairs, the patient's qualify of life has been postulated to be affected. deReuver and colleagues[64] looked at the longitudinal affects of bile duct injuries on 7 aspects of quality of life. Bile duct injuries have a detrimental effect on generic and disease-specific quality of life. In addition, quality of life did not improve over time. Similar declines in the quality of life were not observed in other studies that showed only psychological decline or no statistical differences in all aspects studied.[65,66] The difference in results is due to multiple factors. deReuver was able to show that the quality of life was worse for patients involved in litigation and when the results of the litigation did not favor the patient. These studies also differ in their methods of data collection and subjective interpretations.

SUMMARY

Laparoscopic cholecystectomy has become the standard of care for most gallbladder diseases. Unfortunately, bile duct complication rates for this procedure, although low, have been consistently higher than those of open cholecystectomies, which has resulted in higher rates of morbidity, mortality, and litigation. Bile duct injuries incurred during laparoscopic cholecystectomy are avoidable if the surgeon is vigilant in knowing the risk factors, achieving the critical view of safety, consulting a specialist when appropriate, and knowing when to abort the procedure. Bile duct injuries tend to be more proximal in the biliary system and have the possibility of being associated with vascular injuries. Complete and early diagnosis of the extent of the injury and associated vascular injuries are extremely important for operative planning and better outcomes. The treatment of these injuries is complex and requires expert multidisciplinary teams, therefore it is best to refer patients to centers capable of advanced endoscopic, radiologic, and hepatobiliary surgical techniques. Regardless of the potential superiority of one technique over the other, the most important prognostic factor of morbidity and long-term functional outcome after biliary reconstruction is the surgeon. There is little doubt that the best results for this type of surgery have been achieved in high-volume tertiary referral centers and/or with specialized hepatobiliary surgeons.

REFERENCES

1. Flum DR, Cheadle A, Prela C, et al. Bile duct injury during cholecystectomy and survival in Medicare beneficiaries. JAMA 2003;290(16):2168–73.

2. Nuzzo G, Giuliante F, Giovannini I, et al. Bile duct injury during laparoscopic cholecystectomy: results of an Italian national survey on 56 591 cholecystectomies. Arch Surg 2005;140(10):986–92.

3. Waage A, Nilsson M. Iatrogenic bile duct injury: a population-based study of 152 776 cholecystectomies in the Swedish Inpatient Registry. Arch Surg 2006; 141(12):1207–13.

4. de Reuver P, Busch O, Rauws E, et al. Long-term results of a primary end-to-end anastomosis in peroperative detected bile duct injury. J Gastrointest Surg 2007; 11(3):296–302.

5. Hunter JG. Avoidance of bile duct injury during laparoscopic cholecystectomy. Am J Surg 1991;162(1):71–6.

6. Yaghoubian A, Saltmarsh G, Rosing DK, et al. Decreased bile duct injury rate during laparoscopic cholecystectomy in the era of the 80-hour resident workweek. Arch Surg 2008;143(9):847–51.

7. Way LW, Stewart LM, Gantert WM, et al. Causes and prevention of laparoscopic bile duct injuries: analysis of 252 cases from a human factors and cognitive psychology perspective [article]. Ann Surg 2003;237(4):460–9.

8. Strasberg S, Hertl M, Soper N. An analysis of the problem of biliary injury during laparoscopic cholecystectomy. J Am Coll Surg 1995;180(1):101–25.

9. Strasberg SM. Biliary injury in laparoscopic surgery: part 2. Changing the culture of cholecystectomy. J Am Coll Surg 2005;201(4):604–11.

10. Strasberg S. Error traps and vasculo-biliary injury in laparoscopic and open cholecystectomy. J Hepatobiliary Pancreat Surg 2008;15(3):284–92.

11. Wauben L, Goossens R, Lange J. Evaluation of operative notes concerning laparoscopic cholecystectomy: are standards being met? World J Surg 2010;34(5): 903–9.

12. Yegiyants S, Collins JC. Operative strategy can reduce the incidence of major bile duct injury in laparoscopic cholecystectomy. Am Surg 2008;74:985–7.

13. Traverso L. Intraoperative cholangiography lowers the risk of bile duct injury during cholecystectomy. Surg Endosc 2006;20(11):1659–61.

14. Livingston EH. Intraoperative cholangiography and risk of common bile duct injury. JAMA 2003;290(4):459.

15. Machi J, Johnson J, Deziel D, et al. The routine use of laparoscopic ultrasound decreases bile duct injury: a multicenter study. Surg Endosc 2009;23(2):384–8.

16. Sharp CF, Garza RZ, Mangram AJ, et al. Partial cholecystectomy in the setting of severe inflammation is an acceptable consideration with few long-term sequelae. Am Surg 2009;75:249–52.

17. Lohan D, Walsh S, McLoughlin R, et al. Imaging of the complications of laparoscopic cholecystectomy. Eur Radiol 2005;15(5):904–12.

18. Carroll BJ, Birth M, Phillips EH. Common bile duct injuries during laparoscopic cholecystectomy that result in litigation. Surg Endosc 1998;12(4):310–4.

19. Lee CM, Stewart L, Way LW. Postcholecystectomy abdominal bile collections. Arch Surg 2000;135(5):538–44.

20. Stewart L, Way LW. Bile duct injuries during laparoscopic cholecystectomy: factors that influence the results of treatment. Arch Surg 1995;130(10):1123–8.

21. Fischer CP, Fahy BN, Aloia TA, et al. Timing of referral impacts surgical outcomes in patients undergoing repair of bile duct injuries. HPB (Oxford) 2009;11(1):32–7.

22. de Reuver PR, Grossmann I, Busch OR, et al. Referral pattern and timing of repair are risk factors for complications after reconstructive surgery for bile duct injury [article]. Ann Surg 2007;245(5):763–70.

23. Sicklick JK, Camp MS, Lillemoe KD, et al. Surgical management of bile duct injuries sustained during laparoscopic cholecystectomy: perioperative results in 200 patients [article]. Proceedings of the 116th Annual Meeting of the Southern Surgical Association. December 2004. Ann Surg 2005; 241(5):786–92.

24. Kaldor A, Akopian G, Recabaren J, et al. Utility of liver function tests after laparoscopic cholecystectomy. Am Surg 2006;72:1238–40.

25. Saber A, Laraja R, Nalbandian H, et al. Changes in liver function tests after laparoscopic cholecystectomy: not so rare, not always ominous. Am Surg 2000;66(7): 699–702.

26. Andrei V, Schein M, Margolis M, et al. Liver enzymes are commonly elevated following laparoscopic cholecystectomy: is elevated intra-abdominal pressure the cause? Dig Surg 1998;15(3):256–9.

27. Hakansson K, Leander P, Ekberg O, et al. MR imaging of upper abdomen following cholecystectomy. Normal and abnormal findings. Acta Radiol 2001; 42(2):181–6.

28. McAlister VC. Abdominal fluid collection after laparoscopic cholecystectomy. Br J Surg 2000;87(9):1126–7.

29. Moran J, Del Grosso E, Wills J, et al. Laparoscopic cholecystectomy: imaging of complications and normal postoperative CT appearance. Abdom Imaging 1994; 19(2):143–6.

30. Walker AT, Shapiro AW, Brooks DC, et al. Bile duct disruption and biloma after laparoscopic cholecystectomy: imaging evaluation. Am J Roentgenol 1992; 158(4):785–9.

31. Weber A, Feussner H, Winkelmann F, et al. Long-term outcome of endoscopic therapy in patients with bile duct injury after cholecystectomy. J Gastroenterol Hepatol 2009;24(5):762–9.

32. Branum GD, Schmitt C, Baillie J, et al. Management of major biliary complication after laparoscopic cholecystectomy. Ann Surg 1993;217(5):532–41.

33. Oh HC, Lee SK, Lee TY, et al. Analysis of percutaneous transhepatic cholangioscopy-related complications and the risk factors for those complications. Endoscopy 2007;39(8):731–6.

34. Yeh TS, Jan YY, Tseng JH, et al. Value of magnetic resonance cholangiopancreatography in demonstrating major bile duct injuries following laparoscopic cholecystectomy. Br J Surg 1999;86(2):181–4.

35. Bujanda L, Calvo MM, Cabriada JL, et al. MRCP in the diagnosis of iatrogenic bile duct injury. NMR Biomed 2003;16(8):475–8.

36. Li J, Frilling A, Nadalin S, et al. Management of concomitant hepatic artery injury in patients with iatrogenic major bile duct injury after laparoscopic cholecystectomy. Br J Surg 2008;95(4):460–5.

37. Ragozzino A, Lassandro F, De Ritis R, et al. Value of MRI in three patients with major vascular injuries after laparoscopic cholecystectomy. Emerg Radiol 2007; 14(6):443–7.

38. Halasz N. Cholecystectomy and hepatic artery injuries. Arch Surg 1991;126(2): 137–8.

39. Deziel D, Millikan K, Economou S, et al. Complications of laparoscopic cholecystectomy: a national survey of 4,292 hospitals and an analysis of 77,604 cases. Am J Surg 1993;165(1):9–14.

40. Stewart L, Robinson TN, Lee CM, et al. Right hepatic artery injury associated with laparoscopic bile duct injury: incidence, mechanism, and consequences. J Gastrointest Surg 2004;8(5):523–30.

41. Frilling A, Li J, Weber F, et al. Major bile duct injuries after laparoscopic cholecystectomy: a tertiary center experience. J Gastrointest Surg 2004;8(6):679–85.
42. Laurent AM, Sauvanet AM, Farges OM, et al. Major hepatectomy for the treatment of complex bile duct injury [article]. Ann Surg 2008;248(1):77–83.
43. Buell JF, Cronin DC, Funaki B, et al. Devastating and fatal complications associated with combined vascular and bile duct injuries during cholecystectomy. Arch Surg 2002;137(6):703–10.
44. Schmidt SC, Settmacher U, Langrehr JM, et al. Management and outcome of patients with combined bile duct and hepatic arterial injuries after laparoscopic cholecystectomy. Surgery 2004;135(6):613–8.
45. Lau WY, Lai EC. Classification of iatrogenic bile duct injury. Hepatobiliary Pancreat Dis Int 2007;6(5):457–63.
46. Bismuth H, Majno PE. Biliary strictures: classification based on the principles of surgical treatment. World J Surg 2001;25(10):1241–4.
47. Neuhaus P, Schmidt SC, Hintze RE, et al. Classification and treatment of bile duct injuries after laparoscopic cholecystectomy. Chirurg 2000;71(2):166–73.
48. Gupta N, Solomon H, Fairchild R, et al. Management and outcome of patients with combined bile duct and hepatic artery injuries. Arch Surg 1998;133(2):176–81.
49. Bektas H, Schrem H, Winny M, et al. Surgical treatment and outcome of iatrogenic bile duct lesions after cholecystectomy and the impact of different clinical classification systems. Br J Surg 2007;94(9):1119–27.
50. Winslow ER, Fialkowski EA, Linehan DC, et al. Sideways": results of repair of biliary injuries using a policy of side-to-side hepatico-jejunostomy [article]. Ann Surg 2009;249(3):426–34.
51. Stewart L, Way LW. Laparoscopic bile duct injuries: timing of surgical repair does not influence success rate. A multivariate analysis of factors influencing surgical outcomes. HPB (Oxford) 2009;11(6):516–22.
52. Li J, Frilling A, Nadalin S, et al. Surgical management of segmental and sectoral bile duct injury after laparoscopic cholecystectomy: a challenging situation. J Gastrointest Surg 2010;14(2):344–51.
53. Robinson TN, Stiegmann G, Durham J, et al. Management of major bile duct injury associated with laparoscopic cholecystectomy. Surg Endosc 2001; 15(12):1381–5.
54. Strasberg SM, Picus DD, Drebin JA. Results of a new strategy for reconstruction of biliary injuries having an isolated right-sided component. J Gastrointest Surg 2001;5(3):266–74.
55. Lillemoe KD, Pitt HA, Cameron JL. Postoperative bile duct strictures. Surg Clin North Am 1990;70(6):1355–80.
56. Hepp J, Couinaud C. Approach to and use of the left hepatic duct in reparation of the common bile duct. Presse Med 1956;64(41):947–8.
57. Alves A, Farges O, Nicolet J, et al. Incidence and consequence of an hepatic artery injury in patients with postcholecystectomy bile duct strictures. Ann Surg 2003;238(1):93–6.
58. Ooi LL, Chung YF, Wong WK. Biliary-enteric transanastomotic stenting with Intestofix. ANZ J Surg 2002;72(9):676–7.
59. Mercado MA, Chan C, Orozco H, et al. To stent or not to stent bilioenteric anastomosis after iatrogenic injury: a dilemma not answered? Arch Surg 2002;137(1): 60–3.
60. Bachellier P, Nakano H, Weber JC, et al. Surgical repair after bile duct and vascular injuries during laparoscopic cholecystectomy: when and how? World J Surg 2001;25(10):1335–45.

61. Thurley PD, Dhingsa R. Laparoscopic cholecystectomy: postoperative imaging. Am J Roentgenol 2008;191(3):794–801.
62. Walsh RM, Henderson JM, Vogt DP, et al. Long-term outcome of biliary reconstruction for bile duct injuries from laparoscopic cholecystectomies. Surgery 2007;142(4):450–7.
63. Misra S, Melton GB, Geschwind JF, et al. Percutaneous management of bile duct strictures and injuries associated with laparoscopic cholecystectomy: a decade of experience. J Am Coll Surg 2004;198(2):218–26.
64. deReuver P, Sprangers M, Rauws E, et al. Impact of bile duct injury after laparoscopic cholecystectomy on quality of life: a longitudinal study after multidisciplinary treatment. Endoscopy 2008;40(8):637–43.
65. Hogan AM, Hoti EM, Winter DC, et al. Quality of life after iatrogenic bile duct injury: a case control study. Ann Surg 2009;249(2):292–5.
66. Melton GB, Lillemoe KD, Cameron JL, et al. Major bile duct injuries associated with laparoscopic cholecystectomy: effect of surgical repair on quality of life. Ann Surg 2002;235(6):888–95.

Current Approach to Hepatocellular Carcinoma

Peter Abrams, MD, J. Wallis Marsh, MD, MBA*

KEYWORDS

- Hepatocellular carcinoma • Partial hepatectomy
- Liver transplantation • Locoregional therapy
- Transarterial chemoembolization • Radiofrequency ablation

Hepatocellular carcinoma (HCC), an epithelial tumor derived from hepatocytes, accounts for 80% of all primary liver cancers and ranks globally as the fourth leading cause of cancer-related deaths. Annual mortality rates of HCC remain comparable to its yearly incidence, making it one of the most lethal varieties of solid-organ cancer.[1] A retrospective study using the population-based registries of the Surveillance, Epidemiology, and End Results (SEER) program found that 11,547 cases of HCC were diagnosed in the United States between 1975 and 1998. Attributed at least in part to the hepatitis C (HCV) epidemic beginning in the 1960s, the overall age-adjusted incidence rates of HCC in the United States have steadily increased over the past 2 decades, from 1.3 per 100,000 persons from 1981 to 1983, to 3.0 per 100,000 persons from 1996 to 1998, increasing again to 4.1 per 100,000 persons from 1998 to 2000.[2–4]

Well-established risk factors for the development of HCC include hepatitis B carrier state, chronic hepatitis C infection, hereditary hemochromatosis, and cirrhosis of any etiology, as well as certain environmental toxins. Men are more prone to develop HCC, especially in high-incidence regions such as sub-Saharan Africa and Southeast Asia, with a mean male-to-female ratio of 3.7 to 1.0. Although not completely understood, the disparity in gender distribution is thought to be related to variations in hepatitis carrier states, exposure to environmental toxins, and the trophic effect of androgens.[5] Most cases occur in patients with chronic liver disease or cirrhosis, affecting older persons disproportionately.

DIAGNOSIS

The diagnosis of HCC commonly involves radiology, biopsy, and alpha fetoprotein (AFP) serology testing. Individual evaluations are guided by the context of the patient

Department of Surgery, Thomas East Starzl Transplantation Institute, Montefiore Hospital, University of Pittsburgh School of Medicine, N755.8, 3459 Fifth Avenue, Pittsburgh, PA 15215, USA
* Corresponding author.
E-mail address: marshw@upmc.edu

Surg Clin N Am 90 (2010) 803–816
doi:10.1016/j.suc.2010.04.010
0039-6109/10/$ – see front matter © 2010 Elsevier Inc. All rights reserved.

surgical.theclinics.com

presentation. In almost every instance, some form of high-resolution imaging, usually triphasic CT scan or MRI with gadolinium injection, is indicated to measure the extent of disease. Percutaneous fine-needle biopsy (2%–3% rate of needle tract seeding) may be indicated in the setting of inconclusive imaging.[6,7] At diagnosis, 20% to 60% of small lesions are found to be multifocal and, despite adequate preoperative assessment, up to 30% of tumors in patients with cirrhosis are understaged.[8–10] In the setting of a patient presenting with significant risk factors, the detection of a liver mass requires a high index of suspicion for HCC. The sequence and type of tests used to diagnose HCC depend mainly on the radiologic characteristics and dimensions of the liver mass.

Lesions measuring smaller than 1 cm, particularly in the context of cirrhosis, have a low likelihood of being HCC. If these subcentimeter lesions do not enhance on contrast imaging, their likelihood of being HCC is further diminished.[11] This low likelihood of malignancy, however, is tempered by the ability over time to transform into HCC.[12] Therefore, these lesions must undergo surveillance over the first 1 to 2 years to confirm lack of growth and, by implication, the absence of HCC. The current consensus guidelines regarding surveillance of subcentimeter liver lesions is to perform ultrasound follow-up at intervals from 3 to 6 months over the first 24 months, followed by routine surveillance after documenting no interval growth.[13] Alternative imaging to ultrasound, CT, and/or MRI (such as lipiodol angiography) is not recommended as standalone surveillance in this subset of patients owing to lower sensitivity for small lesions.

Lesions measuring 1 to 2 cm in a cirrhotic liver have been shown to have a significant likelihood of HCC. Many investigators have argued that this size range in the context of chronic liver disease requires biopsy.[14,15] Although obtaining reliable biopsy specimens from these small lesions can be challenging, adequate characterization of lesions smaller than 2 cm by imaging techniques alone appears similarly burdened by likelihood of error. The characteristic arterial-phase enhancement and venousphase wash-out of HCC lesions are more difficult to identify with certainty in nodules smaller than 2 cm. Other non-HCC lesions smaller than 2 cm (eg, dysplastic nodules) may demonstrate similar characteristics to HCC, such as arterial enhancement without venous washout. In cirrhotic livers, it has been estimated that up to 25% of lesions smaller than 2 cm in diameter with arterial uptake but without venous washout will either not increase in size or regress over time and thus do not represent HCC disease.[13,16–18] Biopsy, therefore, remains a critical tool in identifying HCC with sufficient confidence in 1- to 2-cm lesions.

Any liver lesion measuring larger than 2 cm in a cirrhotic liver is HCC until proven otherwise. In the setting of a larger than 2-cm lesion demonstrating characteristic HCC findings on high-resolution, contrast-enhanced imaging along with an AFP higher than 200 ng/ml, the diagnosis of HCC is made with sufficient confidence that biopsy confirmation is rarely indicated.[15,16] Lesions larger than 2 cm with incongruous imaging characteristics in a cirrhotic liver or with classic HCC characteristics in a noncirrhotic liver may require biopsy to achieve sufficient diagnostic confidence.[13] Current consensus guidelines reiterate the lack of necessity for biopsy in patients with cirrhosis with a lesion larger than 2 cm with characteristic HCC findings on 2 high-resolution, contrast-enhanced imaging studies, irrespective of AFP level, as the positive predictive value of the combination of clinical context and imaging findings exceeds 95%.[13,14]

STAGING

The staging of HCC is complicated twofold—by a lack of global consensus on any given HCC staging system and the significant impact of underlying liver function on prognosis. Most US physicians and surgeons use the modified TNM staging system (**Table 1**); however, this system fails as a robust predictor of tumor-free survival after transplantation in patients with HCC.[13,19,20] The United Network for Organ Sharing (UNOS) uses an alternative staging system based on the American Liver Tumor Study Group (ALTSG), allowing certain patients with HCC to be prioritized on the transplant candidate waiting list (**Table 2**).[21] Like the modified TNM system, the ALTSG classification system does not take into consideration the extent of underlying liver disease or tumor biology.

INDICATIONS FOR PARTIAL HEPATECTOMY

Partial hepatectomy (PH) is the standard treatment for resectable HCC in patients without cirrhosis, irrespective of extent of liver fibrosis; however, these criteria are met in only 5% of cases in Western countries, but in up to 40% in Asia. Earlier diagnosis, better patient selection, and advances in operative and postoperative management have increased the long-term survival of patients undergoing PH for HCC, with reported 1- and 5-year survival rates of 55% to 90% and 10% to 50%, respectively.[22,23] Operative mortality rates in patients with cirrhosis and without

Table 1	
TNM staging system for hepatocellular carcinoma	
T	**Primary Tumor**
TX	Primary tumor cannot be assessed
T0	No evidence of primary tumor
T1	Solitary, ≤2 cm, no vascular invasion
T2	Solitary, ≤2 cm, vascular invasion Multiple, one lobe ≤2 cm, no vascular invasion Solitary, >2 cm, no vascular invasion
T3	Solitary, >2 cm, vascular invasion Multiple, one lobe, <2 cm, vascular invasion Multiple, one lobe, >2 cm, with/without vascular invasion
T4	Multiple, more than one lobe Invasion of major branch of portal or hepatic vein Invasion of adjacent organs other than gallbladder Perforation of visceral peritoneum
N	Regional lymph nodes
NX	Regional lymph nodes cannot be assessed
N0	No regional lymph node metastases
N1	Regional lymph node metastases
M	Distant metastasis
MX	Distant metastasis cannot be assessed
M0	No distant metastasis
M1	Distant metastasis
Stage grouping	
Stage I	T1N0M0
Stage II	T2N0M0
Stage IIIA	T3N0M0
Stage IIIB	T1N1M0, T2N1M0, T3N1M0
Stage IVA	T4, any N, M0
Stage IVB	Any T, any N, M1

Table 2
American liver tumor study group modified TNM staging classification

T0, N0, M0	Not Found
T1	1 nodule <1.9 cm
T2	1 nodule 2.0–5.0 cm 2–3 nodules, all <3.0 cm
T3	1 nodule >5.0 cm 2–3 nodules, at least 1>3.0 cm
T4a	≥4, any size
T4b	T2, T3, or T4a plus gross intrahepatic portal or hepatic vein involvement as indicated by CT, MRI, or US
N1	Regional (portal hepatitis) nodes involved
M1	Metastatic disease, including extrahepatic portal or hepatic vein involvement
Stage I	T1
Stage II	T2
Stage III	T3
Stage IVA1	T4a
Stage IVA2	T4b
Stage IVB	Any N1, any M1

Abbreviation: US, ultrasound.

cirrhosis are 7% to 25% and less than 3%, respectively.[8] Recorded deaths after the perioperative period are most frequently associated with tumor recurrence. Patients without cirrhosis but demonstrating compromised hepatic function must be carefully selected for PH to avoid postoperative liver failure and its accompanying high mortality.

A clear departure has occurred from the historical use of the Child-Pugh classification as a predictor of postresection liver function, and most US liver surgeons today use clinical and diagnostic imaging to screen for portal hypertension to determine whether PH is a safe option. Multiple studies have demonstrated that a normal serum bilirubin level and the absence of clinically significant portal hypertension (ie, hepatic vein pressure gradient <10 mm Hg) are the best available indicators of acceptably low risk of postoperative liver failure after PH.[24,25] In the absence of an elevated serum bilirubin and portal hypertension, survival after PH can exceed 70% at 5 years.[24] In patients with an elevated serum bilirubin and significant portal hypertension, survival after PH drops to less than 30% at 5 years, regardless of Child-Pugh score. Survival after PH in patients with significant portal hypertension alone decreases to less than 50% at 5 years.[24] Direct measurement of portal pressure is not necessary in patients with clinical signs of severe portal hypertension, including esophageal varices, ascites, or splenomegaly associated with a platelet count less than 100,000/mL.

Experienced liver centers are now performing advanced laparoscopic liver resections, including right hepatectomy, left hepatectomy, and even extended right and left hepatectomy. A recent review of the international experience with laparoscopic liver resection found that 3- and 5-year survival rates for select patients were comparable with open PH.[26] Reported advantages of laparoscopic liver resection include less analgesic requirements, smaller incisions with preservation of the abdominal wall, shorter inpatient stays, fewer transfusion requirements, accelerated postoperative recovery, and fewer postoperative adhesions. Potential limitations and disadvantages of laparoscopic liver resection include a significant learning curve, delayed control of major bleeding, insufficient assessment of the liver for additional lesions, and increased risk for gas embolism.[26] As liver surgeons become more proficient with laparoscopic liver surgery as a component of the overall approach to HCC in patients without cirrhosis, we anticipate an increasing number of resections will be performed in a minimally invasive fashion. Similar to transitions occurring in the practice of vascular surgery, expertise in performing large open resections will likely contract and eventually be limited to a relatively small number of experienced liver centers.

Exclusion from PH for multiple HCC lesions is a common but not universal practice among US liver surgeons. Notwithstanding evidence that increasing diameter does increase the likelihood of vascular invasion, increased size (>5 cm) of HCC tumors is not an absolute contraindication for PH. A wealth of anecdotal evidence demonstrates that some tumors may grow into very large, single lesions without vascular invasion, and thus represent no increased risk of recurrence after resection as compared with smaller lesions.[25,27]

Despite the many advances in patient selection and management leading to increased rates of long-term survival, the 5-year recurrence rates of HCC following PH range from 60% to 100%.[28] The great majority (>80%) of recurrences are intrahepatic. Multivariate statistical analyses demonstrate the presence of microvascular invasion and multifocal disease as the strongest predictors of recurrence.[25,27,29] These risk factors imply that dissemination, rather than de novo lesions, accounts for most recurrences.[30] Undetected dissemination as the predominant mechanism of early recurrence also explains the preponderance of recurrences occurring within the first 3 years of follow-up.[31] There have been no reports of neoadjuvant or adjuvant therapy causing significant reductions in recurrence rates after PH.[32]

Treatment of recurrence after PH remains an individualized practice with little in the way of outcomes data to support a more or less aggressive approach. Repeat resection may be indicated in the setting of a solitary recurrence. However, as dissemination appears to be the predominant cause of early recurrence, one might reasonably remain skeptical that a single lesion detected on high-resolution imaging does truly represent a solitary recurrence.[33] Nonetheless, repeat resection in selected cases is warranted.

INDICATIONS FOR LIVER TRANSPLANTATION

Although complete surgical resection or ablation can provide cure for select patients, most patients with HCC have underlying cirrhosis, which itself behaves as a premalignant condition.[34,35] Although PH treats localized HCC, it may fail to treat multifocal HCC and has no efficacy in preventing de novo HCC occurring in the remnant cirrhotic liver. Liver transplantation (LT) addresses HCC along with its multifocal potential, and treats the underlying liver disease itself. The accumulation of outcomes data has clearly established LT as the gold standard for early-stage HCC in the setting of cirrhosis. Initially poor outcomes were observed from LT for unresectable HCC in unselected patients (recurrence rates >60% within 2 years and 5-year survival rates <20%).[36–38] Much lower recurrence rates after LT were demonstrated for incidentally detected HCC in pathologic explants, providing the impetus for evaluating the role of LT for patients with small HCC.[39,40] A provocative report by Bismuth and colleagues[39] demonstrated that patients with 3 or fewer tumors each 3 cm or smaller in greatest diameter had a 3-year, disease-free survival of 83% after LT, compared with 18% after PH. A seminal retrospective study by Mazzaferro and colleagues[10] established that favorable results could be achieved in patients with cirrhosis with either a solitary

HCC smaller than 5 cm or with up to 3 nodules smaller than 3 cm, criteria that came to be called "the Milano criteria." The 5-year survival of these early-stage patients exceeded 70%. Recipient age, gender, type of viral infection, or Child-Pugh score did not affect survival after transplantation.

Liver transplantation demonstrates not only the best survival and recurrence-free rates, but also provides the longest recurrence-free survival, which in one retrospective analysis was as high as 77% at 5 years, compared with 20% after PH.[41] In a multivariate analysis of a single-center experience at the University of Pittsburgh involving 307 patients undergoing LT for HCC between 1981 and 1997, the senior investigator of this review (J.W.M) found that independent predictors of tumor-free survival included lymph node status, depth of vascular invasion, greatest tumor dimension, lobar distribution, and tumor number (**Table 3**).[20] There was no direct correlation between the current modified TNM staging system for HCC and tumor-free survival after LT (**Table 4**).

In an effort to prioritize for LT those candidates with the highest short-term risk of mortality, the model for end-stage liver disease (MELD) scoring system was implemented in 2002. Although numerous studies have demonstrated the system's efficacy in predicting mortality in the setting of chronic viral and alcoholic liver disease, others have found that MELD is less robust in predicting mortality related to cholestatic liver disease and has no predictive power for HCC. To impart more urgent access to LT for select patients with HCC (eg, those with early-stage disease), additional points within the scoring system were allotted to patients with HCC to equilibrate their risk of death in comparison with the mortality of end-stage cirrhosis.[42] The original scoring exception, which included lesions smaller than 2 cm, resulted in the overdistribution of donor

Table 3
Univariate analysis of all variables included in the current pathologic TNM staging system

Risk Factor (no.)	Tumor-Free Survival in Months (mean ± SE)	95% CI Significance[a]
Lymph node status		
Neg (231)	140.6 ± 6.8 (127.2–154.0)	P<.00001
Pos (6)	5.3 ± 1.0 (3.3–7.3)	—
Vascular invasion		
None (133)	178.4 ± 7.5 (163.8–192.9)	P_{1-2}<.00001
Micro (67)	112.4 ± 11.2 (90.4–134.4)	P_{1-3}<.00001
Macro (37)	15.3 ± 3.5 (8.5–22.1)	P_{2-3}<.00001
Tumor size (cm)		
≤2 (101)	123.6 ± 6.8 (110.3–137.0)	P_{1-2}<.0001
2–4 (71)	142.7 ± 11.8 (119.5–165.8)	P_{1-3}<.0001
>4 (65)	70.2 ± 9.8 (51.0–89.5)	P_{2-3}<.0001
Lobar distribution		
Unilobar (161)	169.9 ± 7.2 (155.9–183.9)	P<.0001
Bilobar (76)	49.7 ± 6.2 (37.5–61.8)	—
Tumor number		
Single (120)	168.8 ± 9.2 (150.9–186.8)	P<.0001
Multiple (117)	98.2 ± 8.3 (81.9–114.4)	—

Abbreviations: CI, confidence interval; Neg, negative; Pos, positive; SE, standard error; —, failed to reach statistical significance.
[a] P_{x-y} expresses the significance between level x and level y.

Table 4
Multivariate analysis of all variables included in the current pathologic TNM staging system

Risk Factor	Relative Risk[a]	95% CI
Vascular invasion		
None	$\Psi_{3-1} = 14.0$	6.23–31.35
Micro	$\Psi_{3-2} = 3.96$	2.67–6.92
Macro	$\Psi_{2-1} = 3.54$	2.33–4.5
Tumor size (cm)		
<2	$\Psi_{3-1} = 5.37$	1.81–15.9
2–4	$\Psi_{3-2} = 1.55$	0.85–2.81
>4	$\Psi_{2-1} = 3.46$	2.13–5.66
Lymph node status		
Negative	$\Psi_{2-1} = 2.95$	0.98–8.9
Positive	—	
Lobar distribution		
Unilobar	$\Psi_{2-1} = 3.1$	1.80–5.60
Bilobar	—	

Abbreviation: CI, confidence interval; —, failed to reach statistical significance.
[a] Ψ_{x-y} expresses the relative risk of level x to level y.

livers to patients with HCC (with many expected small tumors turning out not to be HCC on explanted pathology) and was therefore modified by a reduction in allocated points for Stage II patients and an elimination of the upgrade for Stage I.[43] Using the American Liver Tumor Study Group Modified TNM staging system (see **Table 2**), current UNOS guidelines do not allow upgrading of candidates with Stage I disease, irrespective of biopsy confirmation; only candidates with Stage II HCC disease are upgraded on the waiting list to a MELD score of 22 (equivalent to a 15% probability of candidate death within 3 months) with the intent to shorten their waiting time. Owing to widely varying degrees of benefit from LT, patients with Stage III to IVa are not allocated extra points while on the UNOS waiting list, a blanket policy with which we disagree. Moreover, we believe that patients with Stage I disease should have the option of undergoing a biopsy, which, if positive for HCC, should qualify for an immediate MELD upgrade, as patients in Stage I are in their most curable stage.

The strict application of the Milano criteria by UNOS for MELD upgrade allocation disadvantages patients with HCC with tumor profiles exceeding the criteria's maximal size or multifocal parameters but in whom favorable outcomes after LT have been demonstrated.[20,44,45] There is an ongoing debate within the liver transplantation community regarding whether and to what extent the indications for LT as primary therapy for HCC should be expanded.[46] For patients with HCC disease beyond standard listing criteria in whom there is no macroscopic evidence of vascular invasion or extrahepatic spread, the survival rates after LT are generally comparable with patients transplanted for disease within the standard listing criteria. Most groups report a 5-year survival of more than 50% in patients transplanted for extended criteria HCC,[41] which many investigators have argued is the minimum acceptable survival rate. In 2001, using explant pathologic data, Yao and colleagues[44] at the University of California, San Francisco (UCSF) defined an expanded set of HCC criteria (solitary tumor ≤6.5 cm, or ≤3 nodules with the largest tumor ≤4.5 cm and total tumor diameter ≤8 cm) for which 1- and 5-year survival rates after LT were 90% and 75%, respectively. Retrospectively evaluating post-LT survival for patients with tumors beyond Milano criteria but within these "UCSF" expanded criteria by pretransplantation imaging and explant pathology, the group at the University of California, Los Angeles (UCLA) confirmed acceptable 1-, 3-, and 5-year survival rates of 82%, 65%, and 52%, respectively.[47] Moreover, the difference in 5-year recurrence-free survival after LT for HCC in the UCLA study did not reach statistical significance between Milano criteria and UCSF expanded criteria tumor groups (74% vs 65%, $P = .09$). The Barcelona Clinic Liver Cancer Group[48–50] has demonstrated 5-year post-LT survival of greater than 50% using expanded criteria including 1 tumor size smaller than 7 cm, 3 tumors smaller than 5 cm, 5 tumors smaller than 3 cm, or downstaging to conventional Milano criteria with pre-LT adjuvant therapies. In the absence of more precise markers of HCC, biologic behavior that might better predict which patients with HCC would benefit from LT, it remains to be seen whether the overly restrictive UNOS tumor size– and number–based criteria for HCC will be expanded to allow access to LT to carefully selected patients who otherwise face certain death.

The major limitation for LT as therapy for early-stage HCC is the insufficient number of donor livers. Without a living donor, there is always a waiting period between candidate listing and transplantation. If the waiting period extends over a sufficient length of time, the tumor will grow and eventually manifest absolute contraindications to LT (eg, macroscopic vascular invasion or extrahepatic spread). In a study by Yao and colleagues[51] of patients with HCC on the waiting list, a 6-month waiting period for LT was associated with a 7.2% cumulative dropout probability, increasing to 37.8% and 55.1% at 12 and 18 months, respectively.

Efforts to address the large waiting list of LT candidates and to decrease the dropout rate have included new strategies such as living donor LT, domino LT, split LT, the use of extended criteria donors, and donors after cardiac death. Living donor LT appears to be an effective option for patients with HCC within the Milano criteria, essentially equivalent in terms of survival to cadaveric LT, and should be especially considered if the anticipated waiting period is sufficient that tumor progression is likely. There are few data to support the use of living donor LT for patients with HCC who exceed the Milano criteria, although its use for this purpose is becoming increasingly common. We disagree with this practice. Because living donation puts a healthy individual at risk, it is our opinion that livers donated from living donors should be reserved for early-stage disease, whereas cadaveric livers should be used for more advanced but acceptable cases.

Some investigators have suggested that patients with recurrent HCC after PH might be candidates for salvage transplantation.[52] This option continues to lack support from clinical outcomes data. Alternatively, because the most strongly predictive factors for recurrence attributable to dissemination (eg, vascular invasion and satellite lesions) can be identified on pathologic examination, other investigators have proposed that a pathology-specific subset of patients lacking these findings on explant pathology be listed for LT immediately after PH, as the results of LT in this population appear favorable.[53]

INDICATIONS FOR ALTERNATIVE THERAPIES

Local regional therapy (LRT) is indicated for select patients who are not candidates for either PH or LT. LRT modalities include percutaneous ethanol injection (PEI), transarterial chemoembolization (TACE), and radiofrequency ablation (RFA), as well as transarterial radioembolization with Yttrium-90 (TARE-^{90}Y). Although PH remains the standard for resectable HCC in the patient without cirrhosis, a growing body of clinical evidence demonstrates LRT survival rates, and outcomes after RFA in particular, are comparable with PH for HCC tumors 3 cm or smaller in diameter.[54] Despite its increasingly common use as "bridge" therapy before LT, it remains to be determined whether LRT provides a survival benefit to those LT candidates facing a prolonged waiting time. Multiple LRT modalities have been used with mixed and controversial efficacy to decrease tumor burden and "downstage" HCC patients to Stage II disease. In the United States, RFA has become the predominant LRT for small HCCs, as it can achieve complete necrosis with fewer treatment sessions compared with PEI.[55] The results of a meta-analysis of published randomized controlled studies indicate that TACE versus conservative management may provide a significant survival benefit to select patients with advanced-stage disease.[50]

In response to improving survival results with LRT, there are many centers outside the United States that offer local ablation as first-line therapy to select patients with small HCC.[56] To date there are no randomized trials comparing PEI or RFA to PH. For treatment of small HCC in patients with cirrhosis, a single European cohort study demonstrated similar overall survival and recurrence rates between PEI and PH.[57] Multicenter outcomes data from Japan demonstrate that Childs A patients with successful tumor necrosis may achieve 50% survival at 5 years, which appears to compare favorably with PH outcomes in nonoptimal surgical candidates.[58]

Reported HCC recurrence rates after LRT vary widely, with most long-term studies involving patients with unresectable disease, but in general are at least as high as for PH.[13,59] Recurrences after ablation occur either from dissemination or the persistence of microscopic satellite nodules outside the ablation zone. With respect to tumor puncture by RFA and PEI, concerns over seeding are restricted mainly to either poorly differentiated HCC or peripheral tumors.[60,61] Apart from reasonable concerns about iatrogenic spread of tumor cells, tumor tract seeding is not synonymous with metastatic disease and has not been found to affect survival.

LRT remains an attractive modality for its ability to induce tumor necrosis and provide temporary control of tumor spread.[14] Preliminary data from several centers have suggested a possible benefit of LRT in reducing rates of candidate drop-out because of tumor progression when the waiting period extends beyond 6 months.[51,62,63] Given the risk of tumor progression, it is the practice of many transplant centers to treat HCC with LRT upon listing and before LT. The most common "bridge" therapy is TACE, as it has been shown to decrease tumor burden and delay tumor progression.[64]

The utility of pretransplant TACE as a means of improving survival after LT remains controversial. A case-control series reported by Decaens and colleagues[65] showed that pre-LT TACE did not impact 5-year survival (59% TACE vs 59% no TACE, $P =$ .7). Olthoff and colleagues[66] similarly showed no difference in survival at 3 years post-LT if patients received pre-LT TACE. However, other centers have studied the outcomes of pathologic stage-specific patients with HCC undergoing TACE followed by LT and reported encouraging preliminary results. In a retrospective analysis of a small number of nonrandomized patients with T2 and T3 HCC within UCSF expanded criteria, treatment with TACE before LT resulted in a significant survival benefit versus no treatment, with 5-year recurrence-free survival rates of 85% versus 51% and 96% versus 87% for T3 and T2 HCC, respectively.[67]

To increase access to LT for patients with HCC, all major modalities of LRT have been used in an attempt to downstage excess tumor burden to within Milano criteria.[67,68] Some investigators have suggested that the process of downstaging helps to identify aggressive disease, providing a window into an individual tumor's probability of dissemination, thereby improving patient selection for LT and potentially post-LT survival.[69] In a prospective study of a small number of patients reported by Yao and colleagues,[70] 70% of patients with tumor burden outside Milano criteria were successfully downstaged using multiple LRT modalities. Which modality or combination of LRT modalities to use and whether downstaging of HCC by any modality leads to better outcomes after LT remain critical questions to be clarified by randomized prospective studies.

SUMMARY

The incidence of HCC in the United States and worldwide continues to increase. Despite many significant advances, most patients continue to face a dismal prognosis, with a median survival after diagnosis of 6 to 20 months. In select patients, PH remains the best treatment option for HCC in the noncirrhotic liver. LT represents the gold standard for patients with HCC and cirrhosis in the absence of extrahepatic spread and macrovascular invasion. The scarcity of liver donors requires that national guidelines ensure outcomes for HCC remain comparable with results for other LT indications; nonetheless, favorable outcomes for patients with HCC exceeding the current national guidelines for LT should motivate expanded access to LT through prospective studies. The inability to offer LT as an immediate treatment option to patients with HCC undoubtedly jeopardizes the outcome in many patients. Living donor LT is emerging as a major strategy to address this dilemma but, in our opinion, should be reserved for patients with early-stage disease given the substantial risk to the donor. In select patients with unresectable HCC, the use of TACE may lead to significant survival benefit. The role of LRT as adjuvant therapy in the setting of LT for HCC continues to evolve and should be further clarified by prospective studies.

REFERENCES

1. Parkin DM. Global cancer statistics in the year 2000. Lancet Oncol 2001;2(9): 533–43.
2. El-Serag HB, Mason AC. Rising incidence of hepatocellular carcinoma in the United States. N Engl J Med 1999;340:745–50.
3. El-Serag HB, Davila JA, Petersen NJ, et al. The continuing increase in the incidence of hepatocellular carcinoma in the United States: an update. Ann Intern Med 2003;139(10):817–23.
4. El-Serag HB. Hepatocellular carcinoma: recent trends in the United States. Gastroenterology 2004;127(5 Suppl 1):S27–34.
5. Okuda K. Epidemiology of primary liver cancer. In: Tobe T, editor. Primary liver cancer in Japan. Tokyo: Springer-Verlag; 1992. p. 3–15.
6. Dumortier J, Lombard-Bohas C, Valette PJ, et al. Needle tract recurrence of hepatocellular carcinoma after liver transplantation. Gut 2000;47(2):301.
7. Huffman GR, Uzar A, Gorgulu S, et al. Preoperative needle biopsy and long-term outcome of patients undergoing resection for hepatocellular carcinoma. Presented at the 48th Annual Meeting of the American Association for the Study of Liver Diseases. Chicago (IL), November 7–11, 1997.
8. Molmenti EP, Klintmalm GB. Liver transplantation in association with hepatocellular carcinoma: an update of the International Tumor Registry. Liver Transpl 2002;8(9):736–48.
9. Barbara L, Benzi G, Gaiani S, et al. Natural history of small untreated hepatocellular carcinoma in cirrhosis: a multivariate analysis of prognostic factors of tumor growth rate and patient survival. Hepatology 1992;16(1):132–7.

10. Mazzaferro V, Regalia E, Doci R, et al. Liver transplantation for the treatment of small hepatocellular carcinomas in patients with cirrhosis. N Engl J Med 1996; 334(11):693–9.
11. Iwasaki M, Furuse J, Yoshino M, et al. Sonographic appearances of small hepatic nodules without tumor stain on contrast-enhanced computed tomography and angiography. J Clin Ultrasound 1998;26(6):303–7.
12. Fracanzani AL, Burdick L, Borzio M, et al. Contrast-enhanced Doppler ultrasonography in the diagnosis of hepatocellular carcinoma and premalignant lesions in patients with cirrhosis. Hepatology 2001;34(6):1109–12.
13. Bruix J, Sherman M. Management of hepatocellular carcinoma. Hepatology 2005; 42(5):1208–36.
14. Bruix J, Sherman M, Llovet JM, et al. Clinical management of hepatocellular carcinoma. Conclusions of the Barcelona-2000 EASL conference. European Association for the Study of the Liver. J Hepatol 2001;35(3):421–30.
15. Torzilli G, Minagawa M, Takayama T, et al. Accurate preoperative evaluation of liver mass lesions without fine-needle biopsy. Hepatology 1999;30(4): 889–93.
16. Levy I, Greig PD, Gallinger S, et al. Resection of hepatocellular carcinoma without preoperative tumor biopsy. Ann Surg 2001;234(2):206–9.
17. Mueller GC, Hussain HK, Carlos RC, et al. Effectiveness of MR imaging in characterizing small hepatic lesions: routine versus expert interpretation. AJR Am J Roentgenol 2003;180(3):673–80.
18. Shimizu A, Ito K, Koike S, et al. Cirrhosis or chronic hepatitis: evaluation of small (<or=2-cm) early-enhancing hepatic lesions with serial contrast-enhanced dynamic MR imaging. Radiology 2003;226(2):550–5.
19. Marsh JW, Dvorchik I, Subotin M, et al. The prediction of risk of recurrence and time to recurrence of hepatocellular carcinoma after orthotopic liver transplantation: a pilot study. Hepatology 1997;26(2):444–50.
20. Marsh JW, Dvorchik I, Bonham CA, et al. Is the pathologic TNM staging system for patients with hepatoma predictive of outcome? Cancer 2000; 88(3):538–43.
21. American Liver Tumor Study Group. A randomized prospective multi-institutional trial of orthotopic liver transplantation or partial hepatic resection with or without adjuvant chemotherapy for hepatocellular carcinoma. Investigators Booklet and Protocol. Richmond (VA): United Network for Organ Sharing; 1998.
22. Fong Y, Sun RL, Jarnagin W, et al. An analysis of 412 cases of hepatocellular carcinoma at a Western center. Ann Surg 1999;229(6):790–9.
23. Grazi GL, Ercolani G, Pierangeli F, et al. Improved results of liver resection for hepatocellular carcinoma on cirrhosis give the procedure added value. Ann Surg 2001;234(1):71–8.
24. Bruix J, Castells A, Bosch J, et al. Surgical resection of hepatocellular carcinoma in cirrhotic patients: prognostic value of preoperative portal pressure. Gastroenterology 1996;111(4):1018–22.
25. Llovet JM, Fuster J, Bruix J. Intention-to-treat analysis of surgical treatment for early hepatocellular carcinoma: resection versus transplantation. Hepatology 1999;30(6):1434–40.
26. Nguyen KT, Gamblin TC, Geller DA. World review of laparoscopic liver resection—2,804 patients. Ann Surg 2009;250(5):831–41.
27. Okada S, Shimada K, Yamamoto J, et al. Predictive factors for postoperative recurrence of hepatocellular carcinoma. Gastroenterology 1994;106(6): 1618–24.

28. Ercolani G, Grazi GL, Ravaioli M, et al. Liver resection for hepatocellular carcinoma on cirrhosis: univariate and multivariate analysis of risk factors for intrahepatic recurrence. Ann Surg 2003;237(4):536–43.
29. Adachi E, Maeda T, Matsumata T, et al. Risk factors for intrahepatic recurrence in human small hepatocellular carcinoma. Gastroenterology 1995;108(3): 768–75.
30. Morimoto O, Nagano H, Sakon M, et al. Diagnosis of intrahepatic metastasis and multicentric carcinogenesis by microsatellite loss of heterozygosity in patients with multiple and recurrent hepatocellular carcinomas. J Hepatol 2003;39(2): 215–21.
31. Imamura H, Matsuyama Y, Tanaka E, et al. Risk factors contributing to early and late phase intrahepatic recurrence of hepatocellular carcinoma after hepatectomy. J Hepatol 2003;38(2):200–7.
32. Schwartz JD, Schwartz M, Mandeli J, et al. Neoadjuvant and adjuvant therapy for resectable hepatocellular carcinoma: review of the randomised clinical trials. Lancet Oncol 2002;3(10):593–603.
33. Poon RT, Fan ST, Lo CM, et al. Long-term survival and pattern of recurrence after resection of small hepatocellular carcinoma in patients with preserved liver function: implications for a strategy of salvage transplantation. Ann Surg 2002;235(3): 373–82.
34. Johnson PJ, Williams R. Cirrhosis and the aetiology of hepatocellular carcinoma. J Hepatol 1987;4(1):140–7.
35. Okuda K. Hepatocellular carcinoma. J Hepatol 2000;32(Suppl 1):225–37.
36. Iwatsuki S, Gordon RD, Shaw BW Jr, et al. Role of liver transplantation in cancer therapy. Ann Surg 1985;202(4):401–7.
37. Macdougal BRD, Williams R. Indications and assessment for orthotopic liver transplantation. In: Calne RY, editor. Liver transplantation. London: Grune & Stratton; 1983. p. 59.
38. Penn I. Hepatic transplantation for primary and metastatic cancers of the liver. Surgery 1991;110(4):726–34.
39. Bismuth H, Chiche L, Adam R, et al. Liver resection versus transplantation for hepatocellular carcinoma in cirrhotic patients. Ann Surg 1993;218(2):145–51.
40. Romani F, Belli LS, Rondinara GF, et al. The role of transplantation in small hepatocellular carcinoma complicating cirrhosis of the liver. J Am Coll Surg 1994; 178(4):379–84.
41. Sotiropoulos GC, Druhe N, Sgourakis G, et al. Liver transplantation, liver resection, and transarterial chemoembolization for hepatocellular carcinoma in cirrhosis: which is the best oncological approach? Dig Dis Sci 2009;54(10): 2264–73.
42. Freeman RB, Wiesner RH, Edwards E, et al. Results of the first year of the new liver allocation plan. Liver Transpl 2004;10(1):7–15.
43. Sharma P, Balan V, Hernandez JL, et al. Liver transplantation for hepatocellular carcinoma: the MELD impact. Liver Transpl 2004;10(1):36–41.
44. Yao FY, Ferrell L, Bass NM, et al. Liver transplantation for hepatocellular carcinoma: expansion of the tumor size limits does not adversely impact survival. Hepatology 2001;33(6):1394–403.
45. Marsh JW, Dvorchik I. Liver organ allocation for hepatocellular carcinoma: are we sure? Liver Transpl 2003;9(7):693–6.
46. Bruix J, Fuster J, Llovet JM. Liver transplantation for hepatocellular carcinoma: foucault pendulum versus evidence-based decision. Liver Transpl 2003;9(7): 700–2.

47. Duffy JP, Vardanian A, Benjamin E, et al. Liver transplantation criteria for hepatocellular carcinoma should be expanded: a 22-year experience with 467 patients at UCLA. Ann Surg 2007;246(3):502–9.

48. Llovet JM, Bruix J, Fuster J, et al. Liver transplantation for small hepatocellular carcinoma: the tumor-node-metastasis classification does not have prognostic power. Hepatology 1998;27(6):1572–7.

49. Llovet JM, Fuster J, Bruix J. The Barcelona approach: diagnosis, staging, and treatment of hepatocellular carcinoma. Liver Transpl 2004;10(2 Suppl 1):S115–20.

50. Llovet JM, Burroughs A, Bruix J. Hepatocellular carcinoma. Lancet 2003; 362(9399):1907–17.

51. Yao FY, Bass NM, Nikolai B, et al. A follow-up analysis of the pattern and predictors of dropout from the waiting list for liver transplantation in patients with hepatocellular carcinoma: implications for the current organ allocation policy. Liver Transpl 2003;9(7):684–92.

52. Majno PE, Sarasin FP, Mentha G, et al. Primary liver resection and salvage transplantation or primary liver transplantation in patients with single, small hepatocellular carcinoma and preserved liver function: an outcome-oriented decision analysis. Hepatology 2000;31(4):899–906.

53. Sala M, Fuster J, Llovet JM, et al. High pathological risk of recurrence after surgical resection for hepatocellular carcinoma: an indication for salvage liver transplantation. Liver Transpl 2004;10(10):1294–300.

54. Lau WY, Lai EC. The current role of radiofrequency ablation in the management of hepatocellular carcinoma: a systematic review. Ann Surg 2009; 249(1):20–5.

55. Livraghi T, Goldberg SN, Lazzaroni S, et al. Small hepatocellular carcinoma: treatment with radio-frequency ablation versus ethanol injection. Radiology 1999; 210(3):655–61.

56. Sato S, Shiratori Y, Imamura M, et al. Power Doppler signals after percutaneous ethanol injection therapy for hepatocellular carcinoma predict local recurrence of tumors: a prospective study using 199 consecutive patients. J Hepatol 2001; 35(2):225–34.

57. Castells A, Bruix J, Bru C, et al. Treatment of small hepatocellular carcinoma in cirrhotic patients: a cohort study comparing surgical resection and percutaneous ethanol injection. Hepatology 1993;18(5):1121–6.

58. Arii S, Yamaoka Y, Futagawa S, et al. Results of surgical and nonsurgical treatment for small-sized hepatocellular carcinomas: a retrospective and nationwide survey in Japan. The Liver Cancer Study Group of Japan. Hepatology 2000; 32(6):1224–9.

59. Wood TF, Rose DM, Chung M, et al. Radiofrequency ablation of 231 unresectable hepatic tumors: indications, limitations, and complications. Ann Surg Oncol 2000; 7(8):593–600.

60. Llovet JM, Vilana R, Bru C, et al. Increased risk of tumor seeding after percutaneous radiofrequency ablation for single hepatocellular carcinoma. Hepatology 2001;33(5):1124–9.

61. Livraghi T, Solbiati L, Meloni MF, et al. Treatment of focal liver tumors with percutaneous radio-frequency ablation: complications encountered in a multicenter study. Radiology 2003;226(2):441–51.

62. Graziadei IW, Sandmueller H, Waldenberger P, et al. Chemoembolization followed by liver transplantation for hepatocellular carcinoma impedes tumor progression while on the waiting list and leads to excellent outcome. Liver Transpl 2003;9(6):557–63.

63. Llovet JM, Mas X, Aponte JJ, et al. Cost effectiveness of adjuvant therapy for hepatocellular carcinoma during the waiting list for liver transplantation. Gut 2002;50(1):123–8.

64. Majno PE, Adam R, Bismuth H, et al. Influence of preoperative transarterial lipiodol chemoembolization on resection and transplantation for hepatocellular carcinoma in patients with cirrhosis. Ann Surg 1997;226(6):688–701.

65. Decaens T, Roudot-Thoraval F, Bresson-Hadni S, et al. Impact of pretransplantation transarterial chemoembolization on survival and recurrence after liver transplantation for hepatocellular carcinoma. Liver Transpl 2005;11(7):767–75.

66. Porrett PM, Peterman H, Rosen M, et al. Lack of benefit of pre-transplant locoregional hepatic therapy for hepatocellular cancer in the current MELD era. Liver Transpl 2006;12(4):665–73.

67. Yao FY, Kinkhabwala M, LaBerge JM, et al. The impact of pre-operative locoregional therapy on outcome after liver transplantation for hepatocellular carcinoma. Am J Transplant 2005;5(4 Pt 1):795–804.

68. Bharat A, Brown DB, Crippin JS, et al. Pre-liver transplantation locoregional adjuvant therapy for hepatocellular carcinoma as a strategy to improve long-term survival. J Am Coll Surg 2006;203(4):411–20.

69. Lewandowski RJ, Kulik LM, Riaz A, et al. A comparative analysis of transarterial downstaging for hepatocellular carcinoma: chemoembolization versus radioembolization. Am J Transplant 2009;9(8):1920–8.

70. Yao FY, Hirose R, LaBerge JM, et al. A prospective study on downstaging of hepatocellular carcinoma prior to liver transplantation. Liver Transpl 2005; 11(12):1505–14.

Intrahepatic Cholangiocarcinoma

George A. Poultsides, MD[a], Andrew X. Zhu, MD[b,c],
Michael A. Choti, MD, MBA[d], Timothy M. Pawlik, MD, MPH[e],*

KEYWORDS

- Peripheral cholangiocarcinoma • Biliary cancer
- Liver cancer • Liver resection • Hepatectomy

Cholangiocarcinoma is a primary cancer of the bile ducts arising from malignant transformation of cholangiocytes, the epithelial cells that line the biliary apparatus. A relatively uncommon malignancy, cholangiocarcinoma has an annual incidence of 5000 new cases in the United States, accounting for 3% of gastrointestinal cancers.[1,2] Cholangiocarcinoma can be classified anatomically into intrahepatic (ICC), hilar (Klatskin tumors), and distal bile duct, according to its location within the biliary tree.[3] Cholangiocarcinoma of the proximal or distal bile duct often presents with features of biliary obstruction. In contrast, ICC occurs within the hepatic parenchyma where it frequently presents as a mass lesion in the absence of jaundice or other constitutional symptoms. Although ICC was historically considered the least common among the bile duct cancers, the incidence of ICC has been increasing. This article reviews the surgical management of ICC, with a particular emphasis on the epidemiology, preoperative workup, and surgical management and outcome of patients with ICC. The current status of adjuvant therapy, including locoregional therapies and systemic chemotherapy options, is also reviewed.

EPIDEMIOLOGY AND RISK FACTORS

ICC is the second most common primary liver malignancy after hepatocellular carcinoma (HCC), accounting for 10% to 15% of all primary liver cancers.[4] Unlike

[a] Department of Surgery, Division of Surgical Oncology, Stanford University School of Medicine, 300 Pasteur drive, H3680, Stanford, CA 94305-5641, USA
[b] Department of Medicine, Division of Medical Oncology, Massachusetts General Hospital Cancer Center, Massachusetts General Hospital, 55 Fruit Street, LH/POB 232, Boston, MA 02114, USA
[c] Department of Surgery, Liver Cancer Research Program, Massachusetts General Hospital, 55 Fruit Street, LH/POB 232, Boston, MA 02114, USA
[d] Department of Surgery, Division of Surgical Oncology, Johns Hopkins Medical Institutions, 600 N Wolfe Street, Blalock 665, Baltimore, MD 21287, USA
[e] Department of Surgery, Johns Hopkins Medical Institutions, 600 N Wolfe Street, Harvey 611, Baltimore, MD 21287, USA
* Corresponding author.
E-mail address: tpawlik1@jhmi.edu

Surg Clin N Am 90 (2010) 817–837
doi:10.1016/j.suc.2010.04.011
0039-6109/10/$ – see front matter © 2010 Elsevier Inc. All rights reserved.

extrahepatic biliary cancers (hilar and distal bile duct), the global incidence of ICC is on the increase.[5] In the United States, the age-adjusted incidence of ICC has increased by 165% over a 30-year period (from 0.32 per 100,000 in 1975 to 0.85 per 100,000 in 1999), and most of this increase in incidence has been observed after 1985 (**Fig. 1**).[6] A similar increase in the incidence of ICC has also been reported in other countries such as the United Kingdom[7] and Japan.[8] The reason for the increasing incidence of ICC in the United States and other low-endemic areas is not entirely understood. While probably multifactorial, one possible reason may be a more accurate recognition of the disease. In the 1970s and 1980s preoperative radiologic and endoscopic workup, as well as pathologic cytokeratin staining, were less sophisticated. As such, patients with adenocarcinoma of the liver with no known primary tumor were often classified as metastatic adenocarcinoma of unknown primary. ICC may therefore have historically been underdiagnosed. Recent epidemiologic evidence, however, has suggested that the rising incidence of ICC may in fact be a true phenomenon.[9]

Several risk factors can predispose an individual to ICC. ICC is more common in women and the risk of ICC increases with age. Additional risk factors include primary biliary cirrhosis, primary sclerosing cholangitis, hepatolithiasis, choledochal cyst disease, the use of the radiological contrast agent Thorotrast, parasitic biliary infestation (*Clonorchis sinensis* and *Opisthorchis viverrini*), and hepatitis B. There has been no ascertainable change in any of these risk factors in the United States to account for the increased incidence of ICC. In contrast, 2 other important risk factors for ICC, hepatitis C and nonalcoholic fatty liver disease (NAFLD), have been increasing in incidence throughout the United States. Specifically, the association between increased hepatitis C and rising ICC incidence has been reported not only in the United States[10,11] but also in Europe[12] and Asia.[13] Obesity-related NAFLD, which is associated with the obesity epidemic in the United States, has also recently been recognized as a risk factor for ICC. As such, the increase in obesity and NAFLD may explain, in part, the observed rising incidence of ICC in North America.[14]

Data on trends in ICC-associated mortality are somewhat conflicted. Some data suggest that mortality from ICC is also on the increase, with an increase in

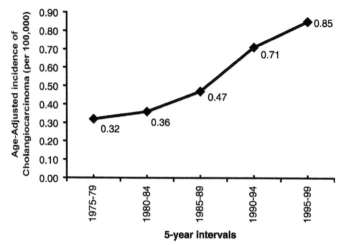

Fig. 1. Graph depicting the rising age-adjusted incidence rate of intrahepatic cholangiocarcinoma in the United States over the last 3 decades. (*From* Shaib YH, Davila JA, McGlynn K, et al. Rising incidence of intrahepatic cholangiocarcinoma in the United States: a true increase? J Hepatol 2004;40(3):474; with permission.)

ICC-related mortality from 0.07 per 100,000 in 1973 to 0.69 per 100,000 in 1997.[15] Other data, however, have suggested a possible improvement in survival after surgery for ICC. Using the Surveillance Epidemiology and End Results (SEER) database, Nathan and colleagues[16] reported on 591 patients with ICC who had undergone cancer-directed surgery from 1973 to 2002. In this study, the 5-year survival of patients who were operated on from 1973 to 1992 was 16.5% compared with 22.9% for those patients undergoing surgery from 1993 to 2002. In multivariate modeling of survival after surgery for ICC, this translated into an improvement in survival only within the last decade studied, resulting in a cumulative 34.4% improvement in survival from 1992 through 2002. While any improvement in ICC survival may be due to advances in imaging, patient selection, and available therapies, the trend in improved survival may also be a result of better classification of ICC. Specifically, with fewer adenocarcinomas of unknown origin being classified as ICC, part of the shift in survival may simply be caused by the exclusion of these patients who traditionally have a poor prognosis.

PREOPERATIVE EVALUATION
Clinical Presentation and Diagnostic Workup

Although extrahepatic (hilar and distal bile duct) cholangiocarcinoma often presents with jaundice, ICC most commonly is detected as an incidental liver mass on imaging performed for other reasons. Not infrequently, patients are discovered to have an indeterminate liver mass found as part of a workup for vague gastrointestinal complaints or other unrelated symptoms. Less frequently, patients with advanced disease may present with symptoms that may include right upper quadrant abdominal pain or constitutional symptoms such as weight loss. Because incidental liver lesions are often of uncertain etiology, a biopsy is often obtained. In turn, the surgeon is not infrequently asked to assess a patient who has a newly discovered liver mass with a biopsy simply revealing adenocarcinoma. Careful pathologic review and immunohistochemistry staining by an experienced pathologist can sometime be helpful in elucidating the etiology of the tumor; however, frequently the exact nature of the malignancy remains unknown. Because most adenocarcinomas of the liver will be metastatic in nature, a careful search to rule out an extrahepatic primary tumor should be performed. Although the extent of the workup is debatable and should be based on sound clinical judgment, most often it should include endoscopy, as well as cross-sectional imaging. An upper and lower endoscopy should be performed to rule out an occult gastrointestinal malignancy. Cross-sectional imaging usually should include a contrast-enhanced computed tomography (CT) of the chest, abdomen, and pelvis to rule out an intrathoracic or intra-abdominal primary. The use of positron emission tomography (PET) may also be helpful to rule out an occult primary and confirm that the liver lesion is the only site of ^{18}F-fluorodeoxyglucose (FDG) avidity. When clinical history dictates, women should also undergo a mammogram and possibly gynecologic screening with pelvic ultrasonography.

As part of the clinical workup of the patient with possible ICC, the aforementioned risk factors should also be assessed. In addition, laboratory examinations, including tumor markers such as carcinoembryonic antigen (CEA), carbohydrate antigen 19-9 (CA19-9), and α-fetoprotein (AFP) should be obtained. The overall accuracy and clinical utility of these tumor markers, however, remain ill defined. Although the diagnostic accuracy and prognostic importance of serum tumor markers have not been extensively studied, CA19-9 is probably the most useful for ICC. One report from the Mayo Clinic noted that serum CA19-9 values greater than 100 U/mL were associated with a sensitivity and specificity of 53% and 75% to 90%, respectively, for the diagnosis of cholangiocarcinoma.[17] An additional finding of the study was that patients with unresectable cholangiocarcinoma had significantly higher CA19-9 levels compared with patients with resectable cholangiocarcinoma.[17] This report, however, included a small number of patients (<50) and was not limited to patients with ICC. In another study of 74 patients undergoing surgical resection of ICC, preoperative CA19-9 values greater than 100 U/mL were found to be independently associated with recurrence-free survival after surgical resection.[18] CA19-9 levels may also be affected by serum bilirubin levels. In the setting of hyperbilirubinemia, it may be helpful to reassess CA19-9 levels after any biliary intervention/drainage procedure because the half-life of CA19-9 is 1 to 3 days.

Cross-Sectional Imaging and Positron Emission Tomography

Cross-sectional imaging includes multidetector, contrast-enhanced helical CT or magnetic resonance imaging/MR cholangiopancreatography (MRI/MRCP). ICC can be classified into 3 types according to the gross morphologic classification system proposed by the Liver Cancer Study Group of Japan (LCSGJ): mass-forming, periductal-infiltrating, and intraductal-growth (**Fig. 2**).[19] On cross-sectional imaging each of these morphologic subtypes may have different characteristics. Periductal-infiltrating ICC is characterized by growth along the dilated or narrowed bile duct without mass formation. Diffuse periductal thickening and increased enhancement can be seen around a dilated or irregularly narrowed intrahepatic duct. Intraductal-growing ICC may manifest with various imaging patterns, including diffuse and marked ductectasia with or without a grossly visible papillary mass, an intraductal polypoid mass with localized ductal dilatation, intraductal cast-like lesions within a mildly dilated duct, or a focal stricture-like lesion with proximal ductal dilatation.[19–21] The mass-forming type is the most common type of ICC (>85% of cases) and usually appears as a homogeneous, low-attenuation mass with irregular peripheral enhancement, accompanied by capsular retraction, satellite nodules, peripheral intrahepatic duct dilatation, and occasionally macroscopic invasion into the hepatic and portal venous vasculature. Specifically, on contrast-enhanced CT mass-forming ICC lesions usually appear with a peripheral irregular rim-like hyperenhancement or with diffuse heterogeneous hypoenhancement.[22] The typical enhancement pattern is often described as an irregular rim-like hyperenhancement at the periphery of the lesion with strip-like enhancement extending to the central portion.[22] When the ICC has abundant fibrous stroma, the lesion can have a hypoenhanced appearance on the arterial phase. Conversely, the tumor might show diffuse hyperenhancement if the major component of the lesion is tumor cells and there is no central necrosis. On MRI, classic mass-forming ICC typically appears hypointense on T1-weighted images, and hyperintense on T2-weighted images with central hypointensity. On dynamic MR images, ICC can show moderate peripheral enhancement followed by progressive and concentric filling in the tumor with contrast material.[23] Maetani and colleagues[24] compared the MRI features of 50 biopsy-proven ICCs with 34 colorectal cancer liver metastases and 234 other hepatic tumors. These investigators reported that 54% of ICC cases and 47% of metastatic colorectal tumors, but only 11% of the remaining hepatic tumors exhibited central areas of hypointensity on T2-weighted images. The areas of T2 hypointensity correlated with fibrosis on pathology. Perhaps more importantly, the study noted that intrahepatic biliary dilatation was associated with the mass lesion in 54% patients with ICC, but only 3% of metastatic colorectal cancer cases. Although neither CT nor MRI are usually definitive, cross-sectional imaging characteristics, including the presence of subtle associated intrahepatic biliary dilatation, can often strongly suggest the diagnosis of ICC.

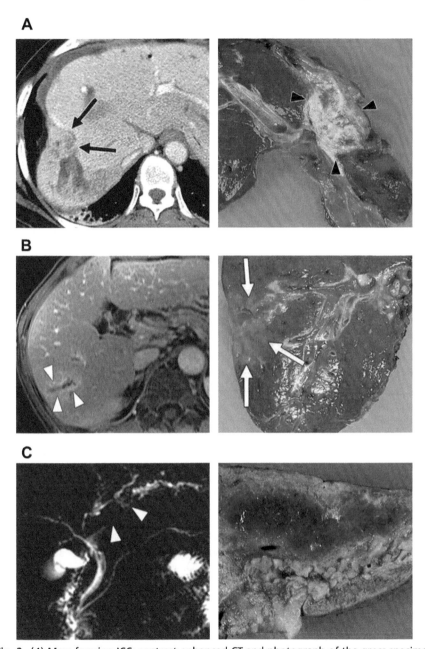

Fig. 2. (*A*) Mass-forming ICC: contrast-enhanced CT and photograph of the gross specimen showing a large, low-attenuated mass (*arrows* and *arrowheads*) with surrounding paren-chymal atrophy, capsular retraction, and bile duct dilatation. (*B*) Periductal-infiltrating ICC: T1-weghted MR image and photograph of the gross specimen showing periductal enhance-ment/tumor around the irregularly dilated intrahepatic duct (*arrowheads* and *arrows*). (*C*) Intraductal-growth ICC: T2-weighted MRCP image showing the mildly dilated duct with irreg-ularities that mimic impacted stones (*arrowheads*). Photograph of the gross specimen reveals a dilated bile duct with innumerable small polypoid lesions representing tubular carcinomas. (*From* Chung YE, Kim MJ, Park YN, et al. Varying appearances of cholangiocarcinoma: radiologic-pathologic correlation. Radiographics 2009;29(3):683–700; with permission.)

The role of FDG-PET in the management of ICC is less clear. Most studies addressing the use of FDG-PET have included few patients and have combined ICC with other biliary cancers, making interpretation of these studies difficult. Nonetheless, these studies suggest a potential benefit of FDG-PET. In one study of 36 patients that evaluated cholangiocarcinoma using FDG-PET, tumors were found to be avid in 85% of ICC cases with a nodular morphology but only in 18% of ICC with an infiltrating morphology.[25] The investigators noted that FDG-PET changed surgical management in 30% of patients through the detection of otherwise unsuspected metastasis. In a separate study, Kim and colleagues[26] evaluated the usefulness of PET in patients with ICC and compared it with conventional CT or MRI; although PET was not beneficial in detecting regional lymph node metastases, it did identify 4 of 11 (36%) patients with occult distant metastases not detected on CT or MRI. Similarly, in a study of 62 patients with cholangiocarcinoma who underwent preoperative PET staging at the Memorial Sloan-Kettering Cancer Center, 78% of the tumors were PET-avid, and PET identified occult metastatic disease that altered management in 24% of patients.[27] PET-CT was compared with conventional contrast-enhanced CT in a study of 61 patients with biliary cancers (gallbladder n = 14, ICC n = 14, hilar n = 33).[28] Although PET-CT was not found to be better in assessing the primary liver lesion, 20% of patients were found to have otherwise occult metastases on PET-CT imaging.[28] In aggregate, PET scanning may be helpful not only to rule out an occult primary but also to confirm that the liver lesion is the only FDG-avid site.

SURGERY FOR ICC
Staging Laparoscopy

Because a subset of patients with upper gastrointestinal tract/biliary malignancies will have unsuspected metastatic disease, some surgeons have advocated for staging laparoscopy at the time of surgery. Data on the role and yield of staging laparoscopy for ICC are lacking. Limited data from previous reports have suggested a potential role for diagnostic laparoscopy. In one series, the investigators reported that staging laparoscopy detected occult peritoneal or intrahepatic metastasis and prevented nontherapeutic laparotomy in 4 of 11 (36%) patients with ICC.[29] In another series, Weber and colleagues[30] reported on a series of 22 patients with ICC who underwent diagnostic laparoscopy. The investigators reported that 6 patients (27%) were found to have previously undetected peritoneal or intrahepatic metastasis. While these reports are interesting, currently there is insufficient evidence to recommend routine staging laparoscopy for patients undergoing surgery for ICC.

Resection and Portal Lymphadenectomy

Surgical resection of ICC represents the only potentially curative therapeutic option. As such, resection should be undertaken in those patients who are appropriate surgical candidates and who have potentially resectable disease. Unfortunately, previous data have shown that only about 40% of patients with potentially operable disease are offered surgical resection.[31] The reason for this is undoubtedly multifactorial, but may be related in part to the fact that patients with ICC often present with large, locally advanced tumors in need of technically complex and challenging operations. As with other hepatic malignancies, the goal of surgical resection is to extirpate all the disease with negative microscopic (R0) margins while preserving an adequate remnant liver volume. Depending on the size and location of the ICC lesion, this may require an extensive resection including adjacent structures such as the extrahepatic biliary tree, vena cava, diaphragm, or bowel (Fig. 3). In one study, the investigators noted that an extended hepatectomy and/or

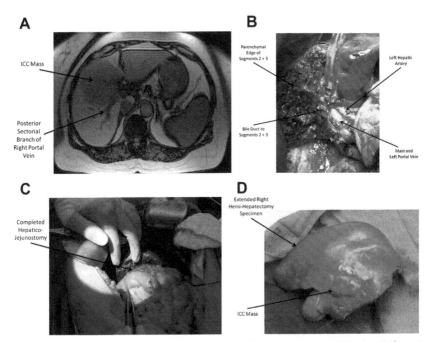

Fig. 3. An extended hepatectomy and/or resection of the extrahepatic bile duct bifurcation is often necessary to obtain an R0 resection for ICC. (*A*) MRI of large, centrally located ICC abutting the portal vein. (*B*) Surgical images depicting remnant liver following extended hepatectomy. (*C*) Completed hepaticojejunostomy to intrahepatic ducts of segments 2 and 3. (*D*) Image of specimen depicting the right hemi-live plus segment 4 with the ICC mass.

resection of the extrahepatic bile duct bifurcation was necessary in 78% and 29% of ICC cases, respectively, to obtain an R0 resection.[32] In a separate report of 82 patients undergoing resection of ICC, 49% of patients required an extended hepatectomy while 21% required a concomitant biliary resection and reconstruction.[33] Extensive resections and biliary reconstruction are therefore frequently necessary for patients with ICC in order to obtain negative microscopic margins. Even though perioperative mortality rates are reported to be less than 2%,[16,33] these operations should probably be performed at high-volume hepatobiliary centers.[18,34–38]

While removal of clinically suspicious nodal disease is mandatory, the role of routine lymphadenectomy for unsuspicious nodes is less defined. In contrast to the practice of many Japanese centers, lymph node dissection is not routinely performed at the time of ICC resection in most Western countries.[39] In the report by Nathan and colleagues[40] only about one-half of patients had at least one lymph node examined, but metastatic nodal disease was found in 32% of such patients. Because lymph node metastasis can occur in up to one-third of patients with ICC, some have advocated for routine lymphadenectomy. Some investigators suggest that routine lymphadenectomy may result in decreased locoregional nodal recurrence and optimizes pathologic staging. Other investigators, however, have argued that routine lymphadenectomy is unnecessary. Shimada and colleagues[37] reported on 68 patients with mass-forming ICC, 36 of whom underwent concomitant lymphadenectomy. These investigators reported that among those patients without lymph node involvement, there was no difference in survival or pattern of recurrence according to the use of lymph node dissection. It was concluded that routine lymphadenectomy was not necessary in patients with mass-forming ICC when lymph node involvement is not clinically apparent. Choi and colleagues[41] reported on 64 patients who underwent resection of ICC; 30 patients also underwent formal portal lymphadenectomy, 21 patients had lymph node sampling, and 13 patients did not undergo any lymph node dissection. Among the 51 patients who had any lymph nodes harvested, the extent of the lymphadenectomy (eg, sampling vs formal lymphadenectomy) did not correlate with overall survival following resection. These studies, however, are difficult to interpret and provide only minimal empirical data to base decisions on whether routine lymphadenectomy should be performed for ICC. In addition to methodological shortcomings, these studies also contained small numbers of patients that may have contributed to the failure to see a difference in the study arms. While leaving microscopically positive nodes behind may not lead to differences in survival, the risk for locoregional recurrence intuitively seems higher. Although the survival benefit of lymphadenectomy for any solid gastrointestinal malignancy is debatable, there has been an established role for lymph node clearance in lowering locoregional recurrence and improving staging of the disease (eg, colon cancer). Given this, as well as the strong prognostic role of lymph node metastasis for ICC, lymphadenectomy should be considered at the time of surgery.

STAGING OF ICC
Japanese Staging Systems

Two staging systems for patients with ICC have been proposed based on data from Japan. Reporting on patients with mass-forming ICC, Okabayashi and colleagues[42] reported that regional lymph node metastasis, a symptomatic tumor, multiple tumors, and the presence of vascular invasion were associated with prognosis. A staging system was devised using these factors: Stage I, a solitary tumor without vascular invasion; Stage II, a solitary tumor with vascular invasion; Stage IIIa, multiple tumors with or without vascular invasion; Stage IIIb, any tumor with lymph node metastasis; Stage IV, any tumor with distant metastasis.[42] In a separate report, Yamasaki[19] proposed a different staging scheme. In this study, Yamasaki proposed using solitary versus multiple tumors, a tumor size cutoff of 2 cm, and the presence or absence of peritoneal, portal/hepatic vein invasion as staging criteria. Each of these 3 factors was considered equivalent and additive in their impact. Regional lymph node and distant metastasis were also considered to be prognostically important (**Table 1**).

American Joint Committee on Cancer/International Union Against Cancer Sixth and Seventh Edition Staging Systems

In the sixth edition of the American Joint Committee on Cancer (AJCC)/International Union Against Cancer (UICC) liver cancer staging system, ICC was staged using a Tumor-Node-Metastasis (TNM) classification scheme that was based on data exclusively derived from HCC patients.[43] The sixth edition AJCC/UICC staging system used tumor size, tumor number, and the presence of vascular invasion as major prognostic criteria to establish the T-classification subgroups. Combining ICC and HCC into a single staging system was seen to be problematic, however, as ICC and HCC have distinct mechanisms of carcinogenesis and biologic behavior.[44–48]

In 2009, Nathan and colleagues[40] published data on 598 patients from the SEER dataset who underwent surgery for ICC, which subsequently has served as the foundation for the seventh edition AJCC/UICC staging of ICC. In this study, the investigators evaluated not only the discriminative abilities of the sixth edition AJCC/UICC staging but also the previously described Japanese staging systems.[19,42] The

Table 1
Comparison of T subclassifications among 4 described staging systems for intrahepatic cholangiocarcinoma (ICC)

	Okabayashi et al,[42] 2001	AJCC/UICC Sixth Edition,[43] 2002	LCSGJ,[19] 2003	Nathan et al,[40] 2009	AJCC/UICC Seventh Edition,[53] 2010
Primary tumor (T)					
T1	Solitary tumor without VI	Solitary tumor without VI, any size	Meets all 3 requirements[a]	Solitary tumor without VI, any size	Solitary tumor without VI
T2	Solitary tumor with VI	Solitary tumor with VI, or multiple tumors all <5 cm	Meets 2 of 3 requirements[a]	Multiple tumors and/or VI, any size	T2a: Solitary tumor with VI; T2: Multiple tumors with or without VI
T3	Multiple tumors with or without VI	Multiple tumors >5 cm or major VI	Meets 1 of 3 requirements[a]	Extrahepatic extension	Direct invasion of adjacent organs (except gallbladder) or with perforation of visceral peritoneum
T4		Direct invasion of adjacent organs (except gallbladder) or with perforation of visceral peritoneum	Meets none of 3 requirements[a]		Periductal invasion[b]

Abbreviations: AJCC, American Joint Committee on Cancer; LCSGJ, Liver Cancer Study Group of Japan; VI, vascular invasion.

[a] Solitary tumor, 2 cm or less, no vascular or capsular invasion.

[b] Pathologic finding of diffuse longitudinal growth pattern along the intrahepatic bile ducts on both gross and microscopic examination (includes the diffuse periductal-infiltrating tumors and the mixed mass–forming and periductal-infiltrating tumors).

presence of multiple lesions and vascular invasion were found to be independent predictors of outcome on multivariate analysis. Of note, the presence of multiple tumors and vascular invasion had similar effects on prognosis, but the presence of both of these factors did not confer additional risk beyond either one alone. Other investigators have similarly noted the prognostic importance of multiple tumors and vascular invasion (Table 2).[18,33,36,37,40,45,49–51] In fact, given the poor prognosis of multifocal ICC, some investigators have argued that the presence of multifocal disease may be a relative contraindication to surgical resection.[36,50] In separate studies, Nakagohri and colleagues[36] and Paik and colleagues[50] reported that the median survival following resection of multifocal ICC was only 5 to 9 months. In another series from the Memorial Sloan-Kettering Cancer Center, the reported median survival of 24 patients who underwent resection of multifocal disease (19 months) was no different from the survival of 28 patients who were treated with only regional, hepatic artery floxuridine (FUDR) chemotherapy (22 months).[33] Other series have similarly reported median survival durations of 17 to 20 months following resection of multifocal ICC.[18,33,51,52] Data on "multifocal" disease, however, can be difficult to interpret. Frequently, patients with satellite lesions, intrahepatic metastasis, and "true" multifocal disease are categorized into a single monolithic group. Such categorization, however, may be inappropriate as patients with satellite lesions may have a very different tumor biology compared with patients who have intrahepatic metastasis or true multifocal disease. In turn, each of these subgroups may derive a different survival benefit from surgical resection. Nonetheless, patients with multifocal ICC need to be selected carefully for surgical resection.

Another important finding of the study by Nathan and colleagues[40] was that tumor size had no independent effect on survival following resection of ICC. The sixth edition of the AJCC/UICC had used tumor size as an important prognostic factor to differentiate T subclassifications. As noted, however, the sixth edition staging scheme had been based exclusively on data from patients with HCC. Previous studies that included only patients with ICC had demonstrated conflicting results regarding the prognostic role of tumor size. While several studies had suggested that tumor size may be prognostically important, these studies were not only limited by insufficient sample size but also failed to separate the effect of tumor size from the effects of other negative prognostic factors (eg, lymph node metastasis, vascular invasion, presence of multiple tumors). The large SEER cohort used by Nathan and colleagues[40] allowed the investigators to demonstrate that tumor size had no effect on survival in both overall and multiple subgroup analyses.

Based on empirical data from their analyses, Nathan and colleagues[40] proposed a simplified staging system for ICC. The simplified staging system was found to have superior discriminatory ability compared with the sixth edition AJCC/UICC scheme, and also had better discriminatory power than the Japanese systems (Fig. 4). The data reported from Nathan and colleagues reflect the seventh edition of the AJCC/UICC staging system for ICC,[53] with some minor modifications (Table 3). In addition, the AJCC/UICC system recognizes 3 morphologic groups of ICC: mass-forming, periductal-infiltrating, and mixed mass–forming and periductal-infiltrating. The presence of any periductal-infiltrating component is used to define a T4 prognostic group.

The seventh edition AJCC/UICC staging system also includes a new stage grouping (IVa) that consists of patients with regional nodal metastasis (upstaged from stage III in the sixth edition). As noted, the presence of lymph node metastasis is a powerful predictor of adverse outcome following surgical resection.[33,37,40,41,45,51,54] In fact, 5-year survival after resection of node-positive ICC has been reported to be as low

Table 2
Select series of outcomes and factors associated with survival following resection of ICC

Authors, year	Study Period	N	Multiple Tumors	Size >5 cm	N1	VI	R1	5-yr OS	Multivariate Predictors of Survival
Weimann et al,[54] 2000	1978–1996	95	47%	–	25%	25%	15%	21%	Jaundice, N1, AJCC Stage
Inoue et al,[45] 2000	1980–1998	52	–	–	40%	63%	31%	36%	R1, N1, VI
Ohtsuka et al,[49] 2002	1984–2001	48	–	–	–	–	–	23%	Multiple tumors, serum CA 19-9 >1000 U/mL
Jan et al,[60] 2005	1977–1997	81	–	–	–	–	39%	14%	Symptoms, absence of mucobilia, R1, AJCC stage
DeOliveira et al,[59] 2007	1973–2004	44	–	–	29%	–	55%	40%	R1
Paik et al,[50] 2008	1994–2005	97	14%	42%	24%	–	7%	31%	Multiple tumors, R1
Konstadoulakis et al,[34] 2008	1991–2005	54	–	–	–	–	22%	25%	–
Nakagohri et al,[36] 2008	1992–2007	56	18%	–	37%	68%	25%	32%	Multiple tumors
Tamandl et al,[18] 2008	1994–2007	74	28%	54%	31%	26%	19%	28%	Size >5 cm, Multiple tumors
Endo et al,[33] 2008	1990–2006	82	29%	65%	9%	26%	15%	–a	Multiple tumors, VI, Bile duct resection, Size >5 cm, N1
Uenishi et al,[51] 2008	1985–2004	133	44%	–b	47%	60%	17%	29%	Multiple tumors, N1, R1
Nathan et al,[40] 2009	1988–2004	598	28%	49%	27%	34%	–	18%	Multiple tumors, VI, N1
Lang et al,[35] 2009	1998–2006	83	53%	84%	34%	41%	36%	21%	Male gender, R1, AJCC Stage
Choi et al,[41] 2009	2000–2007	64	11%	56%	27%	58%	14%	39%	N1
Shimada et al,[37] 2009	1990–2004	104	40%	–	32%	27%	26%	34%	Multiple tumors, N1

Abbreviations: N1, node-positive; VI, vascular invasion; R1, margin-positive; OS, overall survival.

a Median disease-specific survival of 36 months reported.
b 83% of patients in this study had tumors >3 cm in size.

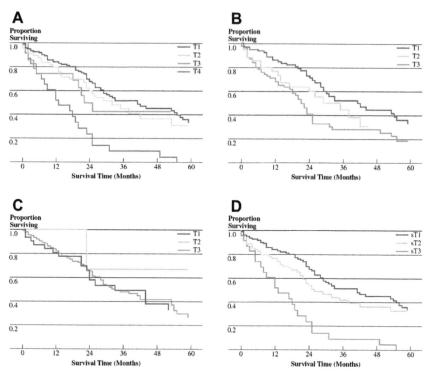

Fig. 4. Comparative performance of the T-stage classification of 4 staging systems for ICC based on analysis of 307 patients without nodal or metastatic disease (N0M0) identified in the SEER database, who underwent surgery for ICC from 1988 to 2004. (*A*) Sixth edition AJCC/UICC liver cancer T classification system. (*B*) Okabayashi ICC T classification system. (*C*) Liver Cancer Study Group of Japan (LCSGJ) ICC T classification system. (*D*) Simplified ICC T classification system proposed by the investigators. (*From* Nathan H, Aloia TA, Vauthey JN, et al. A proposed staging system for intrahepatic cholangiocarcinoma. Ann Surg Oncol 2009;16(1):14–22; with permission.)

as 4% to 11%.[37,40,41] In addition, several studies[39,40,55,56] have noted that the number of lymph nodes with metastatic disease may offer further prognostic information. Nakagawa and colleagues[39] reported that patients with 3 or more lymph nodes with metastatic disease had a worse overall survival than patients who had disease in 1 or 2 lymph nodes (3-year overall survival: 0% vs 50%, respectively). Similarly, Suzuki and colleagues[55] noted that the 5-year survival of patients with a solitary lymph node metastasis was 33% compared with no long-term survivors among the group with 2 or more lymph node metastases. Tamandl and colleagues[56] noted that an increased ratio of positive to examined lymph nodes was associated with recurrence-free and overall survival. Nonetheless, other investigators have reported that long-term survival following resection of ICC even with extensive lymph node metastasis is possible.[57,58]

Resection Margin Status as Prognostic Factor

Margin status is traditionally not included in the various staging systems for ICC; however, the importance of an R0 resection is generally recognized. The data on the relative importance of an R0 resection for ICC has been somewhat conflicting.

Table 3
American Joint Committee on Cancer seventh edition staging for ICC

Characteristics	
TNM classification	
T1	Solitary tumor without vascular invasion[a]
T2a	Solitary tumor with vascular invasion[a]
T2b	Multiple tumors, with or without vascular invasion[a]
T3	Tumor perforating the visceral peritoneum or involving local extrahepatic structures by direct invasion
T4	Tumor with periductal invasion[b]
N0	No regional lymph node metastasis
N1	Regional lymph node metastasis[c]
M0	No distant metastasis
M1	Distant metastasis
Stage groupings	
Stage I	T1 N0 M0
Stage II	T2 N0 M0
Stage III	T3 N0 M0
Stage IVA	T4 N0 M0, Any T N1 M0
Stage IVB	Any T Any N M1

[a] Includes major vascular (portal or hepatic vein) and microvascular invasion.
[b] Includes tumors with periductal-infiltrating or mixed mass–forming and periductal-infiltrating growth pattern.
[c] Nodal involvement of the celiac, periaortic, or caval lymph nodes is considered to be distant metastasis (M1).

Multiple reports have noted that microscopic disease at the surgical margin was associated with a worse outcome on multivariate analysis.[35,45,50,51,59,60] Other studies, however, have reported that margin status was not an independent predictor of adverse outcome.[18,33,36,37,40,41,49,54,61] These latter studies did have some methodological problems, including the inclusion of patients with unresectable disease as well as R0, R1, and R2 patients in the same analysis. Other investigators[18] attributed the lack of association between margin status and outcome to the use of the cavitron ultrasonic dissection device, which the investigators suggested vaporized and aspirated tissue up to 5 mm from cut liver surface.[62] In the same study, patients who underwent an R0 resection that was 1 to 10 mm in width did not experience an increase in intrahepatic or margin recurrences compared with patients who had a negative margin width of greater than 10 mm. Taken together, the surgeon should continue to pursue an operative approach that best ensures a margin clear of microscopic disease. The width of the surgical margin, however, seems of less import and patients should not be excluded from potentially curative surgical resection simply because of an anticipated margin of less than 10 mm.

OUTCOME FOLLOWING SURGERY
Recurrence

Recurrence following surgical resection of ICC remains a concern. Endo and colleagues[33] reported that more than 50% of patients recurred following resection with a median disease-free survival of 26 months. The liver was noted to be the most common site of recurrence (63%) either alone or in combination with one or more extrahepatic sites. Factors associated with an increased risk of recurrence included multiple tumors and lymph node metastasis. While the incidence of recurrence was 47% among patients with solitary tumors and no lymph node metastasis, recurrence was 93% among patients with multiple tumors and lymph node metastasis. Similarly, Choi and colleagues[41] reported a 64% overall risk of recurrence following resection of ICC. In this study the most common site of recurrence was the liver (56%), followed by the portal lymph nodes (31%) and the peritoneum (22%).[41] Yamamoto and colleagues[63] reported a recurrence of 46%, with recurrences occurring in the liver (56%), peritoneum (24%), and lymph nodes (20%). The relatively high rate of recurrence underscores the need for more efficacious adjuvant therapy.

Overall Survival

Five-year overall survival after surgical resection for ICC ranges between 14% and 40% in reported series (see **Table 2**).[18,33–37,40,41,45,49–51,54,59,60] Several studies have documented a trend toward improved overall survival over the last several decades for patients with ICC undergoing surgical resection, both at the national[16] and single-institution level.[33,59] DeOliveira and colleagues[59] recently reported a series of 564 patients with cholangiocarcinoma, 44 of whom had ICC. Five-year survival was better among patients undergoing resection after 1995. One significant shortcoming of this study, however, was that the investigators failed to stratify the analyses according to location of the cholangiocarcinoma. In a separate study, Endo and colleagues[33] did report a similar trend in improved long-term outcome over time among 82 patients with ICC resected from 1990 to 2006.

SYSTEMIC THERAPY FOR ICC

Patients with unresectable ICC have a median survival of between 5 and 8 months.[64] There is a need, therefore, for more effective systemic chemotherapy to treat patients with inoperable disease. Due to the small number of patients and the heterogeneous patient population in biliary tract cancers as compared with other more common malignancies, randomized phase 3 studies examining systemic chemotherapy have been a challenge to conduct. Based on experience from many phase 2 studies, systemic chemotherapy has improved from traditional fluoropyrimidine-based regimens that have response rates of only 10% to 30% to gemcitabine-based combination regimens with response rates in the range of 22% to 50%.[65–68] In 2006, results from a randomized phase 3 study comparing gemcitabine with or without cisplatin in patients with advanced or metastatic biliary tract cancers were presented.[69] This phase 3 study (UK ABC-02 trial), conducted in 410 patients with locally advanced (25%) or metastatic (75%) biliary tract cancers (bile duct, 59%; gallbladder, 36%; ampulla, 5%), demonstrated that the addition of cisplatin to gemcitabine afforded a significant improvement in progression-free (median of 8.4 vs 6.5 months; hazard ratio [HR], 0.72; 95% confidence interval [CI], 0.57–0.90); $P = .003$) and overall survival (median of 11.7 vs 8.3 months; HR, 0.70; 95% CI, 0.54–0.89; $P = .002$). In the exploratory subgroup analysis, the survival benefit persisted when only patients with cholangiocarcinoma were considered. Safety profiles were favorable in the gemcitabine-cisplatin arm without significant added toxicity compared with gemcitabine alone. This trial was the first well-conducted phase 3 study in advanced biliary tract cancers to convincingly demonstrate the improved survival benefits of combining cisplatin with gemcitabine compared with gemcitabine alone. The study also demonstrated the feasibility of conducting a large phase 3 study in an orphan disease such as cholangiocarcinoma.

These data may help to establish combination therapy with gemcitabine and cisplatin as a new standard of systemic treatment for patients with advanced biliary tract cancers. Molecularly targeted agents that inhibit angiogenesis[70,71] and epidermal growth factor receptor pathways[72–74] are also beginning to enter clinical trials for cholangiocarcinoma. It is hoped that further understanding of the molecular mechanism of carcinogenesis coupled with the development of molecular targeted agents in bile duct cancers will improve the outcomes of these patients.

At present, the role of adjuvant therapy for patients with resected cholangiocarcinoma is not established. Because of the relative rarity of ICC, there have been no trials specifically examining the role of adjuvant therapy. Because cholangiocarcinoma has traditionally had a poor response to systemic chemotherapy, systemic chemotherapy is often not employed in the setting of an R0 resection in patients with no lymph node metastasis. Although evidence is lacking, adjuvant chemotherapy using the agents highlighted here should be strongly considered in those patients with lymph node metastasis, given their worse prognosis.

LOCOREGIONAL THERAPY FOR ICC

The use of external-beam radiation therapy in the adjuvant setting is also controversial. While most studies on adjuvant radiation therapy have included only patients with hilar cholangiocarcinoma, Shinohara and colleagues[75] reported a series based on the SEER registry that included only patients with ICC. In this study, the investigators reported an improvement in survival for those patients receiving surgery plus radiation versus surgery alone. Although the difference in survival remained statistically significant even after adjusting for patient and tumor characteristics, selection bias remains a major threat to the validity of this retrospective study. Whereas routine adjuvant radiation therapy is likely unwarranted in patients who undergo an R0 resection, the use of adjuvant radiation therapy in patients undergoing an R1 resection should be strongly considered.

The role of radiation therapy for inoperable ICC disease is also poorly defined. Zeng and colleagues[76] reported a case-control study of 45 patients with unresectable ICC, 22 of whom received external-beam radiation therapy. Patients received a median total dose of 50 Gy in daily doses of 2 Gy per fraction 5 times a week. Objective responses were observed in 36% patients with unresectable ICC, with an associated 1- and 2-year survival of 36% and 19%. The investigators concluded that external-beam radiotherapy may prolong survival among patients with inoperable ICC and deserves further study.

Other locoregional treatment options for unresectable ICC include regional chemotherapy, transarterial chemoembolization (TACE), or thermal ablation. Regional chemotherapy delivered via a hepatic artery pump has mostly been studied among patients with metastatic colorectal cancer.[77] Regional chemotherapy via the hepatic artery has also been examined for primary liver cancer including ICC, with response rates reported to range from 40% to 64%.[78–81] Various chemotherapeutic agents have been used, including FUDR,[79] mitomycin C,[80] epirubicin with cisplatin,[78] and 5-fluorouracil.[81] In the authors' opinion, hepatic artery infusion chemotherapy has limited applicability in patients with ICC, and should only be employed at specialized centers or as part of a clinical trial.

TACE is a treatment modality with more general applicability for patients with unresectable ICC. While TACE has been shown to be associated with an improved survival compared with best supportive care in patients with unresectable HCC,[82,83] the data for TACE in unresectable ICC are much more limited. Gusani and colleagues[84] reported on the use of TACE among 42 patients with unresectable cholangiocarcinoma. In this series, most patients (88%) had a central cholangiocarcinoma while

12% had a peripheral lesion. The median number of TACE treatments per patient was 3.5. TACE was relatively well tolerated, with no periprocedural mortality and limited grade 3 or 4 toxicity. In a separate study, Burger and colleagues[85] reported on 17 patients with unresectable cholangiocarcinoma who were treated with one or more cycles of TACE between 1995 and 2004 at Johns Hopkins Hospital. Follow-up imaging was performed on all patients 4 to 6 weeks after each TACE procedure to determine tumor response and the need for further treatment. The median survival was 23 months. The procedure was well tolerated by 82% of the patients, who experienced no side effects or mild side effects that quickly resolved with conservative therapy alone. Two patients with previously unresectable disease underwent successful resection after TACE. The investigators suggested that TACE was effective at prolonging survival of patients with unresectable cholangiocarcinoma. Other investigators have also suggested that combining TACE with systemic chemotherapy may provide a further improvement in survival. Specifically, Gusani and colleagues[84] noted that patients treated with systemic gemcitabine-cisplatin combined with TACE had a longer survival than patients treated with TACE alone.

In patients who are not candidates for resection due to poor liver function or prohibitive comorbidities, thermal ablation may also be a reasonable option. For thermal ablation to be considered, the ICC lesion needs to be small ($\leq$3–5 cm) and located away from major vascular or biliary structures. Most patients with ICC, however, will usually either be candidates for surgical resection or will present with large tumors, making thermal ablation not a therapeutic option.

SUMMARY

ICC remains a relatively poorly understood malignancy despite its recent increase in incidence in the United States. Patients with ICC should be strongly considered for surgical resection, as this is the only potentially curative therapeutic option. Because many patients with ICC present with large tumors, resection may often require an extended hepatectomy or resection/reconstruction of the extrahepatic biliary tree. Surgery for ICC should therefore be performed by experienced hepatobiliary surgeons. A new pathologic staging system for ICC has been established in the seventh edition of the AJCC/UICC staging manual. ICC staging uses tumor number and the presence of vascular invasion, but not tumor size. Other important prognostic factors include lymph node metastasis and resection margin status. Although adjuvant chemotherapy and radiotherapy is probably not supported by current data, each should strongly be considered in patients with lymph node metastasis or an R1 resection. For those patients with inoperable disease, locoregional therapy with TACE can be considered. ICC remains a complex disease that presents the clinician with a host of diagnostic and therapeutic challenges, and is therefore best managed in the multidisciplinary setting.

REFERENCES

1. Lazaridis KN, Gores GJ. Cholangiocarcinoma. Gastroenterology 2005;128(6): 1655–67.
2. Vauthey JN, Blumgart LH. Recent advances in the management of cholangiocarcinomas. Semin Liver Dis 1994;14(2):109–14.
3. Carpizo DR, D'Angelica M. Management and extent of resection for intrahepatic cholangiocarcinoma. Surg Oncol Clin N Am 2009;18(2):289–305, viii-ix.
4. Aljiffry M, Abdulelah A, Walsh M, et al. Evidence-based approach to cholangiocarcinoma: a systematic review of the current literature. J Am Coll Surg 2009; 208(1):134–47.

5. Patel T. Worldwide trends in mortality from biliary tract malignancies. BMC Cancer 2002;2:10.
6. Shaib YH, Davila JA, McGlynn K, et al. Rising incidence of intrahepatic cholangiocarcinoma in the United States: a true increase? J Hepatol 2004;40(3):472–7.
7. Taylor-Robinson SD, Foster GR, Arora S, et al. Increase in primary liver cancer in the UK, 1979-94. Lancet 1997;350(9085):1142–3.
8. Kato I, Kuroishi T, Tominaga S. Descriptive epidemiology of subsites of cancers of the liver, biliary tract and pancreas in Japan. Jpn J Clin Oncol 1990;20(3):232–7.
9. Welzel TM, McGlynn KA, Hsing AW, et al. Impact of classification of hilar cholangiocarcinomas (Klatskin tumors) on the incidence of intra- and extrahepatic cholangiocarcinoma in the United States. J Natl Cancer Inst 2006;98(12):873–5.
10. El-Serag HB, Engels EA, Landgren O, et al. Risk of hepatobiliary and pancreatic cancers after hepatitis C virus infection: a population-based study of U.S. veterans. Hepatology 2009;49(1):116–23.
11. Shaib YH, El-Serag HB, Davila JA, et al. Risk factors of intrahepatic cholangiocarcinoma in the United States: a case-control study. Gastroenterology 2005; 128(3):620–6.
12. Donato F, Gelatti U, Tagger A, et al. Intrahepatic cholangiocarcinoma and hepatitis C and B virus infection, alcohol intake, and hepatolithiasis: a case-control study in Italy. Cancer Causes Control 2001;12(10):959–64.
13. Kobayashi M, Ikeda K, Saitoh S, et al. Incidence of primary cholangiocellular carcinoma of the liver in Japanese patients with hepatitis C virus-related cirrhosis. Cancer 2000;88(11):2471–7.
14. Welzel TM, Graubard BI, El-Serag HB, et al. Risk factors for intrahepatic and extrahepatic cholangiocarcinoma in the United States: a population-based case-control study. Clin Gastroenterol Hepatol 2007;5(10):1221–8.
15. Patel T. Increasing incidence and mortality of primary intrahepatic cholangiocarcinoma in the United States. Hepatology 2001;33(6):1353–7.
16. Nathan H, Pawlik TM, Wolfgang CL, et al. Trends in survival after surgery for cholangiocarcinoma: a 30-year population-based SEER database analysis. J Gastrointest Surg 2007;11(11):1488–96 [discussion: 1496–7].
17. Patel AH, Harnois DM, Klee GG, et al. The utility of CA 19-9 in the diagnoses of cholangiocarcinoma in patients without primary sclerosing cholangitis. Am J Gastroenterol 2000;95(1):204–7.
18. Tamandl D, Herberger B, Gruenberger B, et al. Influence of hepatic resection margin on recurrence and survival in intrahepatic cholangiocarcinoma. Ann Surg Oncol 2008;15(10):2787–94.
19. Yamasaki S. Intrahepatic cholangiocarcinoma: macroscopic type and stage classification. J Hepatobiliary Pancreat Surg 2003;10(4):288–91.
20. Chung YE, Kim MJ, Park YN, et al. Varying appearances of cholangiocarcinoma: radiologic-pathologic correlation. Radiographics 2009;29(3):683–700.
21. Manfredi R, Barbaro B, Masselli G, et al. Magnetic resonance imaging of cholangiocarcinoma. Semin Liver Dis 2004;24(2):155–64.
22. Chen LD, Xu HX, Xie XY, et al. Enhancement patterns of intrahepatic cholangiocarcinoma: comparison between contrast-enhanced ultrasound and contrast-enhanced CT. Br J Radiol 2008;81(971):881–9.
23. Miller G, Schwartz LH, D'Angelica M. The use of imaging in the diagnosis and staging of hepatobiliary malignancies. Surg Oncol Clin N Am 2007;16(2):343–68.
24. Maetani Y, Itoh K, Watanabe C, et al. MR imaging of intrahepatic cholangiocarcinoma with pathologic correlation. AJR Am J Roentgenol 2001;176(6):1499–507.

25. Anderson CD, Rice MH, Pinson CW, et al. Fluorodeoxyglucose PET imaging in the evaluation of gallbladder carcinoma and cholangiocarcinoma. J Gastrointest Surg 2004;8(1):90–7.
26. Kim YJ, Yun M, Lee WJ, et al. Usefulness of ^{18}F-FDG PET in intrahepatic cholangiocarcinoma. Eur J Nucl Med Mol Imaging 2003;30(11):1467–72.
27. Corvera CU, Blumgart LH, Akhurst T, et al. ^{18}F-fluorodeoxyglucose positron emission tomography influences management decisions in patients with biliary cancer. J Am Coll Surg 2008;206(1):57–65.
28. Petrowsky H, Wildbrett P, Husarik DB, et al. Impact of integrated positron emission tomography and computed tomography on staging and management of gallbladder cancer and cholangiocarcinoma. J Hepatol 2006;45(1):43–50.
29. Goere D, Wagholikar GD, Pessaux P, et al. Utility of staging laparoscopy in subsets of biliary cancers: laparoscopy is a powerful diagnostic tool in patients with intrahepatic and gallbladder carcinoma. Surg Endosc 2006;20(5):721–5.
30. Weber SM, Jarnagin WR, Klimstra D, et al. Intrahepatic cholangiocarcinoma: resectability, recurrence pattern, and outcomes. J Am Coll Surg 2001;193(4):384–91.
31. Tan JC, Coburn NG, Baxter NN, et al. Surgical management of intrahepatic cholangiocarcinoma—a population-based study. Ann Surg Oncol 2008;15(2):600–8.
32. Sotiropoulos GC, Bockhorn M, Sgourakis G, et al. R0 liver resections for primary malignant liver tumors in the noncirrhotic liver: a diagnosis-related analysis. Dig Dis Sci 2009;54(4):887–94.
33. Endo I, Gonen M, Yopp AC, et al. Intrahepatic cholangiocarcinoma: rising frequency, improved survival, and determinants of outcome after resection. Ann Surg 2008;248(1):84–96.
34. Konstadoulakis MM, Roayaie S, Gomatos IP, et al. Fifteen-year, single-center experience with the surgical management of intrahepatic cholangiocarcinoma: operative results and long-term outcome. Surgery 2008;143(3):366–74.
35. Lang H, Sotiropoulos GC, Sgourakis G, et al. Operations for intrahepatic cholangiocarcinoma: single-institution experience of 158 patients. J Am Coll Surg 2009;208(2):218–28.
36. Nakagohri T, Kinoshita T, Konishi M, et al. Surgical outcome and prognostic factors in intrahepatic cholangiocarcinoma. World J Surg 2008;32(12):2675–80.
37. Shimada K, Sano T, Nara S, et al. Therapeutic value of lymph node dissection during hepatectomy in patients with intrahepatic cholangiocellular carcinoma with negative lymph node involvement. Surgery 2009;145(4):411–6.
38. Nathan H, Cameron JL, Choti MA, et al. The volume-outcomes effect in hepato-pancreato-biliary surgery: hospital versus surgeon contributions and specificity of the relationship. J Am Coll Surg 2009;208(4):528–38.
39. Nakagawa T, Kamiyama T, Kurauchi N, et al. Number of lymph node metastases is a significant prognostic factor in intrahepatic cholangiocarcinoma. World J Surg 2005;29(6):728–33.
40. Nathan H, Aloia TA, Vauthey JN, et al. A proposed staging system for intrahepatic cholangiocarcinoma. Ann Surg Oncol 2009;16(1):14–22.
41. Choi SB, Kim KS, Choi JY, et al. The prognosis and survival outcome of intrahepatic cholangiocarcinoma following surgical resection: association of lymph node metastasis and lymph node dissection with survival. Ann Surg Oncol 2009;16(11):3048–56.
42. Okabayashi T, Yamamoto J, Kosuge T, et al. A new staging system for mass-forming intrahepatic cholangiocarcinoma: analysis of preoperative and postoperative variables. Cancer 2001;92(9):2374–83.

43. Greene F, Page D, Flemming I, et al. AJCC cancer staging manual. 6th edition. New York: Springer-Verlag; 2002.
44. Ikeda K, Saitoh S, Koida I, et al. A multivariate analysis of risk factors for hepatocellular carcinogenesis: a prospective observation of 795 patients with viral and alcoholic cirrhosis. Hepatology 1993;18(1):47–53.
45. Inoue K, Makuuchi M, Takayama T, et al. Long-term survival and prognostic factors in the surgical treatment of mass-forming type cholangiocarcinoma. Surgery 2000;127(5):498–505.
46. Parkin DM, Srivatanakul P, Khlat M, et al. Liver cancer in Thailand. I. A case-control study of cholangiocarcinoma. Int J Cancer 1991;48(3):323–8.
47. Srivatanakul P, Parkin DM, Jiang YZ, et al. The role of infection by *Opisthorchis viverrini*, hepatitis B virus, and aflatoxin exposure in the etiology of liver cancer in Thailand. A correlation study. Cancer 1991;68(11):2411–7.
48. Srivatanakul P, Parkin DM, Khlat M, et al. Liver cancer in Thailand. II. A case-control study of hepatocellular carcinoma. Int J Cancer 1991;48(3):329–32.
49. Ohtsuka M, Ito H, Kimura F, et al. Results of surgical treatment for intrahepatic cholangiocarcinoma and clinicopathological factors influencing survival. Br J Surg 2002;89(12):1525–31.
50. Paik KY, Jung JC, Heo JS, et al. What prognostic factors are important for resected intrahepatic cholangiocarcinoma? J Gastroenterol Hepatol 2008;23(5):766–70.
51. Uenishi T, Kubo S, Yamazaki O, et al. Indications for surgical treatment of intrahepatic cholangiocarcinoma with lymph node metastases. J Hepatobiliary Pancreat Surg 2008;15(4):417–22.
52. Shimada M, Yamashita Y, Aishima S, et al. Value of lymph node dissection during resection of intrahepatic cholangiocarcinoma. Br J Surg 2001;88(11): 1463–6.
53. Edge S, Byrd D, Compton C, et al. AJCC cancer staging manual. 7th edition. New York: Springer-Verlag; 2010.
54. Weimann A, Varnholt H, Schlitt HJ, et al. Retrospective analysis of prognostic factors after liver resection and transplantation for cholangiocellular carcinoma. Br J Surg 2000;87(9):1182–7.
55. Suzuki S, Sakaguchi T, Yokoi Y, et al. Clinicopathological prognostic factors and impact of surgical treatment of mass-forming intrahepatic cholangiocarcinoma. World J Surg 2002;26(6):687–93.
56. Tamandl D, Kaczirek K, Gruenberger B, et al. Lymph node ratio after curative surgery for intrahepatic cholangiocarcinoma. Br J Surg 2009;96(8):919–25.
57. Asakura H, Ohtsuka M, Ito H, et al. Long-term survival after extended surgical resection of intrahepatic cholangiocarcinoma with extensive lymph node metastasis. Hepatogastroenterology 2005;52(63):722–4.
58. Murakami Y, Yokoyama T, Takesue Y, et al. Long-term survival of peripheral intrahepatic cholangiocarcinoma with metastasis to the para-aortic lymph nodes. Surgery 2000;127(1):105–6.
59. DeOliveira ML, Cunningham SC, Cameron JL, et al. Cholangiocarcinoma: thirty-one-year experience with 564 patients at a single institution. Ann Surg 2007; 245(5):755–62.
60. Jan YY, Yeh CN, Yeh TS, et al. Clinicopathological factors predicting long-term overall survival after hepatectomy for peripheral cholangiocarcinoma. World J Surg 2005;29(7):894–8.
61. Guglielmi A, Ruzzenente A, Campagnaro T, et al. Intrahepatic cholangiocarcinoma: prognostic factors after surgical resection. World J Surg 2009;33(6): 1247–54.

62. Bodingbauer M, Tamandl D, Schmid K, et al. Size of surgical margin does not influence recurrence rates after curative liver resection for colorectal cancer liver metastases. Br J Surg 2007;94(9):1133–8.

63. Yamamoto M, Takasaki K, Otsubo T, et al. Recurrence after surgical resection of intrahepatic cholangiocarcinoma. J Hepatobiliary Pancreat Surg 2001;8(2):154–7.

64. Chou FF, Sheen-Chen SM, Chen YS, et al. Surgical treatment of cholangiocarcinoma. Hepatogastroenterology 1997;44(15):760–5.

65. Eckel F, Schmid RM. Chemotherapy in advanced biliary tract carcinoma: a pooled analysis of clinical trials. Br J Cancer 2007;96(6):896–902.

66. Huitzil-Melendez FD, O'Reilly EM, Duffy A, et al. Indications for neoadjuvant, adjuvant, and palliative chemotherapy in the treatment of biliary tract cancers. Surg Oncol Clin N Am 2009;18(2):361–79, x.

67. Hezel AF, Zhu AX. Systemic therapy for biliary tract cancers. Oncologist 2008; 13(4):415–23.

68. Verderame F, Russo A, Di Leo R, et al. Gemcitabine and oxaliplatin combination chemotherapy in advanced biliary tract cancers. Ann Oncol 2006;17(Suppl 7):vii, 68–72.

69. Valle J, Wasan H, Palmer DH, et al. Cisplatin plus gemcitabine versus gemcitabine for biliary tract cancer. N Engl J Med 2010;362(14):1273–81.

70. Bengala C, Bertolini F, Malavasi N, et al. Sorafenib in patients with advanced biliary tract carcinoma: a phase II trial. Br J Cancer 2010;102(1):68–72.

71. Zhu AX, Meyerhardt JA, Blaszkowsky LS, et al. Efficacy and safety of gemcitabine, oxaliplatin, and bevacizumab in advanced biliary-tract cancers and correlation of changes in 18-fluorodeoxyglucose PET with clinical outcome: a phase 2 study. Lancet Oncol 2010;11(1):48–54.

72. Malka D, Trarbach T, Fartoux L, et al. A multicenter, randomized phase II trial of gemcitabine and oxaliplatin (GEMOX) alone or in combination with biweekly cetuximab in the first-line treatment of advanced biliary cancer: interim analysis of the BINGO trial [abstract: 4520]. J Clin Oncol 2009;27(Suppl):15s.

73. Philip PA, Mahoney MR, Allmer C, et al. Phase II study of erlotinib in patients with advanced biliary cancer. J Clin Oncol 2006;24(19):3069–74.

74. Ramanathan RK, Belani CP, Singh DA, et al. A phase II study of lapatinib in patients with advanced biliary tree and hepatocellular cancer. Cancer Chemother Pharmacol 2009;64(4):777–83.

75. Shinohara ET, Mitra N, Guo M, et al. Radiation therapy is associated with improved survival in the adjuvant and definitive treatment of intrahepatic cholangiocarcinoma. Int J Radiat Oncol Biol Phys 2008;72(5):1495–501.

76. Zeng ZC, Tang ZY, Fan J, et al. Consideration of the role of radiotherapy for unresectable intrahepatic cholangiocarcinoma: a retrospective analysis of 75 patients. Cancer J 2006;12(2):113–22.

77. Kemeny NE, Niedzwiecki D, Hollis DR, et al. Hepatic arterial infusion versus systemic therapy for hepatic metastases from colorectal cancer: a randomized trial of efficacy, quality of life, and molecular markers (CALGB 9481). J Clin Oncol 2006;24(9):1395–403.

78. Cantore M, Mambrini A, Fiorentini G, et al. Phase II study of hepatic intraarterial epirubicin and cisplatin, with systemic 5-fluorouracil in patients with unresectable biliary tract tumors. Cancer 2005;103(7):1402–7.

79. Jarnagin WR, Schwartz LH, Gultekin DH, et al. Regional chemotherapy for unresectable primary liver cancer: results of a phase II clinical trial and assessment of DCE-MRI as a biomarker of survival. Ann Oncol 2009;20(9): 1589–95.

80. Shitara K, Ikami I, Munakata M, et al. Hepatic arterial infusion of mitomycin C with degradable starch microspheres for unresectable intrahepatic cholangio-carcinoma. Clin Oncol (R Coll Radiol) 2008;20(3):241–6.
81. Tanaka N, Yamakado K, Nakatsuka A, et al. Arterial chemoinfusion therapy through an implanted port system for patients with unresectable intrahepatic cholangiocarcinoma—initial experience. Eur J Radiol 2002;41(1):42–8.
82. Llovet JM, Real MI, Montana X, et al. Arterial embolisation or chemoembolisation versus symptomatic treatment in patients with unresectable hepatocellular carcinoma: a randomised controlled trial. Lancet 2002;359(9319):1734–9.
83. Lo CM, Ngan H, Tso WK, et al. Randomized controlled trial of transarterial lipiodol chemoembolization for unresectable hepatocellular carcinoma. Hepatology 2002;35(5):1164–71.
84. Gusani NJ, Balaa FK, Steel JL, et al. Treatment of unresectable cholangiocarcinoma with gemcitabine-based transcatheter arterial chemoembolization (TACE): a single-institution experience. J Gastrointest Surg 2008;12(1):129–37.
85. Burger I, Hong K, Schulick R, et al. Transcatheter arterial chemoembolization in unresectable cholangiocarcinoma: initial experience in a single institution. J Vasc Interv Radiol 2005;16(3):353–61.

Hepatic Resection for Colorectal Liver Metastases

Russell E. Brown, MD, Matthew R. Bower, MD,
Robert C.G. Martin, MD, PhD*

KEYWORDS

• Liver resection • Metastases • Colorectal cancer

Colorectal adenocarcinoma remains the third most common cause of cancer death in the United States, with an estimated 146,000 new cases and 50,000 deaths annually. Survival is stage dependent, and the presence of liver metastases is a primary determinant in patient survival. Approximately 25% of new cases will present with synchronous colorectal liver metastases (CLM), and up to one-half will develop CLM during the course of their disease.[1–4] The importance of safe and effective therapies for CLM cannot be overstated. Safe and appropriately aggressive multimodality therapy for CLM can provide most patients with liver-dominant colorectal metastases with extended survival and an improved quality of life.[1–14]

OUTCOMES AFTER SURGICAL RESECTION OF CLM

Hepatic resection for metastatic disease has been practiced for decades. Lortat-Jacob and colleagues[15] described right hepatectomy for secondary malignancy in 1952. Initial anecdotal success has been followed by continued improvements in perioperative and long-term survival. The progressive success of CLM resection can be attributed to improvements in multimodality therapy including systemic chemotherapy and targeted therapies, as well as efforts to increase the proportion of patients eligible for resection. Choti and colleagues[16] observed an increase in 5-year survival from 31% to 58% for patients undergoing CLM resection between 1984 and 1992 compared with patients from 1993 to 1999. For solitary CLM, perhaps the most favorable group, 5-year overall survival of 71% has been reported.[17]

Hepatic resection, when feasible, is the only treatment associated with long-term survival.[3–14] Based on a review of 10-year survivors who underwent resection before

Division of Surgical Oncology, Department of Surgery, James Graham Brown Cancer, University of Louisville School of Medicine, 315 East Broadway, Louisville, KY 40202, USA
* Corresponding author.
E-mail address: rcmart03@gwise.louisville.edu

Surg Clin N Am 90 (2010) 839–852
doi:10.1016/j.suc.2010.04.012
0039-6109/10/$ – see front matter © 2010 Elsevier Inc. All rights reserved.

1994 (ie, before the use of modern chemotherapy), current 10-year survival in at least 1 of 6 patients can be postulated after resection of CLM.[18]

With improvements in surgical and anesthetic techniques, as well as postoperative care, hepatic surgery has become a safe procedure in experienced centers. Patients have benefited from improvements in perioperative outcomes after hepatic resection, with reports of mortalities of less than 4% and all-cause morbidity approaching 40%.[4,19–22]

PREOPERATIVE EVALUATION

The central tenets in the preoperative evaluation of patients for potential surgical resection of CLM are: (1) evaluation of the patient's fitness for operation; (2) anatomic and functional determination of tumor respectability; (3) estimation of an individual's tumor biology.[23,24]

All patients with CLM benefit from evaluation by a multidisciplinary team comprising physicians (surgeons, medical oncologists, radiologists, pathologists), nurses, social workers, and research coordinators. In our experience, this approach has been invaluable in terms of reaching efficient consensus on patient treatment plans among specialties. Multidisciplinary conferences and clinics minimize delays in treatment, improve communication between specialties, and allow for the identification of those unresectable patients who may benefit from surgical resection, ablation, or catheter-based therapies.[25–27]

Evaluation of Fitness for Operation

A careful evaluation of a patient's physiologic capability to tolerate hepatic resection is necessary to ensure favorable outcomes after hepatectomy. In addition to a deliberate cardiopulmonary evaluation and the attention to medical comorbidities required for major abdominal surgery, a thorough consideration of the patient's liver function is required. History, physical examination, and routine laboratory studies (complete blood count, liver function testing, and coagulation studies) are relied on to screen for underlying liver dysfunction. Preoperative imaging studies (discussed later) may also help to identify those patients with underlying hepatic disease.

Preoperative biopsy of CLM is rarely indicated or beneficial for assessment of CLM, and has been associated with tumor dissemination and decreased survival.[28] Preoperative biopsy may have usefulness for confirmation of extrahepatic disease when a change in therapy is planned based on the biopsy results.

Anatomic and Functional Determination of Resectability

Resectability of CLM has been well defined by the American Hepato-Pancreato-Biliary Association (AHPBA)/Society of Surgery of the Alimentary Tract (SSAT)/Society of Surgical Oncology (SSO) in a 2006 consensus statement[5] as an expected margin-negative (R-0) resection resulting in preservation of at least 2 contiguous hepatic segments with adequate inflow, outflow, and biliary drainage with a functional liver remnant (FLR) volume of more than 20% (for healthy liver).

Determination of resectability is primarily based on preoperative imaging. High-quality cross-sectional imaging is critical for gauging the extent of disease, response to preoperative therapy, and for operative planning. Patients should be routinely reimaged after any course of systemic therapy; preferably within 4 weeks of planned resection. Currently, we find triple-phase helical computed tomography (CT) to be the most useful modality for defining intrahepatic anatomy and resection planes. We reserve ultrasound and magnetic resonance imaging (MRI) as adjuncts for characterizing small or equivocal lesions by 3-phase CT. Fusion positron emission tomography (PET)-CT imaging has shown high sensitivity (95% on a per patient basis, 76% on a per lesion basis[29]) and we have found it to be beneficial in assessing extrahepatic disease burden.

Meticulous preoperative attention to the relationships of CLM to arterioportal inflow, biliary drainage, and hepatic venous outflow is necessary and allows for an informed and efficient hepatectomy. At present, this level of anatomic detail is only evident using 3-phase CT or dynamic MRI. PET-CT has insufficient resolution to make these preoperative determinations. Vascular and biliary anomalies are common and should be anticipated before resection. If necessary, CT arterial reconstruction and magnetic resonance cholangiopancreatography may be useful in clarifying anatomic variants.

Given the morbidity and potentially devastating consequences of postoperative liver insufficiency, much attention has been given to the future liver remnant (FLR), which remains after extended (≥ 5 segment) hepatectomy. CT volumetry has been used to quantify the FLR by standardized methods.[30–32] Safety of extended hepatectomy has been shown for FLR volumes approaching 20% for patients with normal liver parenchyma. Those patients with underlying liver disease require more conservative limits of FLR (ie, 30% for moderate fibrosis; 40% for cirrhosis[6,33]).

Besides delineating intrahepatic anatomy, preoperative cross-sectional imaging may also help to identify the presence of concomitant parenchymal disease (eg, fibrosis/cirrhosis, portal hypertension, steatohepatitis) or extrahepatic disease. Identification of concomitant hepatic pathology or extrahepatic metastases requires a careful search for the presence of hepatic atrophy, beaking of the liver edge, liver nodularity, splenomegaly, ascites, varices, omental caking, peritoneal nodules, and porta hepatis or aortocaval lymphadenopathy.[34]

Diagnostic laparoscopy has a role in staging those patients in whom preoperative imaging or high-risk scores (see later discussion) suggest a high likelihood for finding intra-abdominal extrahepatic disease[35] or for patients with indeterminate intrahepatic lesions that may be best characterized by intraoperative ultrasound (IOUS). We have occasionally found laparoscopy useful in assessing the status of the remnant liver. In those patients whose history, laboratory studies, or imaging predicts marginal liver function, diagnostic laparoscopy can be used to visually examine the liver as well as to perform biopsies before proceeding with hepatectomy.

Analysis of Tumor Biology

Once tumor resectability and fitness for operation have been confirmed, consideration should be given to an individual patient's tumor biology; that is, whether a patient's disease favors a more indolent or a more aggressive behavior. Consideration of this question is far from an exact science, but valuable information can be gleaned from factors such as the stage of primary disease, number and distribution of CLM, tumor histology, response to chemotherapy (currently best judged by response evaluation criteria in solid tumors [RECIST] criteria based on CT imaging[36]), rate of growth of CLM on serial imaging, or rate of increase in serum carcinoembryonic antigen (CEA). Fong and colleagues,[37] proposed a clinical risk score based on a multivariate retrospective analysis that correlated node-positive primary, disease-free interval of less than 12 months, number of metastases in excess of 1, CEA more than 200 ng/mL, and primary tumor larger than 5 cm with decreased survival (**Table 1**). In an external cohort validation study of multiple prognostic indices,[38] the Fong and Iwatsuki[39] scores were found to be predictive of survival.

Table 1
Clinical risk score based on 5 preoperative risk factors (1 point for each factor): node-positive primary, disease-free interval less than 12 months, more than 1 tumor, size greater than 5 cm, CEA greater than 200 ng/mL

Total	Survival (%)					Median
	1 y	2 y	3 y	4 y	5 y	
0	93	79	72	60	60	74
1	91	76	66	54	44	51
2	89	73	60	51	40	47
3	86	67	42	25	20	33
4	70	45	38	29	25	20
5	71	45	27	14	14	22

(*Data from* Fong Y, Fortner J, Sun RL, et al. Clinical score for predicting recurrence after hepatic resection for metastatic colorectal cancer: analysis of 1001 consecutive cases. Ann Surg 1999;230:309; with permission.)

Although prognostic assessment of individual tumor biology is difficult and inexact at this point, careful evaluation of all patients in a multidisciplinary setting allows for better identification of those patients most likely to benefit from surgical resection as opposed to those who would benefit more from nonoperative therapies, given their particularly aggressive disease.

CONTROVERSIES IN RESECTION OF CLM

The treatment of CLM among institutions is not strictly uniform, and there are multiple controversies that merit discussion.

Timing of Chemotherapy Relative to Hepatectomy

Advances in systemic chemotherapy are largely responsible for the improved outcomes in patients with CLM. Significant debate exists about the timing of chemotherapy administration relative to resection of CLM. Potential downsides of preoperative chemotherapy are largely related to hepatic toxicities that may be clinically relevant. Oxaliplatin has been linked to steatohepatitis and sinusoidal obstruction; irinotecan has been associated with steatohepatitis and periportal inflammation.[40,41] Some groups have noted increases in hepatotoxicity after chemotherapy and have associated this with an increase in perioperative complications.[33,42,43] Other centers have not witnessed an increase in complications with the use of prehepatectomy chemotherapy, despite finding histologic evidence of liver injury.[44–46]

Randomized prospective data from the European Organization for Research and Treatment of Cancer (EORTC) Intergroup trial 40983 showed an absolute increase in 3-year progression-free survival of 9.2% in patients who underwent perioperative (pre- and posthepatectomy) with FOLFOX4 (oxaliplatin, leucovorin, and 5-fluorouracil) compared with surgery alone. A 9% increase in reversible postoperative complications was observed, which reached statistical significance.[47]

Steatohepatitis has also been associated with patient factors including obesity, diabetes, insulin resistance, hypertension, viral hepatitis, alcohol use, and dyslipidemia.[48,49] These patient factors may play an equivalent or larger role in chemotherapy-induced liver injury than chemotherapy itself and should be taken into consideration before hepatic resection.

Potential benefits of prehepatectomy chemotherapy for CLM include the possibility for downstaging liver metastases, in vivo testing of chemotherapeutic efficacy, identification of occult intra- or extrahepatic metastases, and early exposure of subclinical microscopic metastases to systemic therapy. In addition, prehepatectomy chemotherapy, with prudent monitoring and attention to comorbidities, allows for improved patient selection for resection of CLM.[45,46,50]

We find that, in practice, most patients referred to our institution with CLM will have had exposure to systemic chemotherapy before consideration of resection. A recent review of our experience[46] with prehepatectomy chemotherapy did not find an increased risk of postoperative complications or mortality compared with patients without preoperative chemotherapy exposure. In general, we favor up-front chemotherapy administration in close coordination with medical oncologists with interval monitoring for hepatic toxicity. We use 3 to 4 cycles of preoperative chemotherapy, followed by at least 4 weeks for recovery before hepatectomy after oxaliplatin, 5-fluorouracil, irinotecan, or bevacizumab-based regimens. In most cases, we consider progression on systemic chemotherapy a relative contraindication to CLM resection, especially if tumor progression is seen in extrahepatic sites or in the planned remnant liver segments. In such cases, we advocate second-line systemic chemotherapy and consideration of catheter-based therapy (transarterial chemoembolization, irinotecan-eluting beads,[51] or yttrium-90 radioembolization[52]).

Synchronous CLM

Synchronous CLM are noted in 20% to 30% of patients at the time of initial colorectal cancer diagnosis.[53] Surgical management of this group of early metastases has been debated in terms of disease biology, operative approach (staged vs simultaneous colorectal and liver resection), the order of resection, and timing of chemotherapy.[54] Good judgment is required in selection of patients for a simultaneous or a staged resection in close coordination with medical oncologists and collaborating surgeons. Potential benefits of simultaneous CLM resection include avoidance of a second laparotomy and anesthetic, and decreased time to initiation of adjuvant chemotherapy. Perceived risks of simultaneous CLM resection are largely related to the magnitude and complexity of the combined operation.

We favor a selective approach to synchronous CLM based on careful consideration of the technical complexity and risks for the colorectal and liver resections, as well as judicious intraoperative decision making. At our institution, 2 teams of surgeons are commonly used to improve operative efficiency in simultaneous resections. In practice, most simultaneous CLM resections can be performed through a midline laparotomy or (for sigmoid or rectal lesions) a small low-midline incision that can be used for a hand-assisted laparoscopic hepatectomy. For difficult hepatic exposures, a hockey stick (J-shaped) incision is recommended for right lobe mobilization.[55] We favor initial liver resection during simultaneous procedures to take advantage of permissive hypotension and low central venous pressure anesthetic techniques. Our experience supports simultaneous CLM resection in well-selected patients and has shown equivalent morbidity and mortality with reduced hospital stay compared with staged resection.[56]

When a staged approach is planned, a recent decision analysis based on clinical series supports initial hepatectomy followed by colorectal resection.[57]

The role of simultaneous CLM resection using laparoscopic techniques has been reported,[58] but not yet clearly defined. We have successfully performed simultaneous laparoscopic colorectal and liver resections in the setting of CLM in well-selected patients with favorable outcomes. Our expectation is that the advantages of laparoscopic approaches will also extend to this population.

Bilobar Metastases

Bilobar metastases are no longer an absolute contraindication to resection. When feasible, these patients can undergo extended hepatectomy,[59] 2-stage hepatectomy,[60] or combined hepatic resection and ablation.[23] For those patients with insufficient FLR, portal vein embolization (PVE) may be a useful adjunct to increase the size of the FLR and allow for safe extended hepatectomy.[61]

There has been recent interest in 2-stage hepatectomy for patients who present with bilobar metastases not amenable to hepatectomy despite preoperative chemotherapy. This approach generally involves an initial hepatectomy with contralateral portal vein ligation[62] or postoperative PVE,[63] followed by chemotherapy. After restaging, a second hepatectomy is performed based on response to PVE/chemotherapy and ability to achieve resection with an adequate FLR.[60,62–65] This approach requires close coordination with medical oncologists and interventional radiologists for several weeks and demands minimal perioperative complication rates. A proportion of patients (31% according to Wicherts and colleagues[64] and 30% according to Chun and colleagues[63]) will not be eligible for second hepatectomy because of disease progression, inadequate FLR, or perioperative or chemotherapy-associated complications.

In our practice, we have not encountered a large number of patients whose disease is amenable to 2-stage hepatectomy. We attribute this to a close working relationship with our medical oncologist colleagues and referring physicians who recognize the benefits of early referral for consideration of CLM resection. We favor extended hepatectomy in combination with thermal ablation for extensive bilobar metastases, which allows for a single operative intervention and early administration of postoperative chemotherapy without the morbidity of second hepatectomy.[23] Elias and colleagues[66] reported a median survival of 36 months for 63 patients who underwent hepatectomy combined with radiofrequency ablation and perioperative chemotherapy for technically unresectable CLM.

Extrahepatic Colorectal Metastases

In the past, extrahepatic disease has been labeled an absolute contraindication to resection of CLM.[67] However, with the advent of more effective systemic therapies,

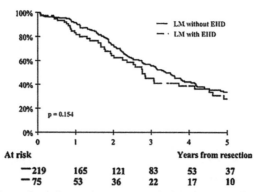

Fig. 1. Influence of extrahepatic metastases on survival in patients who received R-0 resections. EHD, extrahepatic disease; LM, liver metastases. (*From* Elias D, Sideris L, Pocard M, et al. Results of R0 resection for colorectal liver metastases associated with extrahepatic disease. Ann Surg Oncol 2004;11:274; with permission.)

a growing body of literature supports R-0 resection of CLM and extrahepatic metastases (**Fig. 1**).[24,68–71]

All extrahepatic sites of metastases are not equivalent in terms of prognosis. For example, the presence of direct invasion of CLM into adjacent structures (eg, diaphragm) is not equivalent to an extrahepatic metastasis to a separate site (eg, lung, transverse colon, peritoneum, hilar lymph nodes).[11] Further, Jaeck and colleagues[72,73] showed a difference in 3-year survival between patients with nodal involvement of the hepatoduodenal-retropancreatic area compared with nodes in the hepatic artery/celiac axis area (38% vs 0%).

As previously stated, an assessment of tumor biology is critical to selecting patients for resection of CLM as well as extrahepatic metastases. For patients found to have extrahepatic metastases preoperatively, a short course of preoperative chemotherapy followed by reimaging is prudent to better define the disease biology.[24] We do not advocate resection of CLM or extrahepatic metastases in the face of disease progression on chemotherapy.

Intraoperative decision making when faced with previously unrecognized intraabdominal extrahepatic metastases can be difficult. Before proceeding with resection, the following should be considered: (1) the complexity and extent of the R-0 hepatic resection, (2) the complexity of resection of the R-0 extrahepatic metastases, (3) the physiologic age of the patient, (4) availability of postoperative chemotherapeutic options, and (5) the patient's risk of rapid progression with the additional finding of extrahepatic metastases.[24]

OPERATIVE TECHNIQUE

As stated previously, the goal of CLM should be a safe R-0 hepatectomy allowing for preservation of 2 contiguous hepatic segments, with adequate FLR volume to avoid hepatic insufficiency. If possible, anatomic resections may be favored rather than nonanatomic wedge resections, based on improvements in margin width and overall survival.[74] However, given the significant decrease in survival between R-0 and R-1/2 resections (median survival 43 vs 14 months[75]), the ability to achieve R-0 resection, regardless of method, is paramount (**Fig. 2A**). The optimal width of resection margin is unclear, with no clear minimum margin established. Pawlik and colleagues[76] observed that the width of negative margin did not affect survival, recurrence risk, or site of recurrence (see **Fig. 2B**). They conclude that a predicted margin width of less than 1 cm should not be used as an exclusion to resection. An emphasis on the goal of obtaining an R-0 resection rather than striving for a minimal margin width was echoed in the 2006 AHPBA/SSAT/SSO Consensus Statement.[5]

Technical details of liver mobilization and various anatomic hepatectomies have been well described in numerous publications. The complexities of these procedures demand an extensive knowledge of hepatic anatomy and its multiple variations (seen in as many as 45% of patients[77]) as well as flexibility in technique by the surgeon. Furthermore, a thorough knowledge of hepatic ultrasound techniques is required to confirm the disease noted on preoperative imaging, to preemptively identify variant anatomy, and to guide resection planes and margins.

Most procedures can be divided into distinct stages: (1) exploration, (2) liver mobilization, (3) intraoperative ultrasonography, (4) inflow control, (5) outflow control, (6) parenchymal transection, and (7) hemo- and biliostasis.

We use a permissive hypotension (>90 mm Hg)/low central venous pressure (<5 mm Hg) technique[78,79] with active communication with the anesthesia team to minimize blood loss during mobilization and parenchymal transection. Once the specimen is

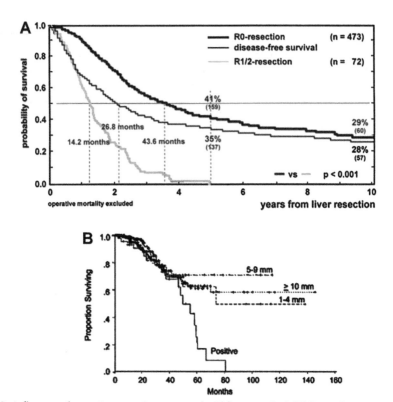

Fig. 2. Influence of resection margin status and width on survival. (*A*) Resection status versus overall survival; R-1/2 resections are associated with significantly poorer overall survival, whereas R-0 resection more closely approximates disease-free survival over time. (*From* Altendorf-Hofmann A, Scheele J. A critical review of the major indicators of prognosis after resection of hepatic metastases from colorectal carcinoma. Surg Oncol Clin N Am 2003;12:165; with permission). (*B*) Margin width versus overall survival. A significant difference exists (*P* = .005) between positive margin and all-width negative margins, whereas no difference exists among margin widths (*P*>.5). (*From* Pawlik TM, Scoggins CR, Zorzi D, et al. Effect of surgical margin status on survival and site of recurrence after hepatic resection for colorectal metastases. Ann Surg 2005;241:715; with permission.)

removed, crystalloid is administered intravenously to achieve euvolemia. Blood transfusions are used sparingly and only if clinically justified.

Most open hepatic resections are performed via a hockey stick (J-shaped) incision[55] for most right hepatectomies or a midline incision for most left hepatectomies. After gross inspection of the liver, a deliberate search for occult intra-abdominal metastases is undertaken. Following exploration, the full liver is mobilized from its diaphragmatic and retroperitoneal attachments. Limited diaphragmatic invasion is dealt with via en bloc resection of full-thickness diaphragm with primary repair and transabdominal evacuation of the pleural space to avoid chest tube thorocostomy.

Once the liver is mobilized, a thorough IOUS examination is performed. Ultrasonic evaluation of the relationship and proximity of intrahepatic metastases to arterioportal, biliary, and hepatic venous structures are reconciled with the preoperative imaging. An active search for occult intrahepatic lesions is undertaken.

Depending on the planned resection, inflow control is most commonly obtained using an intermittent Pringle[80] maneuver or intrahepatic pedicle division using vascular staplers. Outflow control of the hepatic veins is dictated by the nature of the resection and individual hepatic venous anatomy, with extrahepatic ligation before parenchymal division or intrahepatic ligation during parenchymal transection.

Parenchymal transection is undertaken using a clamp-crush technique to expose vascular and biliary structures that are subsequently divided with clips, ties, or staplers as dictated by size and location. We have also found bipolar compression and ultrasonic hemostatic assist devices useful during parenchymal division. Regardless of the transection technique or technology used, flexibility and efficiency are critical to minimizing blood loss and liver ischemic times.

Hemostasis of the cut edge is augmented by direct pressure, topical hemostatics (usually woven oxidized cellulose or gelatin sponge), and argon beam coagulation, followed by a careful search for biliary leakage, with oversewing of any exposed biliary radicals. Viability of the remnant liver is confirmed visually. We routinely leave closed gravity drains near the operative site for 2 to 4 days, based on the amount and character of the drainage.

LAPAROSCOPIC APPROACH

In contrast with many intra-abdominal procedures, the laparoscopic approach to hepatic resection has been slow to be accepted, largely because of concerns regarding difficulty in liver mobilization and parenchymal transaction, and the perceived risks of hemorrhage, carbon dioxide gas embolism, and tumor dissemination. However, hepatobiliary units are increasingly reporting success with this approach.[81–87] Their patients have enjoyed a reduction in blood loss, reduced postoperative morbidities, and shorter hospital stays with demonstrated margin equivalence. We recently compared our experience with laparoscopic lobectomy with a matched group of patients undergoing open hepatectomy and confirmed improvements in blood loss, transfusion requirements, morbidity, and length of stay without compromise of resection margins when using a laparoscopic approach.[88] There is expected to be growth in the use of laparoscopic liver resection for benign, malignant, and transplantation applications. Careful analysis of outcomes and establishment of training paradigms are necessary to benefit the population at large.[89]

The overriding principles of laparoscopic hepatic resection are identical to those described for open hepatectomy. The abdomen is explored laparoscopically and the liver is mobilized and surveyed using laparoscopic ultrasound. The line of transection is identified and marked with electrocautery. Under inflow conditions via intermittent Pringle maneuver, the liver parenchyma is transected using a combination of hemostatic assist devices, clips, and vascular staplers. In most cases, inflow and outflow are controlled intraparenchymally during parenchymal transection.

SUMMARY

The last several decades have seen significant advancements in local and systemic therapies for CLM, but surgical resection remains the cornerstone of definitive treatment in terms of disease-free and overall survival. Careful coordination across multiple disciplines is necessary to maximize the number of patients who can safely undergo resection of CLM and to optimize treatment effectiveness. Future advancements in locoregional and systemic therapies as well as the continued growth of laparoscopic techniques will continue to improve the feasibility and outcomes of CLM resection.

REFERENCES

1. Jemal A, Siegel R, Ward E, et al. Cancer statistics 2009. CA Cancer J Clin 2009; 59(4):225.
2. Steele G Jr, Ravikumar TS. Resection of hepatic metastases from colorectal cancer. Biologic perspective. Ann Surg 1989;210:127.
3. Scheele J, Stangl R, Altendorf-Hofmann A. Hepatic metastases from colorectal carcinoma: impact of surgical resection on the natural history. Br J Surg 1990; 77:1241.
4. Lewis AM, Martin RC. The treatment of hepatic metastases in colorectal carcinoma. Am Surg 2006;72:466.
5. Charnsangavej C, Clary B, Fong Y, et al. Selection of patients for resection of hepatic colorectal metastases: expert consensus statement. Ann Surg Oncol 2006;13:1261.
6. Abdalla EK, Adam R, Bilchik AJ, et al. Improving resectability of hepatic colorectal metastases: expert consensus statement. Ann Surg Oncol 2006;13:1271.
7. Bolton JS, Vauthey JN, Sauter ER. Colorectal cancer: surgical management of recurrent and metastatic disease. J Natl Med Assoc 1988;80:561.
8. Hao CY, Ji JF. Surgical treatment of liver metastases of colorectal cancer: strategies and controversies in 2006. Eur J Surg Oncol 2006;32:473.
9. Donadon M, Ribero D, Morris-Stiff G, et al. New paradigm in the management of liver-only metastases from colorectal cancer. Gastrointest Cancer Res 2007;1:20.
10. Lim E, Thomson BN, Heinze S, et al. Optimizing the approach to patients with potentially resectable liver metastases from colorectal cancer. ANZ J Surg 2007;77:941.
11. Pawlik TM, Schulick RD, Choti MA. Expanding criteria for resectability of colorectal liver metastases. Oncologist 2008;13:51.
12. Shimada H, Tanaka K, Endou I, et al. Treatment for colorectal liver metastases: a review. Langenbecks Arch Surg 2009;394:973.
13. Kopetz S, Chang GJ, Overman MJ, et al. Improved survival in metastatic colorectal cancer is associated with adoption of hepatic resection and improved chemotherapy. J Clin Oncol 2009;27:3677.
14. Martin RC, Eid S, Scoggins CR, et al. Health-related quality of life: return to baseline after major and minor liver resection. Surgery 2007;142:676.
15. Lortat-Jacob JL, Robert HG, Henry C. [Excision of the right lobe of the liver for a malignant secondary tumor]. Arch Mal Appar Dig Mal Nutr 1952;41:662 [in French].
16. Choti MA, Sitzmann JV, Tiburi MF, et al. Trends in long-term survival following liver resection for hepatic colorectal metastases. Ann Surg 2002;235:759.
17. Aloia TA, Vauthey JN, Loyer EM, et al. Solitary colorectal liver metastasis: resection determines outcome. Arch Surg 2006;141:460.
18. Tomlinson JS, Jarnagin WR, DeMatteo RP, et al. Actual 10-year survival after resection of colorectal liver metastases defines cure. J Clin Oncol 2007;25:4575.
19. McLoughlin JM, Jensen EH, Malafa M. Resection of colorectal liver metastases: current perspectives. Cancer Control 2006;13:32.
20. Kostov DV, Kobakov GL. Segmental liver resection for colorectal metastases. J Gastrointestin Liver Dis 2009;18:447.
21. Adam R, Frilling A, Elias D, et al. Liver resection of colorectal metastases in elderly patients. Br J Surg 2010;97(3):366.

22. Lupinacci R, Penna C, Nordlinger B. Hepatectomy for resectable colorectal cancer metastases—indicators of prognosis, definition of resectability, techniques and outcomes. Surg Oncol Clin N Am 2007;16:493.
23. Martin RC, Scoggins CR, McMasters KM. Safety and efficacy of microwave ablation of hepatic tumors: a prospective review of a 5-year experience. Ann Surg Oncol 2010;17:171.
24. Byam J, Reuter NP, Woodall CE, et al. Should hepatic metastatic colorectal cancer patients with extrahepatic disease undergo liver resection/ablation? Ann Surg Oncol 2009;16:3064.
25. Lordan JT, Karanjia ND, Quiney N, et al. A 10-year study of outcome following hepatic resection for colorectal liver metastases — the effect of evaluation in a multidisciplinary team setting. Eur J Surg Oncol 2009;35:302.
26. Nordlinger B, Benoist S. [Liver metastases from colorectal cancer: a multidisciplinary approach is necessary]. Bull Acad Natl Med 2008;192:33 [in French].
27. Wagman LD, Byun TE. Managing colorectal cancer liver metastases. Oncology (Williston Park) 2009;23:1063.
28. Jones OM, Rees M, John TG, et al. Biopsy of resectable colorectal liver metastases causes tumour dissemination and adversely affects survival after liver resection. Br J Surg 2005;92:1165.
29. Bipat S, van Leeuwen MS, Comans EF, et al. Colorectal liver metastases: CT, MR imaging, and PET for diagnosis–meta-analysis. Radiology 2005;237:123.
30. Vauthey JN, Abdalla EK, Doherty DA, et al. Body surface area and body weight predict total liver volume in Western adults. Liver Transpl 2002;8:233.
31. Vauthey JN, Chaoui A, Do KA, et al. Standardized measurement of the future liver remnant prior to extended liver resection: methodology and clinical associations. Surgery 2000;127:512.
32. Kishi Y, Abdalla EK, Chun YS, et al. Three hundred and one consecutive extended right hepatectomies: evaluation of outcome based on systematic liver volumetry. Ann Surg 2009. [Epub ahead of print].
33. Zorzi D, Laurent A, Pawlik TM, et al. Chemotherapy-associated hepatotoxicity and surgery for colorectal liver metastases. Br J Surg 2007;94:274.
34. Martinez L, Puig I, Valls C. Colorectal liver metastases: radiological diagnosis and staging. Eur J Surg Oncol 2007;33(Suppl 2):S5.
35. Yang YY, Fleshman JW, Strasberg SM. Detection and management of extrahepatic colorectal cancer in patients with resectable liver metastases. J Gastrointest Surg 2007;11:929.
36. Therasse P, Arbuck SG, Eisenhauer EA, et al. New guidelines to evaluate the response to treatment in solid tumors. European Organization for Research and Treatment of Cancer, National Cancer Institute of the United States, National Cancer Institute of Canada. J Natl Cancer Inst 2000;92:205.
37. Fong Y, Fortner J, Sun RL, et al. Clinical score for predicting recurrence after hepatic resection for metastatic colorectal cancer: analysis of 1001 consecutive cases. Ann Surg 1999;230:309.
38. Reissfelder C, Rahbari NN, Koch M, et al. Validation of prognostic scoring systems for patients undergoing resection of colorectal cancer liver metastases. Ann Surg Oncol 2009;16:3279.
39. Iwatsuki S, Dvorchik I, Madariaga JR, et al. Hepatic resection for metastatic colorectal adenocarcinoma: a proposal of a prognostic scoring system. J Am Coll Surg 1999;189:291.

40. Karoui M, Penna C, Amin-Hashem M, et al. Influence of preoperative chemotherapy on the risk of major hepatectomy for colorectal liver metastases. Ann Surg 2006;243:1.
41. Vauthey JN, Pawlik TM, Ribero D, et al. Chemotherapy regimen predicts steatohepatitis and an increase in 90-day mortality after surgery for hepatic colorectal metastases. J Clin Oncol 2006;24:2065.
42. Abdalla EK, Vauthey JN. Chemotherapy prior to hepatic resection for colorectal liver metastases: helpful until harmful? Dig Surg 2008;25:421.
43. Reddy SK, Zorzi D, Lum YW, et al. Timing of multimodality therapy for resectable synchronous colorectal liver metastases: a retrospective multi-institutional analysis. Ann Surg Oncol 2009;16:1809.
44. Hubert C, Fervaille C, Sempoux C, et al. Prevalence and clinical relevance of pathological hepatic changes occurring after neoadjuvant chemotherapy for colorectal liver metastases. Surgery 2010;147:185.
45. Benoist S, Nordlinger B. The role of preoperative chemotherapy in patients with resectable colorectal liver metastases. Ann Surg Oncol 2009;16:2385.
46. Scoggins CR, Campbell ML, Landry CS, et al. Preoperative chemotherapy does not increase morbidity or mortality of hepatic resection for colorectal cancer metastases. Ann Surg Oncol 2009;16:35.
47. Nordlinger B, Sorbye H, Glimelius B, et al. Perioperative chemotherapy with FOLFOX4 and surgery versus surgery alone for resectable liver metastases from colorectal cancer (EORTC Intergroup trial 40983): a randomised controlled trial. Lancet 2008;371:1007.
48. Bower MR, Brown RE, Martin RCG. Obesity rather than neoadjuvant chemotherapy predicts for liver injury in patients with colorectal metastasis. HPB (Oxford). [Epub ahead of print].
49. Gentilucci UV, Santini D, Vincenzi B, et al. Chemotherapy-induced steatohepatitis in colorectal cancer patients. J Clin Oncol 2006;24:5467 [author reply: 5467].
50. Kopetz S, Vauthey JN. Perioperative chemotherapy for resectable hepatic metastases. Lancet 2008;371:963.
51. Martin RC, Joshi J, Robbins K, et al. Transarterial chemoembolization of metastatic colorectal carcinoma with drug-eluting beads, irinotecan (DEBIRI): Multi-Institutional Registry. J Oncol 2009;2009:539795.
52. Whitney R, Tatum C, Hahl M, et al. Safety of hepatic resection in metastatic disease to the liver after yttrium-90 therapy. J Surg Res 2009. [Epub ahead of print].
53. Resection of the liver for colorectal carcinoma metastases: a multi-institutional study of indications for resection. Registry of Hepatic Metastases. Surgery 1988;103:278.
54. Elias D, Detroz B, Lasser P, et al. Is simultaneous hepatectomy and intestinal anastomosis safe? Am J Surg 1995;169:254.
55. D'Angelica M, Maddineni S, Fong Y, et al. Optimal abdominal incision for partial hepatectomy: increased late complications with Mercedes-type incisions compared to extended right subcostal incisions. World J Surg 2006; 30:410.
56. Martin RC 2nd, Augenstein V, Reuter NP, et al. Simultaneous versus staged resection for synchronous colorectal cancer liver metastases. J Am Coll Surg 2009;208:842.
57. Van Dessel E, Fierens K, Pattyn P, et al. Defining the optimal therapy sequence in synchronous resectable liver metastases from colorectal cancer: a decision analysis approach. Acta Chir Belg 2009;109:317.

58. Akiyoshi T, Kuroyanagi H, Saiura A, et al. Simultaneous resection of colorectal cancer and synchronous liver metastases: initial experience of laparoscopy for colorectal cancer resection. Dig Surg 2010;26:471.
59. Bolton JS, Fuhrman GM. Survival after resection of multiple bilobar hepatic metastases from colorectal carcinoma. Ann Surg 2000;231:743.
60. Adam R, Laurent A, Azoulay D, et al. Two-stage hepatectomy: a planned strategy to treat irresectable liver tumors. Ann Surg 2000;232:777.
61. Abdalla EK, Hicks ME, Vauthey JN. Portal vein embolization: rationale, technique and future prospects. Br J Surg 2001;88:165.
62. Adam R, Miller R, Pitombo M, et al. Two-stage hepatectomy approach for initially unresectable colorectal hepatic metastases. Surg Oncol Clin N Am 2007;16:525.
63. Chun YS, Vauthey JN, Ribero D, et al. Systemic chemotherapy and two-stage hepatectomy for extensive bilateral colorectal liver metastases: perioperative safety and survival. J Gastrointest Surg 2007;11:1498.
64. Wicherts DA, Miller R, de Haas RJ, et al. Long-term results of two-stage hepatectomy for irresectable colorectal cancer liver metastases. Ann Surg 2008;248:994.
65. Shimada H, Tanaka K, Matsuo K, et al. Treatment for multiple bilobar liver metastases of colorectal cancer. Langenbecks Arch Surg 2006;391:130.
66. Elias D, Baton O, Sideris L, et al. Hepatectomy plus intraoperative radiofrequency ablation and chemotherapy to treat technically unresectable multiple colorectal liver metastases. J Surg Oncol 2005;90:36.
67. Fong Y, Cohen AM, Fortner JG, et al. Liver resection for colorectal metastases. J Clin Oncol 1997;15:938.
68. Nagakura S, Shirai Y, Yamato Y, et al. Simultaneous detection of colorectal carcinoma liver and lung metastases does not warrant resection. J Am Coll Surg 2001;193:153.
69. Ferrero A, Polastri R, Muratore A, et al. Extensive resections for colorectal liver metastases. J Hepatobiliary Pancreat Surg 2004;11:92.
70. Elias D, Sideris L, Pocard M, et al. Results of R0 resection for colorectal liver metastases associated with extrahepatic disease. Ann Surg Oncol 2004;11:274.
71. Elias D, Ouellet JF, Bellon N, et al. Extrahepatic disease does not contraindicate hepatectomy for colorectal liver metastases. Br J Surg 2003;90:567.
72. Jaeck D, Nakano H, Bachellier P, et al. Significance of hepatic pedicle lymph node involvement in patients with colorectal liver metastases: a prospective study. Ann Surg Oncol 2002;9:430.
73. Jaeck D. The significance of hepatic pedicle lymph nodes metastases in surgical management of colorectal liver metastases and of other liver malignancies. Ann Surg Oncol 2003;10:1007.
74. DeMatteo RP, Palese C, Jarnagin WR, et al. Anatomic segmental hepatic resection is superior to wedge resection as an oncologic operation for colorectal liver metastases. J Gastrointest Surg 2000;4:178.
75. Altendorf-Hofmann A, Scheele J. A critical review of the major indicators of prognosis after resection of hepatic metastases from colorectal carcinoma. Surg Oncol Clin N Am 2003;12:165.
76. Pawlik TM, Scoggins CR, Zorzi D, et al. Effect of surgical margin status on survival and site of recurrence after hepatic resection for colorectal metastases. Ann Surg 2005;241:715.
77. Skandalakis JE, Skandalakis LJ, Skandalakis PN, et al. Hepatic surgical anatomy. Surg Clin North Am 2004;84:413.

78. Rees M, Plant G, Wells J, et al. One hundred and fifty hepatic resections: evolution of technique towards bloodless surgery. Br J Surg 1996;83:1526.
79. Melendez JA, Arslan V, Fischer ME, et al. Perioperative outcomes of major hepatic resections under low central venous pressure anesthesia: blood loss, blood transfusion, and the risk of postoperative renal dysfunction. J Am Coll Surg 1998;187:620.
80. Pringle JH. V. Notes on the arrest of hepatic hemorrhage due to trauma. Ann Surg 1908;48:541.
81. Dagher I, Proske JM, Carloni A, et al. Laparoscopic liver resection: results for 70 patients. Surg Endosc 2007;21:619.
82. Rau HG, Buttler E, Meyer G, et al. Laparoscopic liver resection compared with conventional partial hepatectomy–a prospective analysis. Hepatogastroenterology 1998;45:2333.
83. Gigot JF, Glineur D, Santiago Azagra J, et al. Laparoscopic liver resection for malignant liver tumors: preliminary results of a multicenter European study. Ann Surg 2002;236:90.
84. Mala T, Edwin B, Gladhaug I, et al. A comparative study of the short-term outcome following open and laparoscopic liver resection of colorectal metastases. Surg Endosc 2002;16:1059.
85. Lesurtel M, Cherqui D, Laurent A, et al. Laparoscopic versus open left lateral hepatic lobectomy: a case-control study. J Am Coll Surg 2003;196:236.
86. Chang S, Laurent A, Tayar C, et al. Laparoscopy as a routine approach for left lateral sectionectomy. Br J Surg 2007;94:58.
87. Simillis C, Constantinides VA, Tekkis PP, et al. Laparoscopic versus open hepatic resections for benign and malignant neoplasms–a meta-analysis. Surgery 2007; 141:203.
88. Martin R, Scoggins CR, McMasters K. Laparoscopic hepatic lobectomy: advantages of a minimally invasive approach. J Am Coll Surg 2010;210(5):627–33.
89. Buell JF, Cherqui D, Geller DA, et al. The international position on laparoscopic liver surgery: The Louisville Statement, 2008. Ann Surg 2009;250:825.

Neuroendocrine Liver Metastases

Srinevas K. Reddy, MD*, Bryan M. Clary, MD

KEYWORDS

- Neuroendocrine liver metastases • Resection • Ablation
- Liver transplantation • Hepatic arterial infusion • Chemotherapy

The liver is the most common site of metastatic disease for neuroendocrine tumors and ultimately dictates outcomes in most patients. Liver involvement develops in 46% to 93% of patients with neuroendocrine malignancies.[1] The majority of patients with neuroendocrine liver metastases (NLM) have a multiplicity of lesions, with many residing in difficult locations. While the NLM may behave in a relatively indolent manner from an oncologic perspective, additional morbidity and mortality may be caused by excess hormone production when compared with metastatic liver disease from other primaries.[2] Nonoperative therapies for advanced neuroendocrine malignancies are associated with minimal response rates, short durations of disease stability, and no clear survival benefit. For example, ^{131}I-metaiodobenzylguanidine therapy is associated with a mean duration of tumor response of approximately 15 months whereas ^{111}In-octreotide therapy has a mean duration of tumor response of 20 months in patients with progressive unresectable neuroendocrine neoplasms.[3] Tumor progression is common after treatment with lanreotide and/or interferon-α without complete tumor remission.[4] Similarly, chemotherapy is associated with low response rates (15%–56%), short progression-free survival (median 4–5 months), and relatively short overall survival after start of treatment (median 15–26 months)[5,6] when applied to patients with advanced disease. Surgical therapy, on the contrary, offers the only chance at durable survival prolongation and/or improvement in quality of life. The objectives of this review are to summarize regional strategies for management of NLM, including hepatic resection, ablation, liver transplantation, and hepatic arterial embolization/chemoembolization.

RESECTION

Resection of NLM is supported by the favorable long-term outcomes noted in large retrospective series. Because neuroendocrine tumors are often detected after extensive liver metastases are present, complete surgical extirpation via hepatic resection is

Department of Surgery, Duke University Medical Center, Box 3247, Durham, NC 27710, USA
* Corresponding author.
E-mail address: reddy005@mc.duke.edu

Surg Clin N Am 90 (2010) 853–861
doi:10.1016/j.suc.2010.04.016
surgical.theclinics.com

often not possible.[1,7] Consequently, only 10% to 20% of patients with NLM are eligible for resection. Because of the relative rarity and biologic heterogeneity of NLM, there are no prospective randomized controlled trials, cohort studies, or case-control studies comparing liver resection with other treatments in patients with resectable NLM.[8] Designing such a randomized study would be challenging, because to identify a 10% difference in survival (with an alpha of 0.05 and power of 0.8) between surgical debulking over other palliative treatments, 776 patients would be required. Inability to blind patients or health care providers, cross-over to completely resected patients because of down-sizing of liver metastases, and the need for prolonged follow-up due to the indolent nature of disease are all additional obstacles to the development of a prospective randomized trial.[9] Furthermore, the evolving criteria of resectability and recent improvements in the safety of liver resection have complicated comparisons of recent series to older studies.[2] Even when complete resection of NLM is performed, early recurrence is common relative to other common hepatic lesions such as colorectal metastases (**Table 1**).[2,10] However, due to the overall indolent course of neuroendocrine neoplasms, long-term survival is common after even incomplete resection (see **Table 1**). Moreover, initial symptom improvement, particularly for hormonal symptoms, is observed in most patients. These positive results suggest that most patients with disease that can be grossly resected with a sufficient liver remnant with intact biliary and vascular drainage should undergo resection.[2] When complete resection of gross liver disease is not feasible or in the presence of unresectable extrahepatic disease, resection as a tumor debulking strategy should be considered in patients with extreme hormonal symptoms refractory to other treatments or with tumors in locations that would affect short-term quality of life, such as large lesions abutting the hepatic hilum (resulting in biliary obstruction) or the colon/duodenum (resulting in gastrointestinal obstruction).[2,18] Combinations of resection and ablation may be used to achieve complete tumor response when all liver disease cannot be resected. Given the prolonged survival observed following resection of NLM, liver resection should be used as the standard by which all other treatments should be measured.[8,19,20]

Radiofrequency ablation (RFA) can provide local control and short-term symptomatic relief from NLM when resection is not possible. Mazzaglia and colleagues[21] describe the largest experience of ablation in patients with NLM, encompassing a total of 384 lesions in 63 patients via 80 laparoscopic RFA sessions. Eleven and 3 patients underwent 2 and 3 sessions, respectively, and 49% of all patients were treated (medical or radiation) before the first RFA session. The mean number of treated lesions at first session was 6 ± 0.5 lesions with mean tumor size of 2.3 ± 0.1 cm. Thirty-six patients were symptomatic from disease and 94% experienced symptom relief after ablation for a median duration of 11 ± 2.3 months after RFA. After a mean follow-up of 2.8 years, median survival following the first ablation was 3.9 years with a 2-year survival of 77%. Progressive liver disease developed in 80% of patients. Male gender (hazard ratio [HR] 3.1, 95% confidence interval [CI] 1.1–9.1, $P = .04$) and tumor size greater than 3 cm (HR 3.3, CI 1.1–10.1, $P = .03$) were associated with poor survival after ablation. Similarly, Gilliams and colleagues[22] reported results aftr ablation of 189 lesions in 25 patients with median tumor number of 12 and maximum tumor diameter of 3.5 cm. These patients were heavily treated with liver resection, chemotherapy, and/or hepatic arterial embolization. Ablation of at least 90% of the tumor burden was achieved in 26 treatments, 50% to 89% in 33 treatments, and less than 50% in 7 treatments. Sixty-nine percent of patients experienced symptom improvement. Median survival after tumor ablation was 29 months. Elvin and colleagues[23] reported the application of 109 RFA treatment sessions in the management of 198 lesions in 42 patients.

Table 1
Results after resection of neuroendocrine liver metastases

Authors	n	Survival	Symptom Improvement	Comments
Reddy et al[10]	33	3-y 75%	—	Median disease-free survival 13 mo, 3-y disease-free survival 32% 33% with >5 lesions, 58% synchronous disease
Touzious et al[11]	37	—	> 88%	>60% bilobar disease, 79% synchronous disease, 21% with extrahepatic disease Median survival of 96 months after resection ± ablation is better compared with no treatment (median 20 mo, $P<.05$) <50% of liver involvement associated with better survival ($P<.05$)
Sarmiento et al[12]	170	5-y 61% Median 81 mo	96%	44% R_0 resection, 76% with bilateral lesions 5-y recurrence symptom-free rate 84% and 59% Better recurrence-free survival for complete vs incomplete resection (median 30 vs 16 mo, $P = .0004$)
Chen et al[13]	15	5-y 73%	—	All patients with liver-only disease
Osborne et al[14]	61	Mean 50 mo[a]	93%	62% curative resections, 69% complete symptom relief Longer symptom relief with resection compared with embolization (median 56 vs 32 mo, $P = .08$)
Landry et al[15]	23	Median 52 mo	—	16 patients underwent adjunctive therapy 13/23 patients with bilobar disease Performance status better for resected compared with unresected patients
Yao et al[16]	16	5-y 70%	—	Survival better for resected patients (5-y 70% vs 40%, $P<.05$) Better disease-free survival associated with prior resection of primary tumor and <4 metastases
Chamberlain et al[17]	34	5-y 76%	100%	82% curative resections, 62% bilobar disease Curative treatment associated with improved survival Hepatic tumor burden associated with survival among resected patients

[a] For curative resections.

Ninety-eight lesions were successfully treated (as shown by follow-up computed tomography) after a mean follow-up of 3.2 years.

Whereas hormonal treatment alone does not provide durable symptom-free nor reliable long-term survival, adjuvant octreotide and/or interferon α treatment after extirpation does improve symptom relief. Chung and colleagues[24] examined the outcome of 31 patients (90% with hormonal symptoms) with NLM who underwent hepatic resections and/or ablation. Mean duration of symptom relief after surgical therapy was 11 months with symptom recurrence in all patients. Adjuvant octreotide in 10 patients resulted in a median duration of symptom relief of 60 months compared with 16 months with other adjuvant therapies in 21 patients (P = .001). Similarly, Kolby and colleagues[25] described the outcomes of 68 patients who underwent surgical extirpation of the primary tumor followed by hepatic arterial embolization of NLM followed by treatment with octreotide (n = 35) or octreotide + interferon-α (n = 33). Overall 5-year survival was 46.5% with no difference in survival according to treatment after hepatic artery embolization. However, patients treated with octreotide + interferon-α had significantly lower risk of disease progression.

HEPATIC ARTERIAL THERAPY

Hepatic arterial embolization with or without local instillation of chemotherapy may induce disease response, symptomatic improvement, and prolonged survival in patients with unresectable NLM. Because neuroendocrine tumors are prone to produce highly vascular lesions that predominantly derive blood supply from the hepatic artery (as opposed to the normal hepatic parenchyma that derive the majority of blood supply from the portal vein), opportunities exist for selected ischemia of NLM and/or delivery of directed chemotherapy via hepatic artery therapy. Hepatic arterial embolization with cyanoacrylate, gel foam particles, polyvinyl alcohol, and microspheres have all been used to achieve distal embolization without surgical ligation of the hepatic artery.[1] Chemoembolization provides an intratumoral concentration of chemotherapy that is 10 to 20 times higher than systemic administration.[1] Several single-center series report medium-term survival and symptomatic relief after hepatic artery embolization and/or chemoembolization (**Table 2**). Among these studies, carcinoid histology is associated with better outcomes after initiation of therapy. Although in theory synergistic effects can be achieved with ischemia and local chemotherapy, several institutions interestingly report no difference in outcomes between hepatic artery embolization and hepatic artery chemoembolization (see **Table 2**). Of importance is that complete response and long-term survival are not common after hepatic arterial therapy, as the periphery of the tumor is spared from ischemia or chemotherapy. Thus, embolization of lesions close to the hepatic hilum is generally unsuccessful, as the periphery of the tumor will still cause mass-effect associated symptoms. The morbidity of embolization approaches include liver abscess, transient liver failure, pleural effusion, and postembolization syndrome, the latter consisting of fever, abdominal pain, leukocytosis, and a transient increase in liver enzymes and/or bilirubin.[1] Multiple sessions of therapy are often needed with varying intervals between sessions.[1] While not universal, commonly proposed contraindications to hepatic arterial therapy include hepatic failure, portal vein occlusion, uncorrectable coagulopathy, and renal failure.[26–31]

LIVER TRANSPLANTATION

Early disease recurrence, high postoperative mortality, the absence of extensive experience, and lack of universal indications for organ allocation preclude orthotopic

Table 2
Recent large series of hepatic arterial therapy for neuroendocrine liver metastases

Authors	n	Overall Survival	Comments
Pitt et al[26]	49 HACE 51 HAE	Median 25.5 mo, 2-y 52% Median 25.7 mo, 2-y 54%	No difference in survival between HACE and HAE
Gupta et al[27]	74 HAE 49 HACE	PIS: median 23 mo, 2-y 48.7% Carcinoid: median 33.8 mo, 2-y 68.6%	No difference in survival between HACE and HAE Carcinoid histology associated with longer survival, $P = .012$
Vogl et al[28]	48 HACE	3-y 72% and 80% Median 32.9 and 42.8 mo	No systemic chemotherapy or hormonal treatment 19% partial response after therapy
Sward et al[29]	107 HAE	Median 56 mo	71% symptomatic relief Male gender, degree of decline in urinary 5-HIAA and plasma chromogranin A, and postembolized AST levels associated with survival
Christante et al[30]	77 HAI/HACE	Median 39 mo 5-y 27%	Median progression free survival: 19 mo All treated with octreotide Primary tumor resection associated with improved survival
Strosberg et al[31]	84 HAE	Median 36 mo	75% symptomatic, 80% symptom improvement 48% partial response Survival longer for carcinoid vs pancreatic endocrine vs poorly differential histology
Ho et al[32]	46 HAE/HACE	3-y 41%	54% symptomatic, 78% symptom relief Median progression-free survival 563 d

Abbreviations: AST, aspartate aminotransferase; HACE, hepatic arterial chemoembolization; HAE, hepatic arterial embolization; HAI, hepatic arterial infusion; HIAA, 5-hydroxyindoleacetic acid; OS, overall survival; PFS, progression-free survival; PIS, pancreatic islet cell origin.

Table 3
Survival after liver transplantation for neuroendocrine liver metastases

Authors	n	Survival	Comments
Rosenau et al[33]	19	5-y OS: 80% 5-y RFS: 21%	Median RFS: 10.5 mo Ki-67 positivity and E-cadherin staining associated with survival
Lang et al[34]	10	Median OS: 33 mo	All patients symptom-free after transplant 90% tumor recurrence
Le Treut et al[35]	31	3-y OS: 47% 3-y DFS: 29%	23/31 patients treated with medical therapy before transplant 19% postoperative mortality 35% had uncontrolled hormonal and tumor mass effect symptoms, respectively Patients with carcinoid disease had better OS and DFS compared with other patients
van Vilsteren et al[36]	19	1-y OS: 88% 1-y RFS: 77%	All patients had surgical and/or radiologic intervention before transplantation
Florman et al[37]	11	1-y OS: 73% 5-y OS: 36%	10/11 patients with recurrent disease after transplantation
Routley et al[38]	11	1-y OS: 82% 5-y OS: 57%	All patients with symptom relief after transplantation Recurrence in 6/11 patients after transplantation

Abbreviations: OS, overall survival, RFS, recurrence-free survival.

liver transplantation as an option for most patients with unresectable NLM. While transplantation has the benefits of removing all hepatic disease burden, rapid disease recurrence is near universal (**Table 3**). Moreover, long-term actuarial survival among patients transplanted for NLM is poor compared with overall patient and graft survival rates for all indications. Lenhert[39] reviewed the results of 103 patients who underwent liver transplantation for NLM at 23 institutions. Ten and 40 patients underwent antecedent liver resection and chemotherapy treatment, respectively. Postoperative mortality was 14% at 60 days. Three-year overall and recurrence-free survival after transplantation was 53% and 42%. Synchronous upper abdominal operations (HR 4.8, CI 2.3–10.0, $P<.001$) and age greater than 50 (HR 2.1, CI 1.1–4.0, $P = .027$) were associated with poor overall survival. Given these poor initial experiences, liver transplantation cannot be considered a viable option for unresectable NLM.

SUMMARY

The relatively indolent course of many patients with NLM and the lack of randomized controlled trials comparing the various treatment strategies make it difficult to present definitive statements regarding their appropriate roles. Nonetheless, in the current era the following general guidelines represent reasonable approaches to the management of these patients. As resection offers the most effective and durable option for symptom relief and long-term survival, surgical extirpation should be considered for eligible patients. When a curative resection cannot be envisioned, a debulking strategy that removes 80% to 90% of NLM can be beneficial in prolonging survival and improving symptom control. Ablation may be performed in combination with resection or in cases where resection is not possible. Hepatic artery embolization can be used to treat unresectable liver disease or recurrent disease after previous resection, or as a "neoadjuvant" strategy to down-size initially unresectable disease before surgical extirpation is considered.[18] In lieu of data on the relative effectiveness, the choice of embolization strategy (transarterial embolization, transarterial chemoembolization, radioembolization) is largely determined by institutional preference as well as tumor size and distribution. Orthotopic liver transplantation is reserved for very selected patients with isolated, unresectable liver disease and with extreme symptoms refractory to hepatic arterial therapy, immunotherapy, or hormonal suppressive treatments, with recognition that early disease recurrence is common. Patients with widespread unresectable disease are not candidates for liver-directed therapy and should be treated with salvage chemotherapy or hormonal suppression.

REFERENCES

1. Vogl TJ, Naguib NN, Zangos S, et al. Liver metastases of neuroendocrine carcinomas: interventional treatment via transarterial embolization, chemoembolization, and thermal ablation. Eur J Radiol 2009;72:517–28.
2. Clary B. Treatment of isolated neuroendocrine liver metastases. J Gastrointest Surg 2006;10:332–4.
3. Pasieka JL, McEwan AJB, Rorstad O. The palliative role of ^{131}I-MIBG and ^{111}In-octreotide therapy in patients with metastatic progressive neuroendocrine neoplasms. Surgery 2004;136:1218–26.
4. Faiss S, Pape UF, Bohmig M, et al. Prospective, randomized, multicenter trial on the antiproliferative effect of lanreotide, interferon alfa, and their combination for therapy of metastatic neuroendocrine gastroenteropancreatic tumors—the International Lanreotide and Interferon Alfa Study Group. J Clin Oncol 2003;21:2689–96.
5. Sung W, Lipsitz S, Catalano P, et al. Phase II/III study of doxorubicin with fluorouracil compared with streptozocin with fluorouracil or dacarbazine in the treatment of advanced carcinoid tumors: Eastern Cooperative Oncology Group study E1281. J Clin Oncol 2005;23:4897–904.
6. Fjallskog MH, Granberg DPK, Welin SLV, et al. Treatment with cisplatin and etoposide in patients with neuroendocrine tumors. Cancer 2001;92:1101–7.
7. Ishe I, Persson B, Tibblin S. Neuroendocrine metastases of the liver. World J Surg 1995;19:76–82.
8. Guruswamy KS, Ramamoorthy R, Sharma D, et al. Liver resection versus other treatments for neuroendocrine tumours in patients with resectable liver metastases. Cochrane Database Syst Rev 2009;2:CD007060. DOI: 10.1002/14651858. CD007060.pub2.
9. Guruswamy KS, Pamecha V, Sharma D, et al. Palliative cytoreductive surgery versus other palliative treatments in patients with unresectable liver metastases from gastro-entero-pancreatic neuroendocrine tumours. Cochrane Database Syst Rev 2009;1:CD007118. DOI: 10.1002/14651858.CD007118.pub2.
10. Reddy SK, Barbas AS, Marroquin CE, et al. Resection of noncolorectal nonneuroendocrine liver metastases: a comparative analysis. J Am Coll Surg 2007;204:372–82.
11. Touzios JG, Kiely JM, Pitt SC, et al. Neuroendocrine hepatic metastases: does aggressive management improve survival? Ann Surg 2005;241:776–85.
12. Sarmiento JM, Heywood G, Rubin J, et al. Surgical treatment of neuroendocrine metastases to liver: a plea for resection to increase survival. J Am Coll Surg 2003;197:29–37.

13. Chen H, Hardacre JM, Uzar A, et al. Isolated liver metastases from neuroendocrine tumors: does resection prolong survival? J Am Coll Surg 1998;187:88–93.

14. Osborne DA, Zervos EE, Strosberg J, et al. Improved outcome with cytoreduction versus embolization for symptomatic hepatic metastases of carcinoid and neuroendocrine tumors. Ann Surg Oncol 2006;13:572–81.

15. Landry CS, Scoggins CR, McMasters KM, et al. Management of hepatic metastasis of gastrointestinal carcinoid tumors. J Surg Oncol 2008;97:253–8.

16. Yao KA, Talamonti MS, Nemcek A, et al. Indications and results liver resection and hepatic chemoembolization for metastatic gastrointestinal neuroendocrine tumors. Surgery 2001;130:677–85.

17. Chamberlain RS, Canes D, Brown KT, et al. Hepatic neuroendocrine metastases: does intervention alter outcomes? J Am Coll Surg 2000;190:432–45.

18. Sutcliffe R, Maguire D, Ramage J, et al. Management of neuroendocrine liver metastases. Am J Surg 2004;187:39–46.

19. Sarmiento JM, Que FG. Hepatic surgery for metastases from neuroendocrine tumors. Surg Oncol Clin N Am 2003;12:231–42.

20. Que FG, Nagorney DM, Batts KP, et al. Hepatic resection for metastatic neuroendocrine carcinomas. Am J Surg 1995;169:36–42.

21. Mazzaglia PJ, Berber E, Milas M, et al. Laparoscopic radiofrequency ablation of neuroendocrine liver metastases: a 10-year experience evaluating predictors of survival. Surgery 2007;142:10–9.

22. Gilliams A, Cassoni A, Conway G, et al. Radiofrequency ablation of neuroendocrine liver metastases: the Middlesex experience. Abdom Imaging 2005;30:435–41.

23. Elvin A, Skogseid B, Hellman P. Radiofrequency ablation of neuroendocrine liver metastases. Abdom Imaging 2005;30:427–34.

24. Chung MH, Pisegna J, Spirt M, et al. Hepatic cytoreduction followed by a novel long-acting somatostatin analog: a paradigm for intractable neuroendocrine tumors metastatic to the liver. Surgery 2001;130:954–62.

25. Kolby L, Persson G, Franzen S, et al. Randomized clinical trial of the effect of interferon α on survival in patients with disseminated midgut carcinoid tumours. Br J Surg 2003;90:687–93.

26. Pitt SC, Knuth J, Keily JM, et al. Hepatic neuroendocrine metastases: chemo- or bland embolization? J Gastrointest Surg 2008;12:1951–60.

27. Gupta S, Johnson MM, Murthy R, et al. Hepatic arterial embolization and chemoembolization for the treatment of patients with metastatic neuroendocrine tumors. Cancer 2005;104:1590–602.

28. Vogl TJ, Gruber T, Naguib NN, et al. Liver metastases of neuroendocrine tumors: treatment with hepatic transarterial chemotherapy using two therapeutic protocols. AJR Am J Roentgenol 2009;193:941–7.

29. Sward C, Johanson V, Dijkum Nieveen van, et al. Prolonged survival after hepatic artery embolization in patients with midgut carcinoid syndrome. Br J Surg 2009;96:517–21.

30. Christante D, Pommier S, Givi B, et al. Hepatic artery chemoinfusion with chemoembolization for neuroendocrine cancer with progressive hepatic metastases despite octreotide therapy. Surgery 2008;144:885–94.

31. Strosberg JR, Choi J, Cantor AB, et al. Selective hepatic artery embolization for treatment of patients with metastatic carcinoid and pancreatic endocrine tumors. Cancer Control 2006;13:72–8.

32. Ho AS, Picus J, Darcy MD, et al. Long-term outcome after chemoembolization and embolization of hepatic metastatic lesions from neuroendocrine tumors. AJR Am J Roentgenol 2007;188:1201–7.

33. Rosenau J, Bahr M, von Wasielewski R, et al. Ki67, E-Cadherin, and p53 as prognostic indicators of long-term outcome after liver transplantation for metastatic neuroendocrine tumors. Transplantation 2002;73:386–94.
34. Lang H, Schlitt HJ, Schmidt H, et al. Total hepatectomy and liver transplantation for metastatic neuroendocrine tumors of the pancreas—a single center experience with ten patients. Langenbecks Arch Surg 1999;384:370–7.
35. Le Treut YP, Delpero JR, Dousset B, et al. Results of liver transplantation in the treatment of metastatic neuroendocrine tumors: a 31-case French multicentric report. Ann Surg 1997;225:355–64.
36. van Vilsteren FGI, Baskin-Bey ES, Nagorney DM, et al. Liver transplantation for gastroenteropancreatic neuroendocrine cancers: defining selection criteria to improve survival. Liver Transpl 2006;12:448–56.
37. Florman S, Toure B, Kim L, et al. Liver transplantation for neuroendocrine tumors. J Gastrointest Surg 2004;8:208–12.
38. Routley D, Ramage JK, McPeake J, et al. Orthotopic liver transplantation in the treatment of metastatic neuroendocrine tumors of the liver. Liver Transpl Surg 1995;1:118–21.
39. Lehnert T. Liver transplantation for metastatic neuroendocrine carcinoma: an analysis of 103 patients. Transplantation 1998;66:1307–12.

Hepatic Tumor Ablation

David Sindram, MD, PhD, Kwan N. Lau, MD, John B. Martinie, MD,
David A. Iannitti, MD*

KEYWORDS

- Liver • Ablation • Microwave • Radiofrequency • Liver cancer

Primary and metastatic malignancies in the liver have an unfavorable prognosis if left untreated. Resection, or transplantation in select situations, is the ultimate technique resulting in removal of the tumor. This aggressive approach to primary and metastatic liver cancer has been shown to be effective, and survival and disease-free survival have had a positive effect, despite early concerns for significant increases in procedure-related morbidity and mortality. Unfortunately, most liver cancers present at a time when surgical resection is not possible, as a result of anatomic issues, patient-related concerns, or even availability of organs. Moreover, most patients ultimately die from their cancer, despite optimal resection strategies. Patients may still benefit from treatment of these unresectable liver tumors, and in the last several years multiple modalities have been developed to provide liver-directed regional therapy.[1]

Fighting a disease with a surgical knife that microscopically already has disseminated is justified where a reasonable balance between limited morbidity and mortality of the procedure is countered by a significant and sustained benefit in quality of life and survival. An important evolution has taken place in recent decades in this arena. As a result of advances in surgical techniques and care, the indications for liver tumor resection have drastically expanded. Liver surgery was dangerously prohibitive for most of the twentieth century, but in the last 3 decades liver resection for limited unilobar disease has proved to be beneficial in a variety of primary and secondary liver cancers. Further advances resulted in the consensus of a much broader acceptance of hepatic tumor debulking, even in the presence of limited extrahepatic metastatic disease. Now that tumor debulking has been shown to be efficacious in providing patients with significant improvements in quality and quantity of life, the optimal debulking technique has been questioned. Parallel to the expansion of liver resection criteria, new and improved modalities have been discovered to aid in tumor destruction.

Liver ablation was developed for situations were removal of tumors was not feasible, but indications have evolved to complement and even replace resection.[2] Currently, especially in the background of substantial non–cancer-related hepatic parenchymal disease, equivalence of certain ablative strategies to resection is debated. Ongoing

Section of Hepato-Pancreatico-Biliary Surgery, Division of GI and Minimally Invasive Surgery, Department of Surgery, Carolinas Medical Center, 1025 Morehead Medical Drive, Suite 300, Charlotte, NC 28204, USA
* Corresponding author.
E-mail address: David.Iannitti@carolinashealthcare.org

Surg Clin N Am 90 (2010) 863–876
doi:10.1016/j.suc.2010.04.014
0039-6109/10/$ – see front matter © 2010 Elsevier Inc. All rights reserved.

improvements in ablative technology may provide an opportunity to effectively treat liver cancer with significantly reduced procedure-related morbidity and mortality and increased quality and quantity of life. This review describes the current status of ablative technologies as applied to the liver.

ABLATIVE STRATEGIES

Multiple modalities currently exist or are in development to effectively treat tumors in the liver with the ultimate goal of complete tumor destruction. Ablation is therefore defined as the "direct local application of chemicals or energy to achieve tumor destruction." The idea of tumor ablation rather than resection has been around for more than a century,[3] aiming for reduced morbidity, mortality, cost, and improved applicability of ablation compared with resection. Although the aim is to ultimately replace or avoid resection, a less antagonistic approach to ablation is currently advocated. Various modalities aiming for the best possible outcome for patients with resectable and unresectable liver malignancies is summarized by the term liver-directed therapy. An impressive array of technologies and modalities is available to aid in the treatment of liver cancer. As one of such technologies, ablative modalities should therefore be seen as synergistic with other treatment options, including resection. Currently, ablation is achieved in 1 of 3 ways: Chemical ablation, thermal ablation, and novel, mostly investigational techniques such as, irreversible electroporation.

Chemical Ablation

The percutaneous injection of chemicals straight into the tumor had been widely explored in the treatment of mostly small hepatocellular carcinoma (HCC). A significant body of mostly Asian literature has demonstrated the safety and efficacy of percutaneous absolute alcohol injection in the treatment of these tumors. Favorable aspects of HCC, such as hypervascularity and softness in otherwise mostly firm and cirrhotic liver allow for dispersion of the alcohol within the tumor and destruction of the tumor cells.[4] Because tumor necrosis is induced in approximately 70% of the tumor mass, repeated injections are required to complete the ablation. Although this technology is safe, inexpensive, and ultimately fairly effective, percutaneous ethanol injection (PEI) is currently not widely practiced anywhere, in part because of the need for repeated treatments and the emergence of more effective and equally well-tolerated procedures.[5] Other chemicals, such as acetic acid, have been used with similar results and limited application currently.[6]

Thermal Ablation

Most current ablative technologies apply energy into tumors to destroy the cells by either freezing or overheating. Although freezing tissue in itself does not denature proteins or destroy cell structures, repeated quick freeze-thaw cycles are effective in lysing the cell membranes and results in a wide field of tumor necrosis. Heating tumors is more efficacious than freezing in terms of tumor destruction. Tissue that is heated beyond 60°C undergoes almost instant coagulation and denaturing of proteins, with complete and irreversible damage to all cells and cell contents. Higher than 100°C tissue vaporizes and carbonizes.[7] Homogeneous tissue heating to more than 60°C in the area involving the tumor leads to complete destruction of a tumor. However, it is important to recognize the physics underlying the various modalities, as this goal of homogeneous tissue heating is not easily achieved in an inhomogeneous tissue such as the liver. Ideally, a tumor and a suitable margin around the tumor is heated to a temperature between 60 and 100°C. However, heat is not contained to that specific area and conducts into the tissue outside the 60°C zone. All tissue surrounding the ablation zone that is heated between 45 and 60°C as a result of heat conduction undergoes decreasing degrees of thermal injury or coagulative necrosis as the distance from the heating zone increases.[8,9] Because of variations in the heat conductive properties of structures in the liver, cancer cells may survive in the heat conduction zone.[10,11] Predicting the exact size of the ablation zone and the conduction zone depends largely on the type of energy that is applied and the physics of the energy modality. With excellent understanding of the process, real-time image guidance of applicator placement, and thorough knowledge of anatomy, complete tumor destruction can be achieved in a manner equivalent to resection.

Cryoablation

One of the first ablation technologies is cryoablation.[12] The basic premise of this technology is the use of liquid nitrogen or other coolant to rapidly freeze the tumor by inserting a cooling rod into the mass. Destruction takes place by allowing the mass to quickly thaw by instilling helium gas, and repetition of this process using multiple freeze-thaw cycles to increase efficacy. This technology is effective in ablating lesions in the liver, and currently still has some niche applications, especially when attempting to freeze large tumors, adjacent to large and important vascular or biliary structures.[13-22] Because of continued blood flow through the blood vessels that need to be spared, the cold is carried away by the blood stream and the vessels are relatively spared. Logically, this may also represent a nidus for tumor recurrence and this is believed to be one of the downfalls of this technology. In addition, other issues such as cracking of the liver and a modality known as cryoshock have largely resulted in cryoablation becoming out of favor by liver surgeons because of this unfavorable complication profile. Cryoablation of liver tumors may still have niche application for tumors near major vascular structures. The advantage of excellent ultrasound visualization of the ice ball formation and the heat sink effect around large blood vessels may allow for precise deployment and sparing of such structures.

Radiofrequency Ablation

Radiofrequency ablation (RFA) is based on the interaction of an alternating electric current with tissue. Agitation of ions results from high frequency (460–480 kHz) currents traversing through the tissue. The agitated ions cause frictional heat that then conducts into the tissues. The current density is determined by current concentration from large pads on the patients' skin to and from the small tips of the probe inserted in the tumor. Ohms law ($I = V/R$) dictates that current (I) is dependent on voltage (V) and resistance (R) (impedance). The main intrahepatic factor influencing the current through the liver (and thereby the amount of energy delivered) is the impedance. Impedance of liver tissue changes as the tissue undergoes coagulation and desiccation. The electrical current finds the path of least resistance avoiding areas that have higher impedance, and this may constitute one of the major issues with RFA. Blood vessels coursing through or around the tumor may preferentially carry away the current. Blood vessels (and bile ducts to a lesser degree) have up to 10 times lower impedance than surrounding tumor or liver. Electrical current preferentially follows the route of least resistance and, as a result, much less electrical energy is converted into heat. This effect is called "current sink" or "electrical sink." Some modern systems try to overcome some of these issues by providing an output-based generator, which may be less sensitive to the changes in tissue impedance as a fixed amount of electrical energy is delivered, and the use of multipronged applicators with sequential current application, forcing tissue heating and subsequent coagulation in a larger area. Regardless of such adjustments, the resultant ablation zone may not be perfectly homogeneous and be small. The ultimate size of the ablated area is largely dependent on heat conduction. In the heat conduction zone, similar to the issues described for cryoablation, blood flow through vessels may carry heat away resulting in relative cooling and less efficacious ablation.[23] As long as the small ablation zone and large heat conduction zone have a large enough overlap with the tumor, tumor destruction should be complete.[24] However, imprecise placement, or the presence of an unanticipated large current or heat sink, may allow tumor cells or tumor margins to inadvertently survive. Currently, RFA is the most widely used ablation technology in the treatment of liver cancer. Various generators and probe designs exist, with focus on either impedance- or output-based systems. Because current can only go from one point to another, switching technologies are needed to rotate the current from one probe to the next when applying multiple probes simultaneously.

As a result of carrying the concentrated electrical current and the direct effect of the heat generated in the ablation zone, the probes may become very hot, and char may form at the tips of the probes. Charring of the tips results in a dramatic increase of local impedance, resulting either in significantly diminished current through the probe (impedance-based systems) or excessive heating of the probes themselves (output-based systems). Various technologies are used in an attempt to avoid overheating of the probes, such as saline cooling of the shafts and probe. Bipolar radiofrequency electrodes are also used to obviate the need for large grounding pads and minimize current through the patient. This RFA system may be a more efficient modality. Ultimately, in their current form, RFA technologies can ablate tumors up to about 5 cm. However, heat sink effects in the conduction zone and current sink effects in the ablation zone may limit the actual ablation size.

Microwave Ablation

Microwave ablation (MWA) uses electromagnetic radiation, much higher on the spectrum of electromagnetic waves than RFA. Clinically, microwaves are transmitted into tissue at in the 300-MHz to 10-GHz range depending on the system. Microwaves do not require point-to-point currents, much like a radio station broadcasting into the ether. There is no current through the patient, and no grounding pads are required. As a result of antenna design and wavelength, the broadcast area is small and the energy concentration is extremely high in the area immediately surrounding the antenna. The microwaves resonate with polarized water molecules, resulting in movement of the water molecules. Heating of the tissues occurs from friction of the oscillating water molecules with their surrounding molecules. Coagulative necrosis and resultant tumor ablation occurs from the heat that is generated. A crucial difference compared with RFA is that the oscillation of water molecules occurs in the entire field in which the microwaves are transmitted. Instantaneous and homogeneous heating occurs in the entire microwave field.[25] The generated heat is uniformly distributed until the microwave field is turned off. The size of this microwave field is ultimately determined by the wavelength and the antenna design. The speed at which the tissue heats within the microwave field is a function of the energy that is deposited into the tissue The energy delivered is in turn a function of the output wattage generated by the microwave generator and the field size dictated by the antenna design. The ultimate ablation size is next determined by the sum of the microwave field and the conductive heat zone away from the microwave field. Within the microwave field, heat sink and current sink effects are not present.[26] Outside the microwave field there will be a heat sink effect of larger blood vessels in the conduction zone, similar to RFA and cryoablation. Suboptimal placement may allow tumor cells to fall into the conduction zone with a theoretic potential for survival. With precise placement of microwave antennae, complete destruction of tumor is guaranteed as long as the tumor is covered by the microwave field.

As a result of their electromagnetic properties, microwaves are not impeded by charring, or gaseous (vapor) barriers, which are electrical insulators. Consequently, temperatures may be allowed to get much higher in MWA compared with RFA because charring or boiling does not need to be avoided. The higher temperatures yield greater tumor necrosis and significantly reduced likelihood of local tumor recurrence. On the other hand, because there is no physical barrier to microwaves, surrounding tissues and structures may be affected and need to be carefully protected.

Earlier iterations of microwave technology have been used clinically in Japan. However, generator and antenna designs were suboptimal and resulted in small ablation volumes that were clinically impractical. Various systems are currently in use in the United States. These more recent microwave systems have been in clinical use since 2002 and commercially available since 2008. They are optimized for use in tissue. Ablation volumes of 3 to 4 cm, to 8 cm and larger with single applications have been achieved. Multiple antennae can be used to achieve large volume ablations, and they can be used simultaneously. The number of antennae is theoretically only limited by the number of generators that are available. Currently, systems are used at 2 distinct frequencies: 915 MHz and 2.45 GHz. These wavelengths have distinct physical properties related to tissue permeability and antenna design. The 915-MHz system generally allows for deeper tissue penetration of the microwaves. As a result of the deeper penetration, a generally lower energy density within the microwave field is achieved, with subsequent longer ablation times, compared with higher frequencies. Increasing the power that is broadcast through the 915-MHz antenna overcomes this issue. However, the amount of energy that can be delivered is limited by antenna and cable design. At high energy levels the energy losses in the system and the charring of the antenna tip caused by excessive heating diminishes the efficacy of the energy delivery. A smaller ablation volume per antenna is the result. Conversely, the 2.45-GHz microwaves have less tissue penetration, but a much higher energy density within the field. As a result of the antenna and cable design of this system, a large ablation can be achieved with a single antenna.[27,28] We use both systems in a complementary fashion, as smaller lesions and lesions near vital vascular structures are more appropriately treated with the 915-MHz system, and larger lesions are more efficiently ablated with the 2.45-GHz system. Currently, only the 915-MHz system has a percutaneous antenna available. Advances in microwave technology are ongoing and new antenna and generator designs are likely going to augment treatment opportunities in the near future.

Emerging Ablation Technologies

Several technologies with varied clinical applicability are currently under investigation in preclinical and phase I trials. Thermocoagulative systems such as laser-interstitial thermotherapy and high-intensity focused ultrasound are currently finding limited clinical application, mostly in Europe.[29–35] These technologies rely on different wavelengths along the electromagnetic spectrum to generate heating of tissue and embedded tumors. Laser-interstitial therapy revolves around inserting high-intensity laser light-emitting fibers into tissue to allow for slow tissue heating. Ablation volumes up to 7-cm diameter, with acceptable survival rates in metastatic disease, have been reported in single-center series. However, the technology has not been enthusiastically adopted, largely because of the cumbersome nature of the currently available prototypes. High-intensity focused ultrasound uses high-energy ultrasound waves that are subsequently focused on a small area. The technique results in tremendous local sound pressure with resultant generation of heat caused by absorption of acoustic energy. This technology has resulted in early adaptation demonstrating feasibility and safety in animals and patients.[36,37] The combination of imaging and ablation may hold promise for precise energy delivery and tumor destruction. A nonthermal form of tumor ablation is currently being developed using high-voltage currents to effectively create micropores in cell membranes. This technique can be applied at a nonlethal level and is experimentally used to insert protein fragments into cells. When the process is exaggerated, the effect is lethal to the cell. The technique of irreversible electroporation is being investigated in the tumor ablation arena, but has not yet found clinical application.[38–43]

INDICATIONS FOR ABLATION
Ablation of HCC

Hepatocellular carcinoma constitutes a tremendous growing health problem in the United States with increasing incidence of liver disease as a result of increased incidence of obesity and viral hepatitis.[44] As part of a multimodality treatment strategy, resection for anatomically and medically resectable disease historically offered the best option, short of transplanting the liver.[45–49] A liver transplant currently provides the optimal treatment of cancer and underlying liver disease. Therefore patients that fall within the transplant criteria receive an important point allocation in their Mayo End-Stage Liver Disease (MELD) score, aimed at shortening their time on the transplant waiting list. HCC, however, poses significant and unique challenges because of the frequent presence of moderate to severe underlying liver parenchymal disease, the complex tumor biology, and the scarcity of livers for transplantation.

The biology of the tumor and underlying liver disease are important factors to take into consideration in the treatment of HCC. The cancer can be classified as local, regional, or metastatic disease within the liver, and extrahepatic metastatic disease. However, underlying liver disease cannot be separated from this classification. Complex staging schemes have been devised. No current staging modality is able to provide the complete picture, demonstrating the complex nature of HCC. Treatment decisions have to be made based on the expected course of the disease. The treatment approach that we advocate largely follows the classification into local versus regional versus metastatic disease. We next fine-tune this approach with the choice for individual treatment modalities based on the degree of underlying liver disease. For example, a small 2-cm HCC should be considered local tumor disease. This tumor ideally is removed from the liver. In the absence of underlying parenchymal disease the optimal removal of this tumor is achieved by resection. In a severe cirrhotic liver, however, the same 2-cm local tumor may best be removed by MWA. In both cases, transplantation would achieve the ultimate removal of tumor and diseased liver. Unfortunately, most of the patients in our practice do not meet transplant criteria for a variety of tumor- and patient-related reasons.

The same approach is taken with larger tumors. Increased tumor size results in increased risk of vascular invasion, regional microscopic, or intrahepatic metastases. The approach of regional disease should foremost focus on the region. Short of transplantation, optimal regional liver treatments involve transarterial chemoembolization (TACE) (or radioembolization), followed by removal or ablation of the tumor itself, with the choice of removal modality dictated by the degree of underlying disease. Larger tumors still, outside current transplant (Milan) criteria, put the whole liver at risk. In these situations, local therapies such as ablation should be seen as neoadjuvant strategies; tumor volume reduction may either allow return of the patient to within transplant criteria or modify their susceptibility to chemo- or radioembolization. The degree of liver tumor involvement and parenchymal disease dictates the maximum treatment the patient can undergo, in a difficult balance between quality and quantity of life. Because systemic treatment options are limited in number and in their ability to significantly prolong life, aggressive local and regional treatment strategies are warranted. Most patients ultimately succumb to progression of the tumor in the liver in combination with progression of underlying disease, so that local and regional treatment options may affect survival more than systemic therapy. Ablation of liver tumors is an important modality in this light, as it offers maximal treatment of the tumor and is generally well tolerated allowing patients to quickly (in days) return to their baseline functioning.

Ablation is particularly studied in this HCC patient population, and good results are obtained with modern ablation technologies. Multiple case series demonstrate excellent results in small (<3 cm), medium (3–5 cm) and large (>5 cm) HCC treated with RFA.[50–53] Most studies report that ablative treatment of tumor returns the patient to their underlying disease survival curve, particularly in the case of the smaller tumors. One aspect that surfaced in a recent large meta-analyses of RFA for HCC is the issue of local recurrence, which may be as high as 14% with RFA.[54,55] In part this may be because of the inclusion in these meta-analyses of percutaneous ablation studies on very small HCC, which is technically challenging. Recurrence in those studies may be reflective of missed lesions rather than represent true recurrence. The importance of exact placement of ablation probes and theoretic inferiority of RFA compared with MWA have been discussed earlier. It remains to be shown whether MWA overcomes this problem of high local recurrence, in conjunction with improved imaging and targeting modalities, but initial studies show important promise.[28,56–59] Microwave has replaced RFA in our practice, and early follow-up data show drastically reduced local recurrence.

There are some important annotations to be made to ablative strategies for HCC. First, there are 2 randomized reports in the literature directly comparing resection and ablation in small hepatocellular carcinomas. Although at first glance these studies suggested equivalence of RFA to resection, they have received some scrutiny and are currently believed to show proof of concept but not proof of noninferiority or equivalence because of high cross over of patients from one group to the other and additional design issues. Second, the studies applied an ablative technology (RFA) that theoretically does not offer the best ablative modality. With this in mind, the results are essentially outdated at the time of writing this review, as future investigations studying equivalency should be performed comparing the most efficacious modality available. Unfortunately, in a field in which new and improved modalities are constantly just around the corner, designing randomized studies and enrolling patients continues to be inherently difficult.

Treatment strategies in transplantable HCC warrant further discussion. Patients awaiting transplantation for advanced liver disease currently receive 22 additional MELD points when they develop HCC. This favors their chances of receiving a transplant, and shortens their time on the transplant waiting list. Because of organ shortage, time on the waiting list may be considerable, with some geographic variation. An ongoing practical debate has ensued regarding the treatment of cancer while on the waiting list for transplantation. Removing the cancer by means of resection voids the additional points on the waiting list. In light of the superior outcome of transplantation compared with resection as measured by overall survival, it seems to be a significant disadvantage to undergo resection, as it practically results in the inability to receive a transplant. At the same time, allowing cancer to progress while waiting for a transplant that may never arrive, either because of progression of the cancer to beyond current transplant criteria or to the absence of timely organs, seems a debatable ethical approach. At this time, ablation of tumors does not void the extra points patients receive toward their waiting list status. Ablation of tumors is therefore not negatively affecting the patients waiting time on the transplant list. It does raise an additional dilemma: these recommendations are based on studies demonstrating significant residual tumor burden in patients undergoing RFA ablation. Thus, a potentially more effective therapy (resection) is still being withheld in a trade-off for transplant points. Conversely, newer modalities such as MWA may be far superior in treating the cancer. Our own unpublished early experience with MWA and subsequent transplantation demonstrates complete absence of residual tumor in the explanted livers. As a consequence of more effective treatment of the cancer, we are perhaps unduly maintaining their favorable position on the transplant list in lieu of other transplant candidates.

Aside from the transplant dilemma, long-term survival data have been reported with RFA, often in combination with TACE. Although the underlying liver disease remains untreated in this subgroup, 3-year survival rates of 83% to 88% and 5-year survival rates of more than 70% for patients meeting the Milan criteria have been reported, rivaling the survival of transplanted patients, and surpassing resection-only strategies in terms of survival.[60,61] With current technology, those numbers stand to be improved, and our initial data suggest that MWA significantly improves at least the early outcomes in patients with HCC. Currently, MWA of tumors within and beyond Milan criteria offers patients outcomes equivalent to or better than resection. Because patients loose their additional points on the waiting list after resection, MWA offers the patient the best treatment of their cancer, although not eliminating their transplant potential. If the equivalence of MWA to resection can be proved, at least in a retrospective fashion, there may be a need to review how those results affect treatment strategies for stage II, T2 HCC. At this point, long-term outcome data are not yet available because of the novelty of the technology. However, it is clear that older ablative strategies such as PEI and cryoablation have been shown to be inferior to RFA, and in the case of cryoablation to carry a significantly worse complication profile. These modalities should be considered obsolete.

Large HCC (>5 cm) outside transplant criteria require a multimodality approach in most instances, including resection, ablation, and TACE. Larger tumors are at significantly increased risk of vascular invasion and intrahepatic micro- or macrometastatic disease. Underlying liver disease frequently prevents patients from undergoing large volume liver resection. Although resection may still offer a benefit to some select patients, we generally offer neoadjuvant therapies such as TACE or radioembolization followed by local therapy (resection, ablation). To ablate tumors of such size with RFA, multiple applications are required. Local control of the cancer can be achieved effectively. Initial reports show the feasibility of achieving excellent tumor control with MWA as well.[1] Early data demonstrate improved outcome in terms of local recurrence with MWA, but data are largely preliminary. Further studies, ideally randomized and controlled, are needed to establish the role of MWA ablation in the treatment of HCC.

Ablation of Colorectal Metastases

Approximately two-thirds of patients with colorectal cancer develop metastatic disease, and one-third of those patients have isolated metastases to the liver. With the total number of new colorectal cancer diagnoses approaching 150,000 cases a year, liver-directed therapy is an important aspect of colon cancer care in the United

States.[62,63] In the past decades, the treatment strategy for liver-only metastatic disease has evolved to include resection of all tumors when feasible, allowing for sufficient liver parenchyma to survive.[64] Significant improvement in 5- and 10-year survival rates have been shown for single lesions, as well as for multiple lesions, compared with no treatment or chemotherapy alone. Despite this broad recommendation, a significant number of patients are unresectable because of anatomic constraints as a result of multiplicity, multicentricity, or the presence of underlying liver disease. In those cases, alternative ablative strategies have been investigated. PEI and cryoablation have largely been replaced by RFA. In experienced hands, excellent results can be achieved, with 1-, 2- and 3-year survival rates reported of 87%, 77%, and 50%, respectively.[50] Multiple studies demonstrate feasibility and acceptable survival.[65-67] Although most centers are cautious in choosing RFA over resection in patients who are suitable for both,[68,69] some are arguing noninferiority to resection.[70,71] MWA may significantly improve on these outcomes, with improved local control of the tumors after ablation. Only limited studies report feasibility.[58,72-76] Heterogeneity of the study groups in unresectable colorectal liver metastases makes comparison of outcomes difficult outside a strict randomized controlled trial. Currently, we are investigating the role of MWA in colorectal liver metastases. We use MWA in conjunction with various other liver-directed therapies where indicated, including resection, to optimally debulk tumor burden. Initial unpublished data suggest that this is an effective strategy in the treatment of unresectable colorectal metastases to the liver, with improved local control and disease-free interval. Long-term data are currently unavailable.

Metastatic colorectal cancer is a disease with a wide spectrum of presentations. The biologic behavior of the cancer, the timing of presentation, and the response to chemotherapy agents all influence the ultimate outcome. Although true surgical cure can be achieved in rare scenarios, most patients eventually die from progression of disease despite multimodality liver-directed therapy. Fong and colleagues[77] tried to encompass various contributing factors leading to a high probability of early recurrence of cancer in a predictive score, with higher scores predicting early recurrence. Apart from surgical margins, the predictors were all related to the state of the disease at presentation (eg, multicentricity, size, and node positivity of the primary), or to the rapidity of the appearance of tumor metastases (eg, disease-free interval, extrahepatic metastases). All these parameters essentially are reflective of the biologic behavior of the tumor. Similar to the decision difficulties with HCC described earlier, the dilemma facing contemporary hepatobiliary surgeons is striking the balance between morbidity and mortality of aggressive tumor removal strategies versus the quality and quantity of life. Cytoreductive strategies are generally advantageous for the patients, if morbidity and mortality are low. Even in the presence of extrahepatic metastatic disease, carefully planned liver-directed therapy provides patients with improved outcome greatly surpassing the effects of systemic therapy alone.[78] It is clear that MWA provides a treatment option that is well tolerated and can completely destroy a liver tumor. It is the estimation of the biologic behavior of the tumor, however, that should dictate the treatment strategy and modality. The optimal treatment strategy for patients with metastatic colorectal cancer should be individualized based on risk assessment and requires a multimodality approach, and may include resection, ablation, chemo- or radioembolization and multitiered chemotherapeutic options.

PRACTICAL GUIDELINES FOR ABLATION

Modern ablative strategies can be applied in 3 ways: percutaneous, laparoscopic, and during open surgery. It is our opinion based on our previous and ongoing studies, that the optimal ablative technology currently is MWA. Theoretically and practically, MWA should account for a significantly reduced local recurrence rate, regardless of tumor type compared with RFA. Regardless of the mode of application, the technology can only be used effectively with optimal image guidance of probe or antenna placement. Real-time ultrasound guidance is currently the most precise modality to aid in the insertion of probes and antennae. CT-guided systems exist and are currently confined for use during percutaneous ablations, in the hands of interventional radiologists. Although CT scans aid in planning the trajectory, CT currently lacks a real-time guided application. Expert use of intra-operative ultrasound is therefore paramount for precise placement of the ablation antennae or probes into the tumor. Novel three-dimensional and virtual reality guidance systems are being developed to aid the surgeon in real-time with placement, by adding a virtual trajectory predicting the future location of the probe or antenna, irrespective of the angle of approach. This is particularly important when keeping outside of the immediate ultrasound plane. The combination of expert knowledge of anatomy, improved image guidance, and optimized ablation technology will provide the best possible surgical ablation, and may prove to be equivocal to resection in the near future. Currently, we are treating large, unresectable tumors with MWA and are able to limit hospital stay to 1 to 2 days, providing a tremendous impetus to continue to aggressively pursue advances in this arena.

SUMMARY

In the treatment of primary or secondary hepatic malignancies, a multimodality liver-directed strategy is currently used. Ablation of liver tumors is an important part of this strategy. Various methods for tumor ablation are currently available. Each ablation method has its own merit, and should be chosen carefully in the appropriate clinical setting. The most efficacious ablation method is MWA, but niche application for other methods such as RFA and cryoablation still exist. Image guidance is of paramount importance, as ablation can only be effective if precise and accurate placement of ablation instruments can be achieved. Currently, multimodality strategies, including ablation, are used where resection alone is not curative. With increasing effectiveness of ablation methods, as suggested by ongoing research efforts, ablation offers an alternative to resection with significantly reduced morbidity and mortality.

REFERENCES

1. Yamane B, Weber S. Liver-directed treatment modalities for primary and secondary hepatic tumors. Surg Clin North Am 2009;89(1):97–113.
2. Padma S, Martinie JB, Iannitti DA. Liver tumor ablation: percutaneous and open approaches. J Surg Oncol 2009;100(8):619–34.
3. Halsted WS. I. The results of operations for the cure of cancer of the breast performed at the Johns Hopkins Hospital from June, 1889, to January, 1894. Ann Surg 1894;20(5):497–555.
4. Shiina S, Tagawa K, Unuma T, et al. Percutaneous ethanol injection therapy for hepatocellular carcinoma. A histopathologic study. Cancer 1991;68(7):1524–30.
5. Livraghi T. Radiofrequency ablation, PEIT, and TACE for hepatocellular carcinoma. J Hepatobiliary Pancreat Surg 2003;10(1):67–76.
6. Fartoux L, Arrive L, Andreani T, et al. Treatment of small hepatocellular carcinoma with acetic acid percutaneous injection. Gastroenterol Clin Biol 2005;29(12):1213–9.
7. Goldberg SN, Gazelle GS, Mueller PR. Thermal ablation therapy for focal malignancy: a unified approach to underlying principles, techniques, and diagnostic imaging guidance. AJR Am J Roentgenol 2000;174(2):323–31.

8. Hope WW, Arru JM, McKee JQ, et al. Evaluation of mulitprobe radiofrequency technology in a porcine model. HPB (Oxford) 2007;9(5):363–7.
9. Hope WW, Schmelzer TM, Newcomb WL, et al. Guidelines for power and time variables for microwave ablation in a porcine liver. J Gastrointest Surg 2008; 12(3):463–7.
10. Prakash P, Converse MC, Mahvi DM, et al. Measurement of the specific heat capacity of liver phantom. Physiol Meas 2006;27(10):N41–6.
11. Stauffer PR, Rossetto F, Prakash M, et al. Phantom and animal tissues for modelling the electrical properties of human liver. Int J Hyperthermia 2003;19(1): 89–101.
12. Gage AA. History of cryosurgery. Semin Surg Oncol 1998;14(2):99–109.
13. Bayjoo P, Jacob G. Hepatic cryosurgery: biological and clinical considerations. J R Coll Surg Edinb 1992;37(6):369–72.
14. Heniford BT, Arca MJ, Iannitti DA, et al. Laparoscopic cryoablation of hepatic metastases. Semin Surg Oncol 1998;15(3):194–201.
15. Iannitti DA, Heniford T, Hale J, et al. Laparoscopic cryoablation of hepatic metastases. Arch Surg 1998;133(9):1011–5.
16. Kane R. Ultrasound-guided hepatic cryosurgery for tumor ablation. Semin Intervent Radiol 1993;10(2):132–44.
17. Mala T. Cryoablation of liver tumours—a review of mechanisms, techniques and clinical outcome. Minim Invasive Ther Allied Technol 2006;15(1):9–17.
18. McMasters KM, Edwards MJ. Liver cryosurgery. J Ky Med Assoc 1996;94(6): 222–9.
19. Steele G Jr. Cryoablation in hepatic surgery. Semin Liver Dis 1994;14(2):120–5.
20. Weber SM, Lee FT Jr. Expanded treatment of hepatic tumors with radiofrequency ablation and cryoablation. Oncology (Williston Park) 2005;19(11 Suppl 4):27–32.
21. Zhou XD, Tang ZY, Yu YQ, et al. The role of cryosurgery in the treatment of hepatic cancer: a report of 113 cases. J Cancer Res Clin Oncol 1993;120(1–2):100–2.
22. Clavien PA, Kang KJ, Selzner N, et al. Cryosurgery after chemoembolization for hepatocellular carcinoma in patients with cirrhosis. J Gastrointest Surg 2002; 6(1):95–101.
23. Kim SK, Rhim H, Kim YS, et al. Radiofrequency thermal ablation of hepatic tumors: pitfalls and challenges. Abdom Imaging 2005;30(6):727–33.
24. Dodd GD 3rd, Frank MS, Aribandi M, et al. Radiofrequency thermal ablation: computer analysis of the size of the thermal injury created by overlapping ablations. AJR Am J Roentgenol 2001;177(4):777–82.
25. Simon CJ, Dupuy DE, Mayo-Smith WW. Microwave ablation: principles and applications. Radiographics 2005;25(Suppl 1):S69–83.
26. Yu NC, Raman SS, Kim YJ, et al. Microwave liver ablation: influence of hepatic vein size on heat-sink effect in a porcine model. J Vasc Interv Radiol 2008; 19(7):1087–92.
27. Ong SL, Gravante G, Metcalfe MS, et al. Efficacy and safety of microwave ablation for primary and secondary liver malignancies: a systematic review. Eur J Gastroenterol Hepatol 2009;21(6):599–605.
28. Bhardwaj N, Strickland AD, Ahmad F, et al. Microwave ablation for unresectable hepatic tumours: clinical results using a novel microwave probe and generator. Eur J Surg Oncol 2010;36(3):264–8.
29. Amin Z, Donald JJ, Masters A, et al. Hepatic metastases: interstitial laser photocoagulation with real-time US monitoring and dynamic CT evaluation of treatment. Radiology 1993;187(2):339–47.

30. Boppart SA, Herrmann J, Pitris C, et al. High-resolution optical coherence tomography-guided laser ablation of surgical tissue. J Surg Res 1999;82(2): 275–84.
31. Denecke T, Steffen I, Hildebrandt B, et al. Assessment of local control after laser-induced thermotherapy of liver metastases from colorectal cancer: contribution of FDG-PET in patients with clinical suspicion of progressive disease. Acta Radiol 2007;48(8):821–30.
32. Giorgio A, Tarantino L, de Stefano G, et al. Interstitial laser photocoagulation under ultrasound guidance of liver tumors: results in 104 treated patients. Eur J Ultrasound 2000;11(3):181–8.
33. Isbert C, Roggan A, Ritz JP, et al. Laser-induced thermotherapy: intra- and extra-lesionary recurrence after incomplete destruction of experimental liver metastasis. Surg Endosc 2001;15(11):1320–6.
34. Pacella CM, Bizzarri G, Magnolfi F, et al. Laser thermal ablation in the treatment of small hepatocellular carcinoma: results in 74 patients. Radiology 2001;221(3):712–20.
35. Puls R, Langner S, Rosenberg C, et al. Laser ablation of liver metastases from colorectal cancer with MR thermometry: 5-year survival. J Vasc Interv Radiol 2008;20(2):225–34.
36. Zhang L, Zhu H, Jin C, et al. High-intensity focused ultrasound (HIFU): effective and safe therapy for hepatocellular carcinoma adjacent to major hepatic veins. Europe 2009;19(2):437–45.
37. Haar GT, Coussios C. High intensity focused ultrasound: physical principles and devices. Int J Hyperthermia 2007;23(2):89–104.
38. Miller L, Leor J, Rubinsky B. Cancer cells ablation with irreversible electroporation. Technol Cancer Res Treat 2005;4(6):699–705.
39. Al-Sakere B, Andre F, Bernat C, et al. Tumor ablation with irreversible electroporation. PLoS One 2007;2(11):e1135.
40. Lee EW, Loh CT, Kee ST. Imaging guided percutaneous irreversible electroporation: ultrasound and immunohistological correlation. Technol Cancer Res Treat 2007;6(4):287–94.
41. Lencioni R, Cioni D, Pina CD, et al. Hepatocellular carcinoma: new options for image-guided ablation. J Hepatobiliary Pancreat Surg 2009. [Epub ahead of print].
42. Neal RE 2nd, Davalos RV. The feasibility of irreversible electroporation for the treatment of breast cancer and other heterogeneous systems. Ann Biomed Eng 2009;37(12):2615–25.
43. Rubinsky B, Onik G, Mikus P. Irreversible electroporation: a new ablation modality–clinical implications. Technol Cancer Res Treat 2007;6(1):37–48.
44. El-Serag HB. Hepatocellular carcinoma: an epidemiologic view. J Clin Gastroenterol 2002;35(5 Suppl 2):S72–8.
45. Llovet JM, Burroughs A, Bruix J. Hepatocellular carcinoma. Lancet 2003; 362(9399):1907–17.
46. Bruix J, Llovet JM. Prognostic prediction and treatment strategy in hepatocellular carcinoma. Hepatology 2002;35(3):519–24.
47. Nagorney DM, van Heerden JA, Ilstrup DM, et al. Primary hepatic malignancy: surgical management and determinants of survival. Surgery 1989;106(4):740–8 [discussion: 8–9].
48. Choi TK, Edward CS, Fan ST, et al. Results of surgical resection for hepatocellular carcinoma. Hepatogastroenterology 1990;37(2):172–5.
49. Mazzaferro V, Regalia E, Doci R, et al. Liver transplantation for the treatment of small hepatocellular carcinomas in patients with cirrhosis. N Engl J Med 1996; 334(11):693–9.

50. Iannitti DA, Dupuy DE, Mayo-Smith WW, et al. Hepatic radiofrequency ablation. Arch Surg 2002;137(4):422–6.
51. Chen MS, Li JQ, Zheng Y, et al. A prospective randomized trial comparing percutaneous local ablative therapy and partial hepatectomy for small hepatocellular carcinoma. Ann Surg 2006;243(3):321–8.
52. Lu MD, Kuang M, Liang LJ, et al. [Surgical resection versus percutaneous thermal ablation for early-stage hepatocellular carcinoma: a randomized clinical trial]. Zhonghua Yi Xue Za Zhi 2006;86(12):801–5 [in Chinese].
53. Livraghi T, Meloni F, Di Stasi M, et al. Sustained complete response and complications rates after radiofrequency ablation of very early hepatocellular carcinoma in cirrhosis: is resection still the treatment of choice? Hepatology 2008;47(1):82–9.
54. Siperstein A, Garland A, Engle K, et al. Local recurrence after laparoscopic radiofrequency thermal ablation of hepatic tumors. Ann Surg Oncol 2000;7(2):106–13.
55. Mulier S, Ni Y, Jamart J, et al. Local recurrence after hepatic radiofrequency coagulation: multivariate meta-analysis and review of contributing factors. Ann Surg 2005;242(2):158–71.
56. Bhardwaj N, Strickland AD, Ahmad F, et al. A comparative histological evaluation of the ablations produced by microwave, cryotherapy and radiofrequency in the liver. Pathology 2009;41(2):168–72.
57. Gravante G, Ong SL, Metcalfe MS, et al. Hepatic microwave ablation: a review of the histological changes following thermal damage. Liver Int 2008;28(7):911–21.
58. Martin RC, Scoggins CR, McMasters KM. Microwave hepatic ablation: initial experience of safety and efficacy. J Surg Oncol 2007;96(6):481–6.
59. Iannitti DA, Martin RC, Simon CJ, et al. Hepatic tumor ablation with clustered microwave antennae: the US Phase II trial. HPB (Oxford) 2007;9(2):120–4.
60. Graziadei IW, Sandmueller H, Waldenberger P, et al. Chemoembolization followed by liver transplantation for hepatocellular carcinoma impedes tumor progression while on the waiting list and leads to excellent outcome. Liver Transpl 2003;9(6):557–63.
61. Porrett PM, Peterman H, Rosen M, et al. Lack of benefit of pre-transplant locoregional hepatic therapy for hepatocellular cancer in the current MELD era. Liver Transpl 2006;12(4):665–73.
62. Jemal A, Murray T, Ward E, et al. Cancer statistics, 2005. CA Cancer J Clin 2005;55(1):10–30.
63. Cummins ER, Vick KD, Poole GV. Incurable colorectal carcinoma: the role of surgical palliation. Am Surg 2004;70(5):433–7.
64. Abdalla EK, Adam R, Bilchik AJ, et al. Improving resectability of hepatic colorectal metastases: expert consensus statement. Ann Surg Oncol 2006;13(10):1271–80.
65. Siperstein AE, Berber E, Ballem N, et al. Survival after radiofrequency ablation of colorectal liver metastases: 10-year experience. Ann Surg 2007;246(4):559–65 [discussion: 65–7].
66. Sorensen SM, Mortensen FV, Nielsen DT. Radiofrequency ablation of colorectal liver metastases: long-term survival. Acta Radiol 2007;48(3):253–8.
67. Jakobs TF, Hoffmann RT, Trumm C, et al. Radiofrequency ablation of colorectal liver metastases: mid-term results in 68 patients. Anticancer Res 2006;26(1B):671–80.
68. Aloia TA, Vauthey JN, Loyer EM, et al. Solitary colorectal liver metastasis: resection determines outcome. Arch Surg 2006;141(5):460–6 [discussion: 6–7].
69. Pereira PL. Actual role of radiofrequency ablation of liver metastases. Eur Radiol 2007;17(8):2062–70.

70. Abitabile P, Hartl U, Lange J, et al. Radiofrequency ablation permits an effective treatment for colorectal liver metastasis. Eur J Surg Oncol 2007;33(1):67–71.

71. Mulier S, Ni Y, Jamart J, et al. Radiofrequency ablation versus resection for resectable colorectal liver metastases: time for a randomized trial? Ann Surg Oncol 2008;15(1):144–57.

72. Tanaka K, Shimada H, Nagano Y, et al. Outcome after hepatic resection versus combined resection and microwave ablation for multiple bilobar colorectal metastases to the liver. Surgery 2006;139(2):263–73.

73. Evans J. Ablative and catheter-delivered therapies for colorectal liver metastases (CRLM). Eur J Surg Oncol 2007;33(Suppl 2):S64–75.

74. Koshariya M, Jagad RB, Kawamoto J, et al. An update and our experience with metastatic liver disease. Hepatogastroenterology 2007;54(80):2232–9.

75. Garcea G, Ong SL, Maddern GJ. Inoperable colorectal liver metastases: a declining entity? Eur J Cancer 2008;44(17):2555–72.

76. Jagad RB, Koshariya M, Kawamoto J, et al. Laparoscopic microwave ablation of liver tumors: our experience. Hepatogastroenterology 2008;55(81):27–32.

77. Fong Y, Fortner J, Sun RL, et al. Clinical score for predicting recurrence after hepatic resection for metastatic colorectal cancer: analysis of 1001 consecutive cases. Ann Surg 1999;230(3):309–18 [discussion: 18–21].

78. Elias D, Benizri E, Pocard M, et al. Treatment of synchronous peritoneal carcinomatosis and liver metastases from colorectal cancer. Eur J Surg Oncol 2006; 32(6):632–6.

Fulminant Hepatic Failure: When to Transplant

Ajai Khanna, MD, PhD[a],*, Alan W. Hemming, MD[a,b]

KEYWORDS

- Liver failure • Liver transplantation • Fulminant liver failure
- Live donor liver transplantation

Fulminant hepatic failure (FHF) is a syndrome characterized by grossly impaired liver function in an acute setting. By definition, it is the onset of hepatic encephalopathy (HE) and liver failure within 8 weeks of development of jaundice.[1] O'Grady and colleagues[2] reported a modified definition to classify acute liver failure based on the interval between jaundice and encephalopathy into hyperacute (onset within 1 week), acute (between 8 and 28 days), and subacute (between 29 days and 12 weeks). The mainstay of diagnosis is the presence of HE, coagulopathy, hypoglycemia, and increased liver numbers. For all practical purposes, especially when evaluating a patient for transplantation, patients with preexisting subclinical disease who present with acute liver decompensation are also included in this category.

There have been recent elaborate reviews and publications on the causal factors, diagnosis, and management of this complex and life-threatening syndrome.[3–8] This article focuses on the pathophysiology, prognostic criteria, liver transplant options, and measures of outcome in patients with FHF. Various therapeutic transplant surgical options are also discussed.

INCIDENCE

FHF is an uncommon but lethal condition with an average annual incidence of approximately 2000 cases in the United States.[9] Because of its varying mode of presentation, it is associated with a high morbidity or mortality in the absence of timely intervention. Liver injury and hepatocyte necrosis lead to multisystem organ dysfunction including renal, respiratory and circulatory failure, and superimposed infection. The central causative process leading to multisystem organ failure results from tissue hypoxia from

---

No grant funding for this work.
[a] Abdominal Transplant and Hepatobiliary Surgery, Department of Surgery, University of California San Diego School of Medicine, 200 West Arbor Drive, San Diego, CA 92103-8401, USA
[b] Abdominal Transplant and Hepatobiliary Surgery, Department of Surgery, University of California San Diego School of Medicine, 200 West Arbor Drive, San Diego, CA 92103-8401, USA
* Corresponding author.
E-mail address: akhanna@ucsd.edu

doi:10.1016/j.suc.2010.04.013
surgical.theclinics.com

microcirculatory changes consequent on endotoxemia. Macrophage activation and release of cytokines due to an early failure of host defenses lead to end-organ damage.[10]

CAUSES

A prospective study conducted by the US Acute Liver Failure Study Group at 17 tertiary care centers[11] found acetaminophen overdose as the commonest cause of FHF in the United States with an incidence of 39%, followed by idiosyncratic drug reactions (13%), hepatitis A and B infection (4% and 7%, respectively), along with other viral infections like cytomegalovirus (CMV), herpes simplex virus (HSV), adeno- and paramyxoma viruses; ischemic hepatitis (6%), autoimmune hepatitis (4%), Wilson disease (3%), and Budd-Chiari syndrome (2%). Other causes included pregnancy associated FHF, metastatic lymphoma, toxins, and heat stroke. In 17% of these patients, a causative agent was not found.

Fulminant viral hepatitis is the most frequent cause worldwide because it is the commonest causative agent in the Far East where population density is high and viral hepatitis is endemic.[10]

Ninety-three percent (n = 286) of the patients reported by the US Acute Failure Study group had a definitive outcome: death, transplantation, or hospital discharge at 3 weeks, with overall survival of 67% with or without liver transplantation. This finding highlights the rapidity of pathophysiologic processes involved in FHF patients. Twenty-nine percent of the patients in the study group (89 out of 308) received a liver transplant. This study also highlighted poor overall survival rates in patients who were elderly (>65 years), those who presented with subacute (jaundice to encephalopathy>28 days) liver failure, and grade III or IV coma.

PATHOPHYSIOLOGY

Hepatocellular injury is central to FHF, irrespective of the causative agent. The initial insult and interplay of cytokines lead to hepatocyte necrosis or apoptosis. Hepatocyte apoptosis involves 2 signaling pathways: a death receptor–mediated extrinsic pathway or a mitochondria-mediated intrinsic pathway.[12] Death-inducing signaling complex is formed as a result of fatty acid synthetase (FAS) ligand–receptor binding. Caspases are activated resulting in cell death. The intrinsic mitochondrial pathway is activated by oxidative stress, production of reactive oxygen species, and activation of apoptosis genes. Tumor necrosis factor (TNF)-α and FAS ligand (FasL) stimulate hepatocyte apoptosis leading to liver failure. Other mechanisms, especially implicated in hemorrhagic shock, sepsis, and drug-induced liver failure, include accumulation of activated neutrophils and subsequent injury in response to inflammatory cytokines. Dead hepatocytes serve as a good culture medium, leading to local and systemic sepsis syndrome. Regeneration is associated with ductular reaction and proliferation of cholangiocytes, progenitor cells (oval cells, stem cells, and fetal liver cells), and ductular hepatocytes. Cytokines and growth factors involved in regeneration include interleukin (IL)-6, hepatocyte growth factor (HGF), epidermal growth factor, insulin, and epinephrine.[13,14] Successful replacement of necrotic liver by transplantation halts the inflammatory process and provides functioning and healthy hepatocytes, thereby reversing the inflammatory process and restoring the opsonization capacity of the liver (**Fig. 1**). The clinical picture is that of gradually deteriorating liver function as shown by encephalopathy, increased transaminases, coagulopathy, hypoglycemia, and multiorgan dysfunction; these are reversed by successful liver transplantation (**Fig. 2**).

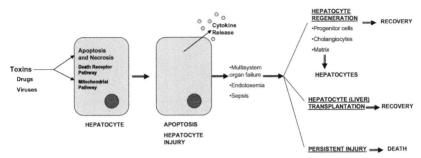

Fig. 1. Pathways in hepatocyte injury: regeneration and outcome: The figure shows the role of death receptor and mitochondrial pathways in apoptosis and necrosis of hepatocytes in fulminant liver failure. Release of cytokines and humoral factors results in multisystem organ failure that can rapidly lead to decompensation and death if not salvaged by timely intervention or liver transplantation.

DIAGNOSIS

The diagnosis is essentially clinical and depends on the stage in which patients present. Mental status change with varying degrees of encephalopathy, nonspecific gastrointestinal (GI) symptoms, fever, respiratory complaints, and edema related to renal failure are some of the common symptoms. HE can present as slight alteration in mental status (stage I); confusion, drowsiness, and asterixis (stage II); stupor, incoherence, and agitation (stage III); or frank coma, unresponsiveness, and decerebration (stage IV). Patients with stage III or IV encephalopathy may present with features of multisystem organ failure and might require endotracheal intubation and renal support.

Laboratory tests show hypoglycemia, increased prothrombin time (PT), international normalization ratio (INR), serum alanine aminotransferase (ALT), and aspartate aminotransferase (AST) levels, metabolic acidosis, hypoglycemia, and increased blood urea nitrogen and serum creatinine. Serum phosphate concentrations have limited clinical usefulness as prognostic markers; however, persistently increased arterial blood lactate levels despite adequate fluid resuscitation are indicators of a poor prognosis in FHF.

Gross appearance of the liver shows a shiny yellow or pale, often enlarged liver (**Fig. 3**). Transjugular liver biopsy can help to evaluate the degree of liver injury and

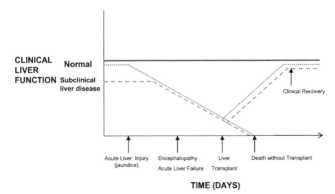

Fig. 2. Clinical course of FHF and outcome following liver transplantation.

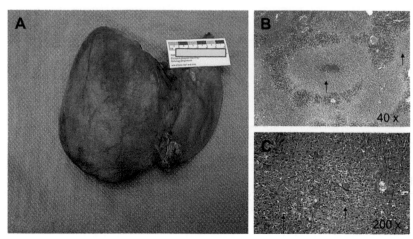

Fig. 3. Fulminant liver failure: gross and histopathologic features. (*A*) Explant from a patient with fulminant liver failure. Note the pale, enlarged, and swollen liver, suggestive of hepatocyte swelling and necrosis. (*B*) Liver biopsy (40×) showing massive centrilobular necrosis (*small arrows*) (*C*) Liver biopsy (200×) showing massive centrilobular necrosis (*small arrow*) and ballooning and vacuolization of remaining viable hepatocytes (*large arrow*).

necrosis, but not all centers use this. Liver biopsy shows diffuse centrilobular hemorrhagic necrosis depending on the extent of hepatocellular damage, and vacuolization of remaining viable hepatocytes (see **Fig. 3**). For neonates in acute liver failure, an open liver biopsy is often helpful.

A careful history and list of medications can give essential diagnostic clues. Diagnostic workup includes viral serologies for hepatitis A to E viruses, CMV and Herpes. A full liver transplant workup should be initiated for patients in FHF.

MANAGEMENT

The essentials of management have been discussed in detail in several recent publications.[3,5–7] These include admission to an intensive care unit, placement of monitoring lines, close monitoring of clinical signs, symptoms, neurologic status, and laboratory tests. Nutrition, treatment of hypoglycemia, hydration, electrolyte imbalance, coagulopathy, and prevention of infection are mainstays of supportive care.

Rapid evaluation of treatable causes of FHF helps to institute specific therapy. These include antiviral therapy for patients with hepatitis B and D (lamivudine, entecavir), CMV hepatitis (ganciclovir, valganciclovir), Epstein-Barr virus (EBV), and HSV hepatitis (acyclovir); chelating agents for patients with Wilson disease, corticosteroids for autoimmune hepatitis, *N*-acetylcysteine for patients with acetaminophen toxicity, 2-(2-nitro-4-trifluoromethylbenzoyl)-1,3-cyclohexanedione (NTBC) for tyrosinemia, and heparin therapy for patients with Budd-Chiari syndrome.[6] Early imaging studies should include liver ultrasound scan to serve as a baseline, Doppler ultrasound scan of the liver to evaluate vascular flows, and liver texture and computed tomography (CT) scan of the abdomen to evaluate the appearance of the liver and its volume (**Fig. 4**).

Involvement of the multidisciplinary transplant team to include transplant surgeon, intensivist, hepatologist, social worker, transplant coordinator and pharmacist is critical in the management of these patients. Serial laboratory tests are done every 6 to

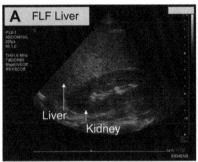 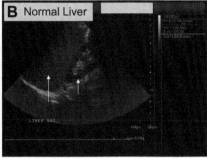

Fig. 4. (*A*) Ultrasound appearance of liver parenchyma with heterogenous architecture and increased echogenicity in a patient with fulminant liver failure, compared with (*B*) normal liver following liver transplantation in the same patient. Compared with renal echogenicity (*small arrows*), the liver looks more echogenic in a patient with fulminant liver failure (*large arrow A*).

8 hours depending on the patient's condition include blood gases and lactate, INR, liver chemistry, and factor V levels. Close monitoring of neurologic status and blood sugar level is essential. A sudden change in mental status in this setting portends acute decompensation and helps the transplant team decide on the need for urgent liver transplantation. A major dilemma for clinicians managing these patients is that the interval between intervention being too early or too late can be short.

Cerebral edema is managed by head elevation, avoiding unnecessary movement or stimuli, close monitoring of pupils and papilledema, cooling to lower patient's core temperature, mannitol, hyperventilation, and use of propofol for sedation. Intracranial pressure monitoring using intracranial probes is not being practiced in all units because of its invasive nature in coagulopathic patients. Near-infrared spectrophotometry (NIRS) has been used to evaluate changes in cerebral perfusion in patients with FHF.[15] However, its use is currently limited to certain pediatric units.

Prompt use of renal replacement therapy in patients with renal compromise helps to keep the patient euvolemic and prevents cerebral edema. Antibiotics and antifungal treatment are instituted for infection prophylaxis. Coagulopathy is corrected with fresh frozen plasma only if a procedure is planned because INR and PT are used as measures of liver function during FHF.

PROGNOSTIC CRITERIA AND PREDICTORS OF OUTCOME

The decision to proceed with a liver transplant is important and has to be timely. Premature transplantation could take away the possibility of spontaneous recovery and expose the patient to a major procedure with accompanying potential complications and lifelong immunosuppression. Late referrals, listing, and transplantation for a patient who is in multisystem organ failure carries a high mortality. A delay in diagnosis, management, and transplantation could result in worsening cerebral edema and brain death. Early transfer to a liver transplant center is critical. The patient has to be monitored closely, preferably in a liver intensive care unit. Because these patients give a narrow window, timely listing for liver transplantation is critical.

Bernuau and colleagues[16] described the Clichy criteria for patients with FHF due to hepatitis B. Predictors of outcome included patient age, absence of hepatitis B surface antigen (HBSAg), serum α-fetoprotein (AFP) level, and factor V level. Bismuth and colleagues[17] recommended liver transplantation for patients with grade 3 or 4 encephalopathy and factor V levels less than 20% (patients with age <30 years) to 30% (patients >30 years). The King's College criteria reported by O'Grady and colleagues[18] in 1989 were a retrospective multivariate analysis of variables in patients with FHF. These included patient age, cause of FHF, duration of icterus, bilirubin level, arterial pH, PT, and serum creatinine. These criteria are used by most liver transplant units to triage and identify patients who need expedited listing for liver transplantation. For patients with acetaminophen-induced liver failure, an arterial pH of less than 7.3 or a combination of grade III to IV encephalopathy, serum creatinine more than 300 μmol per liter (>3.4 mg/dL) and PT more than 100 seconds (INR>6.5) are indications for liver transplantation. For non–acetaminophen-induced liver failure the presence of PT more than 100 seconds (INR>6.5) or a combination of any 3 of the following predicts the need for urgent transplantation: age less than 10 or more than 40 years, period of jaundice to encephalopathy more than 7 days, non-A/non-B hepatitis, drug-induced hepatitis or Wilson disease, PT more than 50 seconds (INR>3.5), and serum bilirubin more than 300 μmol/L (17.5 mg/dL). The importance of these factors has been validated in several series.[19,20] Shakil and colleagues[4] showed that patients who did not meet King's College criteria still had poor prognoses. This finding is because of variability in presentation and listing and transplantation of patients with FHF.

The need for liver transplantation in patients with acetaminophen poisoning and prognostic criteria have been studied by various investigators.[21,22]

In a retrospective analysis of 144 patients with FHF due to viral hepatitis, Dhiman and colleagues[23] showed that Mayo End-Stage Liver Disease (MELD) score greater than 33, King's College Hospital criteria, and any 3 clinical prognostic indicators of age, duration of jaundice, jaundice-encephalopathy interval, grade of encephalopathy, presence of cerebral edema, bilirubin, PT, and creatinine have a high positive predictive value but low negative predictive value.[23] This indicates that these models have the greatest applicability in predicting a more negative outcome than survival. Kremers and colleagues[24] showed that FHF without acetaminophen toxicity has the poorest survival probability while awaiting liver transplant compared with other status I candidates (FHF due to acetaminophen toxicity, primary graft nonfunction, and hepatic artery thrombosis). There was a negative correlation between status I survival probability and MELD scores.

A cross-validated risk-stratified scoring system to predict survival probability following liver transplantation for FHF has been proposed by Barshes and colleagues.[25] They identified history of life support, recipient age greater than 50 years, recipient body mass index (BMI) 30 kg/m², and serum creatinine more than 2 mg/dL as risk factors associated with poor posttransplant survival.

Perkins[26] reported on the role of serum bilirubin and liver volumetry in determining the extent of liver disease. Serum bilirubin, computed tomography–derived liver volume (CTLV), and standardized liver volume (SLV) of 30 adult patients with acute liver failure were calculated at the time of diagnosis. The median CTLV/SLV ratios of patients who recovered without surgical intervention and those who were transplanted or died of liver failure were 1.019 and 0.757, respectively ($P = .0009$), with a sensitivity and specificity of 76.5% and 92.3%, respectively.

Acute deterioration in mental status, stage III/IV coma, persistently increased PT and INR despite replacement with fresh frozen plasma, development of respiratory or renal dysfunction, need for pressors to maintain hemodynamics, and hypoglycemic spells are absolute indications to list and proceed with liver transplantation. Development of multisystem organ failure is a sign of acute decompensation, which can rapidly lead to cerebral edema and brain death. The decision to list and transplant is preferably made in a multidisciplinary setting to ensure that all facts of a particular patient have been considered. A delay in decision to transplant is associated with increased morbidity and mortality. Patients with bad prognostic indicators and severe liver injury are likely to die of sepsis before the liver can regenerate and recover. Some of the patients in this category who recover will eventually develop liver cirrhosis and portal hypertension. This possibility should be considered when deciding on the need for liver transplantation.

NONTRANSPLANT INTERVENTIONS FOR FHF

As a result of high mortality associated with FHF, and in the absence of a readily available donor, several bridging devices have been developed. These include nonbiologic and biologic devices and hepatocyte transplantation.

Nonbiologic devices that have been used to treat FHF include charcoal hemoperfusion, hemofiltration, and molecular adsorbent recirculating systems. Biologic systems include the bioartificial liver (BAL) and an extracorporeal liver assist device.[27] Several investigators have reported on the use of these devices with temporary or partial success because of issues arising from cell availability and viability and regulatory constraints.[28,29] However, no controlled trials have been conducted to justify the use of these devices as standards of care.

HEPATOCYTE TRANSPLANTATION

This modality has worked in several experimental models.[30] In the clinical setting, there are isolated series and reports of the use of isolated hepatocyte transplantation in patients with liver failure.[31–34] However, further controlled clinical trials are needed for hepatocyte transplantation to be adopted as an established therapy for patients with FHF. Advances in regenerative medicine and tissue engineering have prompted investigators to develop models of engineered liver tissue, but their clinical applicability is presently lacking.[35]

LIVER TRANSPLANTATION
Indications for Liver Transplantation in FHF

Acute deterioration in mental status
Stage III/IV encephalopathy
Persistently increased PT and INR
Development of multisystem dysfunction
Hypoglycemic episodes.

Patients who meet established criteria are listed as status I according to United Network for Organ Sharing (UNOS) guidelines are listed as priority candidates for liver transplant. Priority listing for these patients has gone through several changes since UNOS was established.[36,37] Current UNOS listing criteria (http://unos.org/PoliciesandBylaws2/policies/pdfs/policy_8.pdf) for patients at status I include (1) fulminant liver failure, defined as the onset of HE within 8 weeks of the first symptoms of liver disease. The absence of preexisting liver disease is critical to the diagnosis. One of 3 criteria must be met to list a pediatric candidate with fulminant liver failure: (a) ventilator dependence, (b) requiring dialysis or continuous venovenous hemofiltration (CVVH) or continuous venovenous hemodialysis (CVVD), or (c) INR greater than 2.0; (2) primary nonfunction (3) hepatic artery thrombosis; (4) acute decompensated Wilson disease; and (5) chronic liver disease. Candidates meeting criteria (1) (2), (3), or (4) may be listed as a status 1A; those meeting criteria (5) may be listed as a status 1B.

Adam and colleagues[38,39] reported European Liver Transplant Registry data that showed survival following deceased donor liver transplantation for FHF at 5 years is worse than for non-FHF (5-year survival at 59% and 70%, respectively).

LIVER TRANSPLANT OPTIONS

Deceased donor
  Whole liver
  Split liver
  Auxiliary liver
Live donor
  Orthotopic
  Auxiliary.

WHOLE LIVER TRANSPLANTATION

This is the gold standard for liver transplantation. It involves explanting the diseased liver and performing an orthotopic liver transplantation. It is associated with the best results, although no randomized trials exist to compare the different liver transplant options because the choice of this life-saving procedure depends on organ availability and whether deceased donation laws exist in the patient's country.

Status I patients usually have shorter waiting times resulting in low rates of death while on waiting lists. Status I patients account for approximately 5% to 8% of the liver transplant waiting list. The overall 1-year patient and graft survival following liver transplantation for FHF is 81% and 75%, respectively.[40] Farmer and colleagues[41] analyzed 35 variables to determine their effects on patient and graft survival in a cohort of 204 FHF patients who underwent liver transplant. They reported 1- and 5-year patient survival of 73% and 67%, respectively. The advantages of whole organ liver transplantation include availability of large hepatocyte mass providing the recipient with enough functioning hepatocyte, thereby maximizing chances of recovery (**Fig. 5**). The option

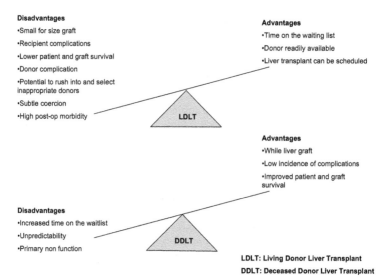

Fig. 5. Advantages and disadvantages of live donor liver transplantation (LDLT) and deceased donor liver transplantation (DDLT) in patients with fulminant liver failure.

of deceased donor transplantation is not available in countries where there are no brain death laws. These places have popularized live donor liver transplantation (LDLT) for FHF because this is the only available option.

The downside of deceased donor transplant is its unpredictable availability and timing; duration of cold ischemia; and donor factors such as use of pressors, hypotension, hypernatremia, and sepsis that lead to a compromised organ. In addition, deceased donor liver transplantation is associated with a higher incidence of primary nonfunction.[41] Transplantation of critically ill patients with a marginal graft can result in a bad outcome. On multivariate analysis, Farmer and colleagues[41] found pretransplant creatinine and conjugated bilirubin to be significant predictors of outcome following liver transplantation. In a similar analysis, Bismuth and colleagues[17] found that segmental donor grafts, donor liver steatosis, and degree of encephalopathy on admission adversely affected patient survival. Deceased donor liver transplant also commits the patient to lifelong immunosuppression.

AUXILIARY LIVER TRANSPLANTATION

Auxiliary liver transplantation was developed to serve as a bridge and to provide liver function while the injured liver regenerates and hypertrophies. Auxiliary graft can be placed heterotopically or as auxiliary partial orthotopic liver transplantation (APOLT).

Auxiliary heterotopic liver transplant is rarely practiced because it is associated with high technical complications (primary nonfunction, vascular thrombosis). APOLT consists of removing part of the native liver, right or left lobe, and performing an orthotopic liver transplant using a lobe from the donor (deceased or live). The advantages of APOLT include the possibility of immunosuppression withdrawal.[42,43] However, it is technically more challenging and could be associated with a high incidence of small-for-size syndrome, portal vein thrombosis, and graft failure.[44] The transplanted liver volume may not provide enough hepatocyte function, resulting in the need for retransplantation and associated morbidity and neurologic injury.[45] Hence the allograft should be at least 1% of the recipient weight. Compared with conventional liver transplantation, APOLT is associated with more postoperative complications such as bile leak, nonfunction, and retransplantation.

There is also a theoretical risk of reduction in portal flow to the native liver or the graft, which can lead to impaired liver regeneration in fibrosis and cirrhosis. Optimal results with APOLT can be expected in younger patients with increased regenerative capacity following liver injury, and patients with viral or acetaminophen-induced FHF.[46] An added advantage is that APOLT from a live donor can be performed in countries where brain death laws are not in place.

LDLT FOR FHF

The lack of deceased donors in countries where brain death laws are not in place for religious, political, or cultural reasons[47] has made live donation the only option for liver transplantation.[48] However, this is an ethical issue in European countries and in the United States where deceased donation is an option.[49]

A recent report by Faraj and colleagues[50] reported results of APOLT performed in 20 children with FHF. The patients were evaluated prospectively with radiologic and nuclear medicine imaging and histopathology. Patients were followed for a 10-year period. Of 17 survivors, 14 have successfully regenerated their native liver and 11 underwent immunosuppression withdrawal at a median time of 23 months after transplantation. There were no biliary or technical complications in this series. Therefore, the results of APOLT seem more promising in children than in adults.

LDLT FOR FHF

Most of the reports of LDLT for FHF come from the Asian countries where this operation is a necessity because of the lack of deceased donors. LDLT accounts for more than 90% of transplants in Asia, compared with 5% in the Western world. LDLT for children using the lateral segment is associated with low donor morbidity. However, applying this for adults is associated with increased donor morbidity and raises an ethical question of subtle and psychological donor coercion in the midst of possibly preventable and imminent death of a loved one. The advantages of LDLT include a readily available graft, hence the opportunity to wait to see whether the patient improves without the transplant; predictability of timing of the operation; and better and predictable allograft function due to minimal cold ischemia time (see **Fig. 5**). However, following the death of a live liver donor in New York, the Advisory Committee on Organ Transplantation recommended that LDLT should be contraindicated in FHF.[51]

Lee and colleagues[52] reported 57 LDLT in patients with FHF. Donor selection was according to strict criteria ensuring that the donor's remnant liver volume was greater than 30% of total liver volume and liver steatosis was minimal (<10%). Dual grafts from 2 donors were used (15 patients) when the expected remnant liver volume was less than 30% of total liver volume or small-for-size graft for recipients. At 11 to 107 months after LDLT, 47/57 recipients were alive and well. Graft survival at 1 year for large-for-size grafts with graft volume to standard liver volume ratio greater than 50% was 87.1%, compared with 50% for small-for-size grafts with graft volume/standard liver volume ratio less than 40%, emphasizing the importance of graft to recipient volume ratio. Theoretically, FHF patients could tolerate small grafts because of the absence of preexisting portal hypertension. With improved techniques and the increasing awareness of the importance of reconstructing the anterior sector vein when it drains into the middle hepatic, the outcome of LDLT for FHF has improved. The interplay of graft volume, portal hypertension, and outflow capacity has to be factored in when evaluating the prospective live donor and recipient (**Fig. 6**).

The outcomes of LDLT for FHF as part of adult-to-adult living donor liver transplantation cohort study were reported in 2008. Fourteen of the 1201 recipients had FHF. Five of the 10 live donors had 7 posttransplant complications, leading the group to conclude that LDLT is rarely performed for FHF. In carefully selected recipients and donors, it can have acceptable recipient and donor morbidity. LDLT recipient survival

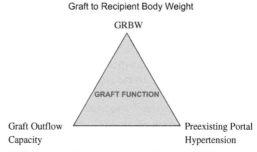

Graft to Recipient Body Weight

GRBW

GRAFT FUNCTION

Graft Outflow Capacity

Preexisting Portal Hypertension

Fig. 6. Live donor/split liver transplantation: physiologic considerations. Allograft survival in split or live donor liver transplant depends on the functioning liver mass transplanted and successful interplay of graft to recipient body weight, graft outflow capacity, and presence of preexisting portal hypertension. (*Adapted from* Marcos A.)

rate was comparable with that of those who underwent deceased donor liver transplantation (70% compared with 82%). Therefore, LDLT maybe an option for some patients with FHF.

SUMMARY

Fulminant liver failure is a complex medical and surgical emergency that is associated with high morbidity and mortality. Timely intervention with supportive care and medical management at a tertiary care center is essential. Liver transplantation with an appropriate size-matched graft is the treatment of choice for patients who show signs of liver failure and decompensation.

ACKNOWLEDGMENTS

The authors gratefully acknowledge the following for their contributions to this article: Denise M. Malicki MD, PhD, Associate Pathologist and Director Blood Bank Rady Children's Hospital San Diego for providing the illustrations in **Fig. 3**; Mary O' Boyle MD, Attending Radiologist, University of California, San Diego, Medical Center for providing the illustrations in **Fig. 4**; and Katharine Anderson PA-C, University of California, San Diego for her assistance with the illustrations.

REFERENCES

1. Trey C, Lipworth L, Chalmers TC, et al. Fulminant hepatic failure. Presumable contribution to halothane. N Engl J Med 1968;279(15):798–801.
2. O'Grady JG, Schalm SW, Williams R. Acute liver failure: redefining the syndromes. Lancet 1993;342(8866):273–5.
3. Sass DA, Shakil AO. Fulminant hepatic failure. Liver Transpl 2005;11(6):594–605.
4. Shakil AO, Kramer D, Mazariegos GV, et al. Acute liver failure: clinical features, outcome analysis, and applicability of prognostic criteria. Liver Transpl 2000; 6(2):163–9.
5. Craig DG, Lee A, Hayes PC, et al. Review article: the current management of acute liver failure. Aliment Pharmacol Ther 2010;31(3):345–58.
6. Fontana RJ. Acute liver failure including acetaminophen overdose. Med Clin North Am 2008;92(4):761–94, viii.
7. Kelly DA. Managing liver failure. Postgrad Med J 2002;78(925):660–7.
8. Stravitz RT, Kramer AH, Davern T, et al. Intensive care of patients with acute liver failure: recommendations of the U.S. Acute Liver Failure Study Group. Crit Care Med 2007;35(11):2498–508.
9. Lee WM. Acute liver failure. N Engl J Med 1993;329(25):1862–72.
10. Williams R. Classification, etiology, and considerations of outcome in acute liver failure. Semin Liver Dis 1996;16(4):343–8.
11. Ostapowicz G, Fontana RJ, Schiodt FV, et al. Results of a prospective study of acute liver failure at 17 tertiary care centers in the United States. Ann Intern Med 2002;137(12):947–54.
12. Liu Q. Role of cytokines in the pathophysiology of acute-on-chronic liver failure. Blood Purif 2009;28(4):331–41.
13. Michalopoulos GK. Liver regeneration. J Cell Physiol 2007;213(2):286–300.
14. Karp SJ. Clinical implications of advances in the basic science of liver repair and regeneration. Am J Transplant 2009;9(9):1973–80.

15. Nielsen HB, Tofteng F, Wang LP, et al. Cerebral oxygenation determined by near-infrared spectrophotometry in patients with fulminant hepatic failure. J Hepatol 2003;38(2):188–92.
16. Bernuau J, Goudeau A, Poynard T, et al. Multivariate analysis of prognostic factors in fulminant hepatitis B. Hepatology 1986;6(4):648–51.
17. Bismuth H, Samuel D, Castaing D, et al. Orthotopic liver transplantation in fulminant and subfulminant hepatitis. The Paul Brousse experience. Ann Surg 1995; 222(2):109–19.
18. O'Grady JG, Alexander GJ, Hayllar KM, et al. Early indicators of prognosis in fulminant hepatic failure. Gastroenterology 1989;97(2):439–45.
19. Pauwels A, Mostefa-Kara N, Florent C, et al. Emergency liver transplantation for acute liver failure. Evaluation of London and Clichy criteria. J Hepatol 1993;17(1):124–7.
20. Donaldson BW, Gopinath R, Wanless IR, et al. The role of transjugular liver biopsy in fulminant liver failure: relation to other prognostic indicators. Hepatology 1993; 18(6):1370–6.
21. Bernal W, Wendon J, Rela M, et al. Use and outcome of liver transplantation in acetaminophen-induced acute liver failure. Hepatology 1998;27(4):1050–5.
22. Bailey B, Amre DK, Gaudreault P. Fulminant hepatic failure secondary to acetaminophen poisoning: a systematic review and meta-analysis of prognostic criteria determining the need for liver transplantation. Crit Care Med 2003; 31(1):299–305.
23. Dhiman RK, Jain S, Maheshwari U, et al. Early indicators of prognosis in fulminant hepatic failure: an assessment of the Model for End-Stage Liver Disease (MELD) and King's College Hospital criteria. Liver Transpl 2007;13(6):814–21.
24. Kremers WK, van IJperen M, Kim WR, et al. MELD score as a predictor of pretransplant and posttransplant survival in OPTN/UNOS status 1 patients. Hepatology 2004;39(3):764–9.
25. Barshes NR, Lee TC, Balkrishnan R, et al. Risk stratification of adult patients undergoing orthotopic liver transplantation for fulminant hepatic failure. Transplantation 2006;81(2):195–201.
26. Perkins JD. Another formula to determine the prognosis of patients with acute liver failure. Liver Transpl 2009;15(8):986–91.
27. Singhal A, Neuberger J. Acute liver failure: bridging to transplant or recovery–are we there yet? J Hepatol 2007;46(4):557–64.
28. Carpentier B, Gautier A, Legallais C. Artificial and bioartificial liver devices: present and future. Gut 2009;58(12):1690–702.
29. Rikker C. Liver support systems today. Orv Hetil 2009;150(51):2299–307.
30. Teng Y, Wang Y, Li S, et al. Treatment of acute hepatic failure in mice by transplantation of mixed microencapsulation of rat hepatocytes and transgenic human fetal liver stromal cells. Tissue Eng Part C Methods 2010. [Epub ahead of print].
31. Strom SC, Fisher RA, Thompson MT, et al. Hepatocyte transplantation as a bridge to orthotopic liver transplantation in terminal liver failure. Transplantation 1997; 63(4):559–69.
32. Horslen SP, Fox IJ. Hepatocyte transplantation. Transplantation 2004;77(10):1481–6.
33. Horslen SP, McCowan TC, Goertzen TC, et al. Isolated hepatocyte transplantation in an infant with a severe urea cycle disorder. Pediatrics 2003;111(6 Pt 1):1262–7.
34. Bilir BM, Guinette D, Karrer F, et al. Hepatocyte transplantation in acute liver failure. Liver Transpl 2000;6(1):32–40.
35. Hoganson DM, Pryor HI, Spool ID, et al. Principles of biomimetic vascular network design applied to a Tissue-Engineered Liver Scaffold. Tissue Eng Part A 2010;16(5):1469–77.

36. Garcia-Gil FA, Luque P, Ridruejo R, et al. Liver transplant, in emergency 0 (UNOS Status 1). Transplant Proc 2006;38(8):2465–7.
37. Wiesner RH. MELD/PELD and the allocation of deceased donor livers for status 1 recipients with acute fulminant hepatic failure, primary nonfunction, hepatic artery thrombosis, and acute Wilson's disease. Liver Transpl 2004; 10(10 Suppl 2):S17–22.
38. Adam R, Cailliez V, Majno P, et al. Normalised intrinsic mortality risk in liver transplantation: European Liver Transplant Registry study. Lancet 2000;356(9230): 621–7.
39. Adam R, McMaster P, O'Grady JG, et al. Evolution of liver transplantation in Europe: report of the European Liver Transplant Registry. Liver Transpl 2003; 9(12):1231–43.
40. Earl TM, Chari RS. Which types of graft to use in patients with acute liver failure? (A) Auxiliary liver transplant (B) Living donor liver transplantation (C) The whole liver. (C) I take the whole liver only. J Hepatol 2007;46(4):578–82.
41. Farmer DG, Anselmo DM, Ghobrial RM, et al. Liver transplantation for fulminant hepatic failure: experience with more than 200 patients over a 17-year period. Ann Surg 2003;237(5):666–75 [discussion: 675–6].
42. Girlanda R, Vilca-Melendez H, Srinivasan P, et al. Immunosuppression withdrawal after auxiliary liver transplantation for acute liver failure. Transplant Proc 2005; 37(4):1720–1.
43. Jaeck D, Pessaux P, Wolf P. Which types of graft to use in patients with acute liver failure? (A) Auxiliary liver transplant (B) Living donor liver transplantation (C) The whole liver. (A) I prefer auxiliary liver transplant. J Hepatol 2007;46(4):570–3.
44. van Hoek B, de Boer J, Boudjema K, et al. Auxiliary versus orthotopic liver transplantation for acute liver failure. EURALT Study Group. European Auxiliary Liver Transplant Registry. J Hepatol 1999;30(4):699–705.
45. Azoulay D, Samuel D, Ichai P, et al. Auxiliary partial orthotopic versus standard orthotopic whole liver transplantation for acute liver failure: a reappraisal from a single center by a case-control study. Ann Surg 2001;234(6):723–31.
46. Bismuth H, Azoulay D, Samuel D, et al. Auxiliary partial orthotopic liver transplantation for fulminant hepatitis. The Paul Brousse experience. Ann Surg 1996; 224(6):712–24 [discussion: 724–6].
47. Chen SC, Hsu HT, Hwang SL, et al. Attitude toward living donor liver transplantation in Taiwan. Transplant Proc 2006;38(7):2108–10.
48. Lo CM, Fan ST, Liu CL, et al. Applicability of living donor liver transplantation to high-urgency patients. Transplantation 1999;67(1):73–7.
49. Erim Y, Beckmann M, Kroencke S, et al. Psychological strain in urgent indications for living donor liver transplantation. Liver Transpl 2007;13(6):886–95.
50. Faraj W, Dar F, Bartlett A, et al. Auxiliary liver transplantation for acute liver failure in children. Ann Surg 2010;251(2):351–6.
51. Campsen J, Blei AT, Emond JC, et al. Outcomes of living donor liver transplantation for acute liver failure: the adult-to-adult living donor liver transplantation cohort study. Liver Transpl 2008;14(9):1273–80.
52. Lee SG, Ahn CS, Kim KH. Which types of graft to use in patients with acute liver failure? (A) Auxiliary liver transplant (B) Living donor liver transplantation (C) The whole liver. (B) I prefer living donor liver transplantation. J Hepatol 2007;46(4):574–8.

Surgical Shunt Versus TIPS for Treatment of Variceal Hemorrhage in the Current Era of Liver and Multivisceral Transplantation

Guilherme Costa, MD, Ruy J. Cruz Jr, MD, PhD,
Kareem M. Abu-Elmagd, MD, PhD*

KEYWORDS

- Portal hypertension • Portomesenteric venous thrombosis
- Surgical shunt • Transjugular intrahepatic portosystemic shunt
- Multivisceral transplant • Hypercoagulable status

Variceal hemorrhage occurs as a result of portal hypertension due to different underlying diseases such as portal vein thrombosis (prehepatic), liver cirrhosis (hepatic), and Budd-Chiari syndrome (posthepatic).[1,2] The interplay between the portal hemodynamic changes and hepatic reserve (**Table 1**) plays a major role in the short and long-term management of these complex patients. Of the important observed hemodynamic changes, is the increase in the intrahepatic vascular resistance compounded by the vasoconstrictor effect of a deficient state of intrahepatic nitric oxide. Of the major sequelae are the development of portosystemic collaterals, gastroesophageal varices, and a chronic state of systemic hyperdynamic syndrome.[3–7]

The natural history of the underlying liver disease is another major factor that should be considered for the establishment of the management algorithm of these patients. Ethanol abuse, chronic viral hepatitis, and cholestatic/autoimmune disorders are the most common liver diseases that significantly influence the long-term outcome with the currently available different therapeutic modalities that are discussed herein. Another important factor that further complicates the management plan of these complex patients is the presence of extensive splenic and portomesenteric venous

Intestinal Rehabilitation and Transplantation Center, Thomas East Starzl Transplantation Institute, Department of Surgery, University of Pittsburgh Medical Center, UPMC Montefiore – 7 South, 3459 Fifth Avenue, Pittsburgh, PA 15213-2582, USA
* Corresponding author.
E-mail address: abuelmagdkm@upmc.edu

Surg Clin N Am 90 (2010) 891–905
doi:10.1016/j.suc.2010.04.015
0039-6109/10/$ – see front matter © 2010 Elsevier Inc. All rights reserved.

Table 1 Child-Pugh classification			
	1	2	3
Albumin (g/dL)	>3.5	2.8–3.5	<2.8
Bilirubin (mg/dL)	<2	2–3	>3
Prothrombin time[a]	1–3	4–6	>6
Encephalopathy	None	1–2	3–4
Ascites	None	Slight	Moderate

Child-Pugh A = 5–6 points: excellent hepatic reserve; Child-Pugh B = 7–9 points: good hepatic reserve; Child-Pugh C = 10–15 points: poor hepatic reserve.
[a] Seconds prolonged.

thrombosis that develops in cirrhotics and in hypercoagulable patients with normal hepatic parenchyma.

Recent advances in pharmacologic and endoscopic management of gastroesophageal variceal bleeding has significantly shifted the main paradigm of therapy from surgical to medical management.[8–14] However, medical failure does occur with an incidence of 20%, which requires radiologic or surgical intervention to decompress the portal system as a palliative but life-saving procedure. Nonetheless, organ replacement with liver alone or a multivisceral graft is the ultimate and definitive treatment for these patients.[13–15] In this article, a management algorithm is outlined to guide and optimize therapy for acute and recurrent variceal bleeding in these unique patients.

EVALUATION GUIDELINES

The standard evaluation process of patients with variceal bleeding has been comprehensively addressed in the literature.[9–13] However, special emphasis should be placed on the history of the gastrointestinal hemorrhage including the number and severity of episodes. Documentation of the source of bleeding and the location of varices must be established to exclude other sources and guide therapy. The presence of gastric varices in the absence of Food and Drug Administration approval to use cyanoacrylate in the United States limits the therapeutic use of endoscopic therapy and calls for radiologic or surgical intervention.[11] The role of new endoscopic techniques including the recently introduced endoscopic capsule has increased the accuracy of variceal detection, particularly in patients with enteric and ectopic varices. The diagnosis of portal hypertensive gastropathy and/or colopathy, in the absence of gastrointestinal varices, may also shed some light on the source of bleeding and guide further therapy.

The status of portal hypertension can be semiquantitatively assessed by the degree of the pancytopenia, splenomegaly, and radiologic evidence of intra-abdominal visceral collaterals in addition to the endoscopic documentation of gastrointestinal varices, gastropathy, and/or colopathy. Noninvasive radiologic studies could also be helpful as a screening test for the possible coexistence of splenic or portomesenteric venous thrombosis. In persons with radiologic evidence of partial or complete visceral venous thrombosis, a hypercoagulable syndrome must be suspected and thoroughly evaluated. The evaluation process includes measurement of protein C, protein S, antithrombin III, and total homocysteine serum levels. In addition, genetic studies for factor V Leiden, prothrombin G20210A, and JAK-2 gene mutations should be conducted. Equally important are the diagnosis of paroxysmal nocturnal hemoglobinuria and the detection of anticardiolipin, lupus anticoagulant, and antiphospholipid antibodies.

When portomesenteric venous thrombosis is suspected or the pattern of gastroesophageal varices is unusual, particularly in the presence of normal liver parenchyma, patients must undergo visceral angiographic studies to evaluate the extent of thrombosis and to map the collateral circulation, including the assessment of the extent of collateralization and direction of flow (**Fig. 1**). The angiographic studies include superior mesenteric and splenic arterial injections with venous phases. On multiple occasions in their practice, the authors have observed unexpected angiographic findings such as arterial varices, arteriovenous malformations, and intrahepatic arterioportal communications. The old technique of measuring the portal venous pressure through a transsplenic, transhepatic, or transvariceal approach has been abandoned. In selected patients, catheterization of the hepatic veins with measurement of the free and wedged hepatic venous pressure is used, particularly in those with gastroesophageal varices in the absence of significant liver disease or portomesenteric venous thrombosis.

Finally, the etiology and extent of liver disease can be easily assessed in a systematic way, including thorough medical history, biochemical and hematological studies, abdominal imaging and, if necessary, percutaneous or transjugular liver biopsy. The histopathologic examination is of utmost importance, particularly in Child A/B patients who could be managed by radiologic or surgical intervention.

VARICEAL DECOMPRESSION WITHOUT ORGAN REPLACEMENT
Surgical Shunts

With a long-standing history of more than a half of a century, surgical shunts have played a major rule in the management of variceal bleeding by total, partial, selective, or super-selective decompression of the portal, mesenteric, splenic, and gastroesophageal variceal venous system; respectively. Since its peak popularity during the 1960s through the 1980s, surgical shunts have been gradually used with less

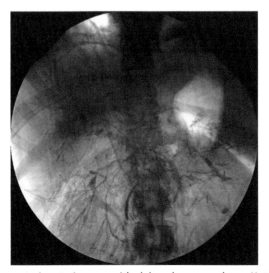

Fig. 1. Superior mesenteric arteriogram with delayed venous phase. Note complete occlusion of the superior mesenteric and portal veins. The patient was hypercoagulable and underwent a multivisceral transplantation.

frequency because of the introduction or revisiting of new nonsurgical therapeutic modalities and the evolution of abdominal organ transplantation.

Total portal systemic shunts are shunts that totally decompress the portal system with surgical anastomosis between the portal vein or one of its major branches, and the vena cava or one of its major tributaries. These shunts have usually been made as a side-to-side shunt with 10 or more millimeters of diameter, with decompression of the whole splanchnic portal hypertensive bed and the high hepatic sinusoidal pressure. Such shunts have a high patency rate, and excellent control of variceal bleeding as well as ascites.[16,17] However, most of the published series document a high incidence of encephalopathy and variable long-term survival outcome, which could be attributed to the differences in the severity and nature of the underlying liver disease among the selected study population.[18]

Because of the potentially prohibitive risk of encephalopathy with total shunts, Sarfeh and colleagues[19] popularized partial portal systemic shunts in the 1980s and 1990s by reducing the diameter of the shunt to 8 mm. The rationale is to maintain some portal flow to the hepatocyte without compromising the therapeutic decompression of the varices.[18–20] Technically, the shunt can be easily performed by placing an 8-mm polytetrafluoroethylene-reinforced graft between the portal vein and inferior vena cava (**Fig. 2**). Data that were published in the 1990s documented excellent control of bleeding with a low risk of encephalopathy and acceptable rate of long-term survival. The shunt has also been compared with the transjugular intrahepatic portosystemic shunt (TIPS) procedure in a randomized trial, as discussed later.

Selective decompression of the gastroesophageal varices was achievable by the clinical introduction of the distal splenorenal shunt (DSRS) by Warren and colleagues.[21–23] The shunt selectively decompresses the gastroesophageal varices through the short gastric veins into the splenic venous system and subsequently into the systemic circulation via the left renal vein. With proximal disconnection of

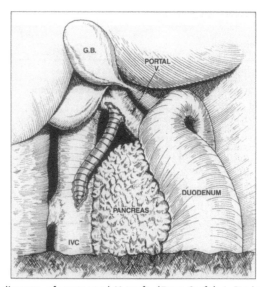

Fig. 2. Schematic diagram of portacaval H-graft. (*From* Sarfeh I, Rypins EB, Mason GR. A systematic appraisal of portacaval H-graft diameters. Clinical and hemodynamic perspectives. Ann Surg 1986;204(4):358; with permission.)

the splenic vein from the portal circulation, the state of portal hypertension is maintained in the superior mesenteric and portal venous system with preservation, in principle, of the portal flow to the cirrhotic liver. However, such a compartmentalization and selective variceal decompression was an enigma because of the gradual development of collateralization between the two, high and low, pressure systems that are contained in one celomic cavity.[24] These collaterals were identified as gastric, colon-splenic, and pancreatic (**Fig. 3**A). Accordingly, technical modification of the procedure was required to minimize the development of collaterals between the portal and shunt circulation by adding a complete splenopancreatic disconnection to the standard operation (see **Fig. 3**B).[25] Nonetheless, most series that were published in the 1980s and 1990s proved the therapeutic efficacy of the procedure, with low incidence of recurrent variceal bleeding (5%–8%), acceptable risk of hepatic encephalopathy (5%–15%), and excellent long-term survival.[22,23,26] These results reflected the outcome in low-risk Child A/B patients with stable liver disease, particularly those with nonalcoholic and nonhepatic cirrhosis. The popularity of the procedure, however, was limited by different anatomic and technical obstacles that imposed significant surgical challenges. With the increased use and popularity of the TIPS procedure during the late 1990s, particularly among Child A/B variceal bleeders, a multicenter randomized trial sponsored by the National Institutes of Health was conducted, which compared the radiologic shunt with the DSRS among variceal bleeders with preserved hepatic functions. The results are discussed in the section Published Data.[26]

With the loss of DSRS selectivity within the first 6 months after surgery, Inokuchi and colleagues[27,28] introduced the coronocaval shunt as a super-selective shunt procedure with direct decompression of the gastroesophageal varices into the systemic circulation. The operation did not gain popularity among the surgical community because of the technical difficulty and the wide variations in the anatomic and hemodynamic pattern of the left gastric venous system among variceal bleeders.

A modification of most of the aforementioned shunt procedures has been used at the authors' center for patients with portomesenteric and splenic venous thrombosis who developed collaterals that are technically amenable for surgical shunting. On multiple occasions, the authors used the coronary, gastroepiploic, and other unnamed collaterals. In these challenging patients, complete gastric devascularization has been

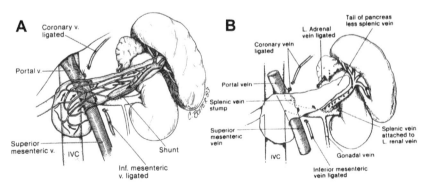

Fig. 3. (*A*) The distal splenorenal shunt with the pancreatic sump that develops in the pancreatic region siphoning the portal blood flow to the distal splenic segment. (*B*) Distal splenorenal shunt with complete splenopancreatic disconnection. (*From* Warren WD, Millikan WJ, Henderson JM, et al. Splenopancreatic disconnection: improved selectivity of distal splenorenal shunt. Ann Surg 1986;204(4):347; with permission.)

a useful surgical alternative, with excellent long-term outcome and very low risk of rebleeding (**Fig. 4**).

Radiologic Shunt

TIPS is a "minimally invasive" procedure that provides direct portal decompression by creating an intrahepatic shunt between the high-pressure portal system and the low-pressure hepatic venous circulation (**Fig. 5**). With advances in technology, the early reported high-shunt thrombosis was significantly reduced by using covered stents, with reduction in the overall reintervention rate resulting from stenosis and/or thrombosis. Overall, TIPS has been associated with increased risk of stenosis and/or thrombosis, with a 20% or more rebleeding rate. Therefore, follow-up and management protocols have been adopted for prompt reintervention to avoid such a life-threatening complication. The therapeutic efficacy of the procedure has been evaluated in two prospective randomized trials comparing TIPS with the commonly used shunt procedures: the Sarfeh 8-mm portacaval H-graft shunt and the Warren DSRS.

Published Data

This section focuses on the most recent results of two major randomized clinical trials that have been conducted comparing the two commonly used surgical shunts with the TIPS procedure.

Portacaval H-graft (8 mm) shunt versus TIPS

With nonconventional randomization, the study was initiated in 1993, with 50% of the study population being Child class C variceal bleeders with a mean age of 54 years.[29] All patients had failed initial therapy with pharmacologic and endoscopic management. The underlying liver disease was alcoholic cirrhosis in 60% of the patients, with a mean Model of End-Stage Liver Disease (MELD) score of 14.

With similar distribution of risk factors among both groups, TIPS was associated with a significantly higher risk of variceal rebleeding (30%) with no single example of recurrent variceal hemorrhage among the surgical shunt group.[20,29] Reintervention, however, was required in both cohorts with a lower rate (11%) after surgical shunt compared with TIPS (48%). The metabolic impairment of both shunt procedures was measured by the development of new-onset hepatic encephalopathy, which

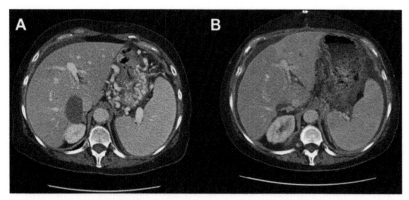

Fig. 4. (*A*) Computed tomography (CT) with visualization of extensive gastric wall collaterals in a patient with life-threatening recurrent episodes of bleeding gastric varices caused by portomesenteric venous thrombosis. (*B*) Radiologic evidence of decompressed gastric wall varices 1 week after complete gastric devascularization.

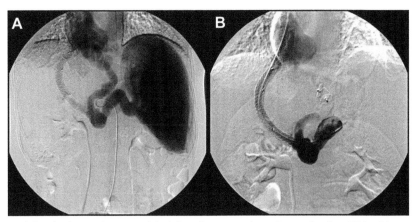

Fig. 5. (*A*) Splenic arteriogram with delayed venous phase 1 month after TIPS with patent shunt. Note preferential flow of the splenic venous return through a large gastroesophageal coronary collateral. (*B*) Successful occlusion of the collateral with an Amplatzer Vascular Plug to reduce the risk of recurrent bleeding and TIPS thrombosis by improving the portal venous flow through the TIPS.

was similar in both groups with an incidence of 3% among the surgical group and 4.5% among the TIPS patients. Ascites, at late follow-up, was also lower in the surgical (28%) compared with the TIPS (40%) patients. These results are summarized in **Table 2**.

As expected, particularly among Child C cirrhotics, the hospital mortality was higher (20%) with surgical shunt compared with the minimally invasive TIPS procedure (15%). Because both procedures are, at best, palliative measures and the study population was mostly alcoholics with Child C cirrhosis, late mortalities with a mean

Table 2
Outcomes at a median follow-up of 8.3 years in trial of 8-mm H-graft portosystemic shunt versus TIPS

	8-mm H-graft (N = 66)	TIPS (N = 66)	*P*
Rebleeding:			
Variceal	0 (0%)	20 (30%)	<.01
Gastric	5 (7.6%)	0 (0%)	
Reintervention	7 (11%)	32 (48%)	<.01
Encephalopathy (new)	2 (3%)	3 (4.5%)	NS
Ascites	18 (28%)	26 (40%)	NS
Mortality:			
Hospital	13 (20%)	10 (15%)	NS
Late	49 (74%)	48 (73%)	NS
Transplants	1	6	

Abbreviation: NS, not significant.

Data from Rosemurgy AS, Bloomston M, Clark WC, et al. H-graft portacaval shunts vs TIPS; 10 year follow-up of a randomized trial with comparison to predicted survivals. Ann Surg 2005;241:238–46.

follow-up of 8.3 years were unacceptably high in both groups, with 74% death rate after surgical shunt and 73% after TIPS (see **Table 2**). Of note, transplantation was used as a rescue therapy in only 7 of the randomized patients, with 1 example after surgical shunt and 6 after TIPS.

DSRS versus TIPS

The study was a well-designed prospective randomized multicenter trial funded by the National Institutes of Health and initiated in 1996.[26,30] There were 5 participating centers, namely Cleveland Clinic, Emory University, University of Wisconsin, University of Miami, and University of Pittsburgh. The study included a total of 140 Child class A (60%) and B (40%) patients, with a mean age of 53 ± 10 years and a male/female ratio of 3:2. Failure of endoscopic or pharmacologic therapy to prevent recurrent variceal bleeding was documented in all of the enrolled patients. The primary liver disease was alcoholic cirrhosis in 60% of the patients, with a mean MELD score of 9.8. The primary end points were rebleeding and hepatic encephalopathy with the secondary end points being death, ascites, need for transplant, progression of liver disease, quality of life, and cost. All these end points and other pertinent related medical information were prospectively reviewed and periodically documented by different specialized review committees and agreed on by consensus. Very strict criteria for reintervention were defined from the outset, which guided the decision-making process for either dilatation or restenting of the shunt particularly of the TIPS procedure.

As shown in **Table 3** and **Fig. 6**, there was no significant difference in the overall incidence and cumulative risk of the two primary end points. However, the rebleeding rate was relatively higher (10.5%) after TIPS compared with DSRS (5.5%). Unexpectedly, the overall incidence of encephalopathy was similar among both groups. However, many of these episodes were isolated single events that were successfully treated with simple medical measures. With no significant difference in the overall incidence, DSRS patients had a higher rate of early postoperative ascites while more of the TIPS

Table 3
Results of the National Institutes of Health Multicenter Randomized Study

Parameter	DSRS (N = 73)	TIPS (N = 67)	Significance
Rebleeding	5.5%	10.5%	NS
Encephalopathy	50%	50%	NS
Survival: 2 years	81%	88%	NS
Survival: 5 years	62%	61%	NS
Thrombosis/stenosis	11%	82%	P<.001
Ascites	21 (29%)	17 (25%)	NS
Need for transplant	6 (8%)	8 (12%)	NS
Quality of life SF36[a]			
Physical component	41.7	42.1	NS
Mental component	44.3	44.2	NS
Costs	$28,734	$21,607	NS

Abbreviation: NS, not significant.
[a] Normal scores for physical and mental components for SF36 are 50.
Data from Henderson JM, Boyer TD, Kutner MH, et al. Distal splenorenal shunt versus transjugular intrahepatic portal systematic shunt for variceal bleeding: a randomized trial. Gastroenterology 2006;130:1643–51.

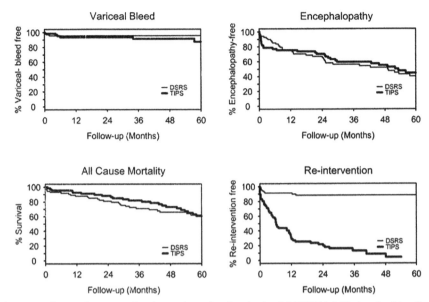

Fig. 6. Kaplan-Meier curves for the main end points in the DIVERT Trial. Variceal rebleeding, first hepatic encephalopathy episode, and survival show no significant difference at any time point to 5 years. The reintervention rate was significantly (*P*<.001) greater in the TIPS group than in the DSRS group at all time points. (*From* Henderson JM, Boyer TD, Kutner MH, et al. Distal splenorenal shunt versus transjugular intrahepatic portal systematic shunt for variceal bleeding: a randomized trial. Gastroenterology 2006;130:1647; with permission.)

patients developed ascites with long-term follow-up, particularly those who experienced progressive liver failure. The transplantation rate was 8% after DSRS and 12% after TIPS.

One of the most important findings in the study, as shown in **Fig. 6**, is the significant higher reintervention rate with TIPS (82%) compared with DSRS (11%). It is obvious from the Kaplan-Meier cumulative reintervention-free curve that the events after DSRS occurred during the early postoperative period, whereas those after TIPS continued to occur throughout the study period. These data support the current recommendation of careful monitoring of long-term TIPS patency.

Both DSRS and TIPS were associated with similar short and long-term survival, as shown in **Fig. 7**, with approximately 2- and 5-year survival of 85% and 62%, respectively. The causes of death were variable and the subset analysis showed no significant difference in mortality by Child-Pugh class score, procedural related, liver disease related, and other causes of death between the DSRS and TIPS groups.[30] The quality of life measured by the Short Form-36 score at 1 year after both procedures is shown in **Table 3**, with similar results. Of note, the preliminary as well as the most recent update of cost analysis showed that TIPS is as cost-effective as DSRS in preventing variceal rebleeding in patients who failed medical therapy.[31]

ABDOMINAL ORGAN TRANSPLANTATION
Liver Transplantation

Hepatic transplantation is no longer used as an emergency procedure for active variceal bleeding.[32] This is mostly because of the current shortage in cadaveric organs and the availability of effective alternative minimally invasive procedures such as

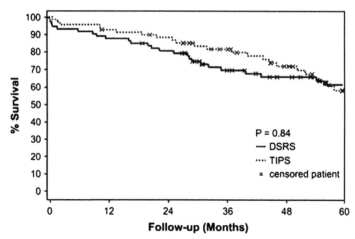

Fig. 7. Survival curves for the DSRS and TIPS DIVERT Study patients. (*From* Henderson JM. Surgery versus transjugular intrahepatic portal systemic shunt in the treatment of severe variceal bleeding. Clin Liver Dis 2006;10:610; with permission.)

endoscopic ablation and TIPS. Both procedures are sometimes complementary, with more use of the TIPS procedure in patients with gastric varices and those who are not amenable for endoscopic treatment. However, emergent surgical intervention may still play a significant role as a life-saving therapeutic modality, particularly in patients with failed TIPS and those with portomesenteric venous thrombosis or Budd-Chiari syndrome. When emergent surgical decompression is required for patients who are transplant candidates, an interposition mesocaval or mesorenal shunt, which can simply be ligated during the transplant operation, is recommended. The conventional total portosystemic shunts, particularly those who require hepatic hilar dissection, can precipitate liver failure and increase the operative risk at the time of surgery or transplantation. In the presence of adequate hepatic reserve and hemodynamic stability, emergent selective shunt can also be used with a high success rate. With

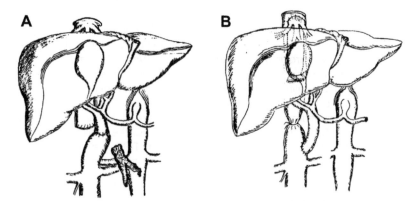

Fig. 8. Cavoportal hemitransposition with end-to-end (*A*) or end-to-side (*B*) anastomosis. Note plication of the inferior vena cava above the anastomosis with the end-to-side anastomosis. (*From* Tzakis AG, Kirkegaard P, Pinna AD, et al. Liver transplantation with cavoportal hemitransposition in the presence of diffuse portal vein thrombosis. Transplantation 1998;65:622; with permission.)

portomesenteric venous thrombosis, gastric devascularization with left gastric vein ligation is probably the only therapeutic option when medical treatment fails. Nonetheless, all of these procedures are palliative measures and are commonly used as a bridge to transplantation.

For elective therapy, the quantity of the functional hepatic reserve is the most important factor to be considered in the decision-making process and timing of transplantation. With Child C cirrhosis, liver transplantation seems to be the only therapeutic option for variceal bleeders. For compensated (Child A/B) cirrhotics with adequate hepatic reserve, a simmering controversy still exists regarding the issue of liver transplantation versus shunt procedures. In these patients, the choice between shunting and transplantation after failure of endoscopic intervention is often difficult. Although long-term survival for this group is probably superior with transplantation, a portal perfusion–preserving operation, preferably DSRS, may serve for several years as an effective bridge to transplantation. Because of its nonsurgical nature, TIPS has recently been promoted to treat patients with good hepatic reserve who may not require liver transplantation for a long time, as discussed earlier.

With better understanding of transplant immunology and allograft tolerance with minimization or discontinuation of immunosuppression, liver transplantation may stand in the near future as the treatment of choice with normal life expectancy. The

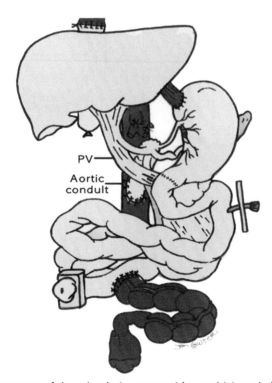

Fig. 9. Total replacement of the splanchnic organs with a multivisceral allograft, including stomach, duodenum, pancreas, intestine, and liver. Note the en bloc total replacement of the thrombosed portomesenteric venous system with the transplanted organs. (*From* Abu-Elmagd K, Costa G, Bond GJ, et al. Five hundred intestinal and multivisceral transplantations at a single center. Major advances with new challenges. Ann Surg 2009;250(4): 569; with permission.)

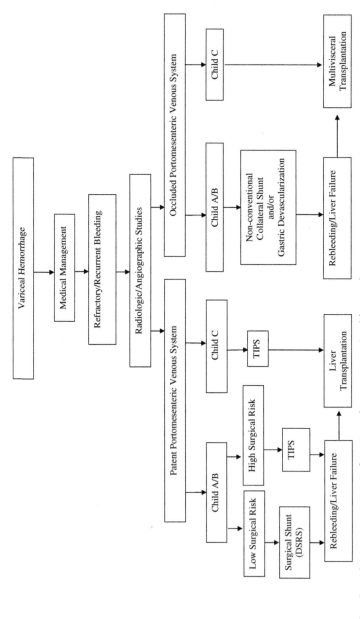

Fig. 10. The algorithmic management of acute and recurrent variceal hemorrhage.

problem of organ shortage has been recently ameliorated by the innovative techniques of cadaveric split and live-donor transplantation. Further evolution of the field has also been recently fueled by the growing knowledge of stem cell biology and gene technology, with the hope for organ engineering and xenotransplantation.

Multivisceral Transplantation

With portomesenteric and splenic venous thrombosis, variceal bleeders with combined parenchymal and vascular decompensation have very limited therapeutic options. These options are commonly dictated by the extent of the thrombotic process and the pattern of collateral development. With isolated portal vein thrombosis, liver transplantation has been used with increasing frequency since the technique of portal thrombectomy and venous jump graft was introduced at the authors' institution during the late 1980s.[33] With extensive portomesenteric venous thrombosis, liver replacement with cavoportal hemitransposition (**Fig. 8**) and multivisceral transplantation (**Fig. 9**) are the only two technically feasible transplant procedures that could be offered to these patients.[34,35] The cavoportal hemitransposition technique was advocated at times when the multivisceral transplant procedure was technically challenging with a poor outcome. With the recent evolution of multivisceral transplantation and continuous improvement in survival, the procedure should be offered to all variceal bleeders with extensive portomesenteric and splenic vein thrombosis.[35] A major disadvantage of the cavoportal hemitransposition technique is the persistent risk of life-threatening variceal hemorrhage, because the procedure usually fails to decompress the thrombosed portomesenteric and splenic venous system. With multivisceral transplantation, the visceral collaterals as well as the gastrointestinal varices are eradicated by replacing the thrombosed portal venous system en bloc with the donor stomach, duodenum, pancreas, intestine, and liver.

SUMMARY

The authors' current policy for the management of variceal bleeders based on the status of the portomesenteric venous system and hepatic reserve is summarized in **Fig. 10**. This new management algorithm requires a multidisciplinary team approach in a tertiary center with the availability of surgical and radiologic expertise in portal hypertension and abdominal organ transplantation. In brief, surgical shunt and TIPS are equally effective in the management of Child A/B variceal bleeders, and organ transplantation should be considered for patients with Child C cirrhosis and those who fail the shunt procedure or develop progressive liver failure.

ACKNOWLEDGMENTS

The authors would like to thank Darlene Koritsky for her extraordinary efforts in preparing the manuscript.

REFERENCES

1. Lebrec D, Moreau R. Pathophysiology of portal hypertension. Hepatogastroenterology 1999;46:1426–8.
2. Boyer TD. Natural history of portal hypertension. Clin Liver Dis 1997;1:31–44.
3. Groszmann R. Hyperdynamic circulation of liver disease forty years later: pathophysiology and clinical consequences. Hepatology 1994;20:1359–63.

4. Pinzani M, Vizzutti F. Anatomy and vascular biology of the cells in the portal circulation. In: Sanyal AJ, Shah VH, editors. Clinical gastroenterology: portal hypertension. Totowa (NJ): Humana Press Inc; 2005. p. 15–35.

5. Rockey DC. Cell and molecular mechanisms of increased intrahepatic resistance and hemodynamic correlates. In: Sanyal AJ, Shah VH, editors. Clinical gastroenterology: portal hypertension. Totowa (NJ): Humana Press Inc; 2005. p. 37–50.

6. Wiest R, Grozsmann RJ. The paradox of nitric oxide in cirrhosis and portal hypertension: too much, not enough. Hepatology 2002;35:478–91.

7. Moreau R, Lebrec D. Molecular and structural basis of portal hypertension. Clin Liver Dis 2006;10:445–57.

8. Rana SS, Bhasin DK. Gastrointestinal bleeding: from conventional to nonconventional. Endoscopy 2008;40(1):40–4.

9. Garcia-Tsao G, Lim JK, Members of Veterans Affairs Hepatitis C Resource Center Program. Management and treatment of patients with cirrhosis and portal hypertension: recommendations from the Department of Veterans Affairs Hepatitis C Resource Center Program and the National Hepatitis C Program. Am J Gastroenterol 2009;104(7):1802–29.

10. Toubia N, Sanyal AR. Portal hypertension and variceal hemorrhage. Med Clin North Am 2008;92:551–74.

11. Sass DA, Chopra KB. Portal hypertension and variceal hemorrhage. Med Clin North Am 2009;93(4):837–53.

12. Kravetz D. Prevention of recurrent esophageal variceal hemorrhage: review and current recommendations. J Clin Gastroenterol 2007;41(3):S318–22.

13. Garcia-Pagan JC, De Gottardi A, Bosch J. Review article: the modern management of portal hypertension: primary and secondary prophylaxis of variceal bleeding in cirrhotic patients. Aliment Pharmacol Ther 2008;28(2):178–86.

14. de Franchis R, Dell'Era A, Primignani M. Diagnosis and monitoring of portal hypertension. Dig Liver Dis 2008;40(5):312–7.

15. Boyer TD, Henderson JM. Portal hypertension and bleeding esophageal varices. In: Zakim D, Boyer TD, editors. Hepatology: a textbook of liver disease. 4th edition. Philadelphia: WB Saunders; 2002. p. 581.

16. Stipa S, Balducci G, Ziparo V, et al. Total shunting and elective management of variceal bleeding. World J Surg 1994;18:200–4.

17. Orloff MJ, Orloff MS, Orloff SL, et al. Three decades of experience with emergency portocaval shunt for acutely bleeding esophageal varices in 400 unselected patients with cirrhosis of the liver. J Am Coll Surg 1995;180:257–72.

18. Collins JC, Ong J, Rypins EB, et al. Partial portacaval shunt for variceal hemorrhage. Longitudinal analysis of effectiveness. Arch Surg 1998;133:590–3.

19. Sarfeh IJ, Rypins EB, Mason GR. A systematic appraisal of portocaval H-graft diameters. Clinical and hemodynamics perspectives. Ann Surg 1986;204:356–63.

20. Rosemurgy AS, Goode SE, Zwiebel BR, et al. A prospective trial of transjugular intrahepatic portosystemic stent shunt vs. small diameter prosthetic H-graft portacaval shunts in the treatment of bleeding varices. Ann Surg 1996;224:378–84.

21. Warren WD, Zeppa R, Fomon JJ. Selective trans-splenic decompression of gastroesophageal varices by distal splenorenal shunt. Ann Surg 1967;166:437–55.

22. Henderson JM, Millikan WJ Jr, Warren WD. The distal splenorenal shunt: an update. World J Surg 1984;8:722–32.

23. Henderson JM, Millikan WJ Jr, Warren WD. Selective variceal decompression: current status and recent advances. Adv Surg 1984;18:81–116.

24. Maillard JN, Flamant YM, Hay JM, et al. Selectivity of the distal splenorenal shunt. Surgery 1979;86(5):663–71.
25. Warren WD, Millikan WJ, Henderson JM, et al. Splenopancreatic disconnection: improved selectivity of distal splenorenal shunt. Ann Surg 1986;204(4):346–55.
26. Henderson JM. Surgery versus transjugular intrahepatic portal systemic shunt in the treatment of severe variceal bleeding. Clin Liver Dis 2006;10:599–612.
27. Inokuchi K, Kobayashi M, Kusaba A, et al. New selective decompression of esophageal varices by a left gastric venous-caval shunt. Arch Surg 1970;100: 157–62.
28. Inokuchi K, Sugimachi K. The selective shunt for variceal bleeding: a personal perspective. Am J Surg 1990;160(1):48–53.
29. Rosemurgy AS, Bloomston M, Clark WC, et al. H-graft portacaval shunts vs. TIPS: ten year follow up of a randomized trial with comparison to predicted survivals. Ann Surg 2005;241:238–46.
30. Henderson JM, Boyer TD, Kutner MH, et al. Distal splenorenal shunt versus trans-jugular intrahepatic portal systematic shunt for variceal bleeding: a randomized trial. Gastroenterology 2006;130(6):1643–51.
31. Boyer TD, Henderson MJ, Heery AM, et al. Cost of preventing variceal rebleeding with transjugular intrahepatic portal systemic shunt and distal splenorenal shunt. J Hepatol 2008;48:407–14.
32. Iwatsuki S, Starzl TE. Liver transplantation in the management of bleeding esoph-ageal varices. Baillieres Clin Gastroenterol 1992;6(3):517–25.
33. Tzakis AG, Todo S, Stieber A, et al. Venous jump grafts for liver transplantation in patients with portal vein thrombosis. Transplantation 1989;48:530–1.
34. Tzakis AG, Kirkegaard P, Pinna AD, et al. Liver transplantation with cavoportal hemitransposition in the presence of diffuse portal vein thrombosis. Transplanta-tion 1998;65:619–24.
35. Abu-Elmagd KM, Costa G, Bond GJ, et al. Five hundred intestinal and multivisc-eral transplantations at a single center. Major advances with new challenges. Ann Surg 2009;250(4):567–81.

Index

Note: Page numbers of article titles are in **boldface** type.

Surg Clin N Am 90 (2010) 907–917
doi:10.1016/S0039-6109(10)00085-X
0039-6109/10/$ – see front matter © 2010 Elsevier Inc. All rights reserved.

surgical.theclinics.com

Moving?

Make sure your subscription moves with you!

To notify us of your new address, find your **Clinics Account Number** (located on your mailing label above your name), and contact customer service at:

Email: journalscustomerservice-usa@elsevier.com

800-654-2452 (subscribers in the U.S. & Canada)
314-447-8871 (subscribers outside of the U.S. & Canada)

Fax number: 314-447-8029

Elsevier Health Sciences Division
Subscription Customer Service
3251 Riverport Lane
Maryland Heights, MO 63043

*To ensure uninterrupted delivery of your subscription, please notify us at least 4 weeks in advance of move.

Printed and bound by CPI Group (UK) Ltd, Croydon, CR0 4YY

03/10/2024

01040457-0011